"What's more delicious than a London broil? *Losing It.*
This is an exposé in the old-fashioned sense; Fraser scores
her points not by preaching but with impressive reportage."
—Susan Faludi, author of
Backlash: The Undeclared War Against Women

"A sound and informative tour through the darkest
recesses of Dietland."
—*Washington Post*

"A persuasive and well-researched case for the
cessation of all dieting."
—*Baltimore Sun*

LAURA FRASER is a freelance writer and contributing editor at
Health magazine. Her articles have appeared in *Vogue*, *Glamour*,
Mirabella, *Mademoiselle*, and the *San Francisco Examiner*. She
lives in San Francisco.

"The sheer breadth of Fraser's research renders
her final arguments convincing."
—*Entertainment Weekly*

"Fraser has written an insightful book that traces
the evolution of society's thin obsession, the health
myths it fuels, the human toll it takes, and the
enormous amount of money it generates."
—*Denver Post*

"Exemplary research . . . a readable and convincing
exposé of the diet industry."
—*Publishers Weekly*

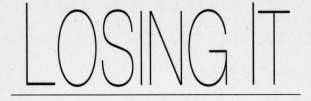

LOSING IT

False Hopes and Fat Profits in the Diet Industry

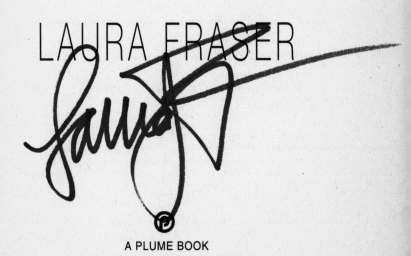

LAURA FRASER

A PLUME BOOK

PLUME
Published by the Penguin Group
Penguin Putnam Inc., 375 Hudson Street, New York, New York 10014, U.S.A.
Penguin Books Ltd, 27 Wrights Lane, London W8 5TZ, England
Penguin Books Australia Ltd, Ringwood, Victoria, Australia
Penguin Books Canada Ltd, 10 Alcorn Avenue, Toronto, Ontario, Canada M4V 3B2
Penguin Books (N.Z.) Ltd, 182–190 Wairau Road, Auckland 10, New Zealand

Penguin Books Ltd, Registered Offices:
Harmondsworth, Middlesex, England

Published by Plume, an imprint of Dutton NAL, a member of Penguin Putnam Inc.
Previously published in a Dutton edition.

First Plume Printing, May, 1998
10 9 8 7 6 5 4 3 2 1

The table on pages 176–177 is reprinted with permission from *Weighing the Options*,
copyright © 1994 by the National Academy of Sciences, courtesy of the
National Academy Press, Washington, D.C.

The definition of "Normal Eating" on page 269 is reprinted with permission
from a handout from the *How to Eat* series. Copyright © 1995 by Ellyn Satter.

Portions of chapters in this book were originally published in a different form
as magazine articles: chapter 3, in *Glamour*; chapters 4, 5, and 6, in *Vogue*; and
chapters 8 and 9, in *Health*.

 REGISTERED TRADEMARK—MARCA REGISTRADA

The Library of Congress catalogued the Dutton edition as follows:

Fraser, Laura.
    Losing it : America's obsession with weight and the industry that feeds on it / Laura
Fraser.
    p.   cm.
    Includes bibliographic references and index.
    ISBN 0-525-93891-5 (hc.)
    ISBN 0-452-27291-2 (pbk.)
    1. Weight loss—Social aspects—United States.   2. Weight loss preparations industry—
    United States.   I. Title
    RM222.2.F696   1997   96-27543
    613.2'5—dc20   CIP

Original hardcover design by Eve L. Kirch
Printed in the United States of America

BOOKS ARE AVAILABLE AT QUANTITY DISCOUNTS WHEN USED TO PROMOTE PRODUCTS OR SER-
VICES. FOR INFORMATION PLEASE WRITE TO PREMIUM MARKETING DIVISION, PENGUIN
PUTNAM INC., 375 HUDSON STREET, NEW YORK, NY 10014.

For my sisters
and
In memory of Lacey Fosburgh

Contents

x / Contents

Preface to the
Paperback Edition

Just over a year ago, when this book was first published I exchanged e-mail with a woman who was taking the popular diet drug combination known as fen-phen. She was one of about six million women who were taking fenfluramine and phentermine in 1996. Like many of them, this woman was completely frustrated trying to get rid of about thirty pounds. She would go on a diet, lose some weight, and then she couldn't help it—something always set her off—she would start overeating again. The drugs made her feel more in control. They calmed her cravings and her anxieties about food. For the first time in many years, she began to lose some weight. She was optimistic, even delighted.

I told her I didn't think the drugs were such a good idea, though, especially since she didn't sound fat enough that her weight was causing or aggravating any medical condition. No one knows whether those drugs are actually *safe* together, I said. The FDA never approved their use together, and doctors are prescribing them "off-label." The only study on the two drugs together, published in 1992 by University of Rochester pharmacologist Michael Weintraub (now with the FDA), looked at how *effective* the drugs were over time, not how *safe*. There were only 121 people in that study, and just 56 left at the end (26 dropped out because of unpleasant side effects)—nowhere near enough to determine what unusual problems might develop. As David Levitsky, a Cornell University psychologist who studies obesity put it, "We have absolutely no idea what the long-term risks of these drugs are."

What researchers did know at the time was that the drugs weren't all that effective for most people. Only a third of the people in the Weintraub study lost more than ten percent of their body weight after four years of therapy. Even those who did lose weight—and there were some for whom the drugs did make a big difference—gained it back again once their prescriptions ran out. More seriously, researchers knew there were concerns about adverse side effects: Studies showed that 1 in 25,000 of the people who took fenfluramine (or its cousin, dexfenfluramine or Redux) would likely get primary pulmonary hypertension, a heart and lung illness that is fatal in about half the cases. Doctors were supposed to balance that risk with a patient's medical need to lose weight, but many of them prescribed the drugs to people with only cosmetic weight problems. Obesity researchers also knew at the time that fenfluramine and phentermine cause brain damage in laboratory animals, fizzling the neural axons that produce serotonin, the calming, feel-good chemical in their brains. What tangled neurons in monkeys, rats, and dogs meant for human beings, no one knew. But clearly, the drugs were not to be taken lightly.

The responses to my on-line warnings about the drugs were heated. The woman said I was trying to burst her bubble. These drugs were the only promising obesity treatment to emerge in years, and why did I want to ruin it? Others in the chat group chimed in. Obesity is a terrible health problem, they said, and all drugs carry some risks. It's worth it to lose weight.

Recently, I met the woman I chatted with on-line in person at a book fair. In her forties, she was not particularly heavy, but seemed to be in ill health, moving slowly and breathing with some difficulty. In fact, she had recently had a heart attack. Did I know, she wondered, whether other fen-phen users had suffered similar cardiac events? Her doctor also found that she had leaky heart valves after taking the drugs; she had been perfectly healthy before. The woman told me she's had to quit working temporarily because of her heart problems, and her lawyer is now suing the pharmaceutical company. All she wishes is that she'd never tried fen-phen; her life will never be the same.

She isn't alone. Aside from the nearly 100 people who—as predicted at the Redux FDA hearings—have developed primary pulmonary hypertension as a result of taking the drugs (more than a dozen have died), many others now have heart valve abnormalities. After researchers at the Mayo Clinic reported, in July 1997, that there was an association between fen-phen use and valvular heart disease in 24 users—many of which have required surgery to be repaired—more and more of these unusual cases came to light. Subsequent studies showed that between a fourth and a third of fen-phen users developed heart-valve irregularities, particularly if they'd been on the drugs more than six months. In September the FDA requested a voluntary recall of fenfluramine and dexfenfluramine, and the manufacturer, Wyeth-Ayerst, complied. The drugs have now been recalled all over the world. In November the FDA urged patients who had used the drugs to have an echocardiogram if they developed any symptoms of heart-valve disease—shortness of breath and heart murmurs. It remains unclear who will pay for these procedures; if everyone on fen-phen had an echocardiogram, the bill would be more than $3 billion.

It's easy, in hindsight, to say that fen-phen was a public health disaster waiting to happen, and that patients should have been more cautious before swallowing their doctors' advice. We have ample precedents in this country for diet pill disasters, particularly with the millions of women who became addicted to amphetamines in the 1960s. But the desire to be thin is so intense in the United States that it not only clouds the judgment of patients, but of their doctors, too. And the financial interests backing these drugs are so strong that researchers are effectively bought, studies are skewed, and the FDA lowers the bar when it judges the safety and efficacy of obesity treatments. The fen-phen fiasco should be a cautionary tale to avoid future diet drug disasters. Instead, it seems likely to be a story that will be repeated again and again as people try to lose weight at any cost.

Other players in the diet industry were quick to try to fill the void left behind by fen-phen. As some physicians pulled up stakes in their fen-phen pill mills, others, including ones who work for the commercial weight-loss center Nutri/System, immediately began prescribing "phen-Pro," a combination of phentermine and the antidepressant Prozac, which is similarly untested together. Medeva Pharmaceuticals, which makes phentermine—the amphetamine-like part of the fen-phen combination that was not pulled by the FDA—sent letters to physicians offering them $10 off monthly prescriptions.[1] Companies that make dietary supplements reported phenomenal sales in "herbal fen-phen," which contains ephedrine, a stimulant herb that the FDA is trying to regulate because of numerous reports of deaths and adverse effects. Weight Watchers launched a half-million-dollar campaign for former diet pill users, and claims its membership is up 50 percent over the year before.

In November 1997, the FDA approved sibutramine, the first obesity drug to emerge in the wake of fen-phen. The agency approved it in spite of the fact that the committee reviewing the drug voted against its approval, mainly because it can cause high blood pressure in some patients. Many researchers believe that obesity itself is not dangerous until people get extremely fat and have mobility problems; what's dangerous are the conditions that typically go along with obesity, and obesity treatment should be aimed at improving those conditions. Hypertension is one of the main problems for obese people, and sibutramine—which, in any case, causes on average only 5 percent body weight loss—makes that problem worse for many patients. But the FDA approved the drug nevertheless, in part because now that fen-phen and Redux are banned, people who took the drugs are gaining weight again. To the FDA, that's a public health concern; to the pharmaceutical companies pushing drug approval, it's an enormous market hungry for a new drug.

It may be that sibutramine will be helpful for an as yet undefined subgroup of obese people, but recent history shows that many doctors will prescribe it to anyone who walks into their clinics worried about their big thighs. Neither the FDA, medical organizations, nor certainly the pharmaceutical companies are doing anything to put the brakes on the problem of physicians over-prescribing the drugs, exploiting their patients' fears of being fat. The fen-phen disaster doesn't seem to have dampened anyone's enthusiasm for using people who are worried about their weight as guinea pigs for new combinations of herbs and drugs. It may only be lawsuits brought by people who have developed heart and lung problems on fen-phen that will eventually slow down the pharmaceutical companies' and physicians' eagerness to categorize heavy people as "obese" in order to make huge profits prescribing them pills.

In the meantime, millions of people who have taken fen-phen, many of them unaware of the risks, wait and wonder whether they'll be one of the ones who will end up with a serious heart condition as a result of wanting to lose some weight—to improve their health.

—December, 1997
San Francisco

Introduction

Adventures in Dietland

Late one afternoon after school, I was sitting in a brown padded chair in a dimly lit office. Across the room, a psychologist with domino-sized sideburns was speaking softly. "Wouldn't you like to be thin, Laurie?" he asked me. "You'd be a pretty girl, you know, if you lost some of that weight."

I had just turned thirteen. I was going through that awful period when it seemed as if everyone was focusing on my body when all I wanted was to be invisible. But like most other girls, I couldn't hide my changing body and forget about it. Nor could I skip out on what seemed to be America's favorite rite of female passage: Dieting.

Actually, I'd been practicing this feminine ritual ever since I started counting calories in kindergarten; I can't remember a time when I wasn't on a diet. But at thirteen, when my already chubby body was growing more curves, it was time to get serious. It was getting more and more clear to me that becoming a woman—at least an attractive and successful woman—meant being able to lose weight. Nothing else seemed to matter more.

My parents sent me to this psychologist—I've repressed his name—to figure out why I was overeating. I had always been chubby, near the top of the growth charts since the age of two, but my parents were worried that my eating and weight were getting out of hand.

They had tried everything they could think of to keep me from getting fat: They served low-calorie meals, banished peanut butter and potato chips from the house, encouraged me to be active, and kept a watchful eye on my weight. They did the best they could, but somehow their strategy backfired.

Years later, I learned, in part, why it did. Children whose parents worry about their weight and control how much they eat, according to studies, tend to be fatter than kids whose parents are more relaxed. That's because kids who are put on diets don't learn to eat when they're hungry and stop when they're full, as normal kids do, but learn instead to eat according to someone else's rules.[1] Often they break those rules, out of rebellion, as I did, sneaking into the kitchen pantry for handfuls of Cap'n Crunch, and eating huge bowls of ice cream or potato chips at friends' houses, where the cupboards were stocked with forbidden foods.

For kids like me, the pleasure in eating was the taste of independence, but the aftertaste was one of shame. We got called "fat face" in preschool and were told by our dance teachers, at the age of five, that ballerinas never have such big tummies. In grade school, we were mocked in gym class, where we couldn't climb the ropes or run very fast. By junior high, the boys had ruled us out as potential love interests. And so we ate some more, to console ourselves, and what might have been only a slight tendency toward pudginess turned into real fat.

In the mid 1970s, though—at the time I was sitting in that psychologist's office—no one dreamed that putting kids on diets would end up making them fatter. My parents thought, sensibly, that a psychologist would not only put me on a diet but also help me sort out the feelings that led me to overeat. And so I went every week, while the shrink—who, it turned out, never asked me much about my feelings at all—charted my progress on yet another thousand-calorie-a-day diet. I was supposed to weigh myself twice a day and walk a mile every morning, using an early power-walking technique that I knew would greatly amuse the neighborhood kids. I didn't do the jog-walk, for fear of humiliation; I'd already been called a "whale" once on the way to school and didn't want to risk attracting attention to myself. When the psychologist's diet, like every other diet I had tried, didn't work, I simply lied, made up the numbers, and felt guilty.

Did I want to be thin and pretty? the psychologist had asked. Of course I did, more than almost anything. I had all kinds of fantasies about life as a thin teenager. I'd be popular at school, especially with the guys, who would ask me to dances and stop being so quick to announce that they wanted to be "just friends." I would feel smug next to the cheerleaders, knowing I could be one of them if I wanted to, but I'd rather not. I'd get chosen for teams, and run the fifty-yard dash as fast as the kid in gym class who made fun of me for being slow. I would eat like a normal person, wear colorful clothes (I always dressed in dark brown to look thinner), and make my parents happy. The desire to be thin, and the knowledge that I was falling short, was the soundtrack to my childhood, always playing somewhere in the background.

"Yes," I whispered to the psychologist. "I want to be skinny."

He nodded approvingly, and told me we were going to try something different that day. My parents said he practiced something called "behavior modification," which I gathered had to do with changing people's eating habits. I'd heard that these behavior modification shrinks gave people little shocks when they ate something wrong, the way you might experiment on rats in a maze. I was scared, imagining that this psychologist, whom I didn't like or trust, would hook me up to an electric machine and give me some sort of shock treatment for being fat. I told myself to be brave: It would be worth it to lose weight.

Instead, to my great relief, he said we'd try hypnosis. Before we began, he asked me to tell him all the "bad" foods I liked to eat. I knew which ones he was talking about, because at the time I believed there were only two food groups: "good" and "bad." Good food included cottage cheese, D-Zerta Jell-O, and celery sticks. Bad food meant just about anything else. Whatever tasted good seemed to be fattening and made you feel bad about yourself for eating it. So I gave the shrink a really good list of bad food: Sugar Babies, hot tamales, cookie dough, long john doughnuts, Hostess fruit pies, and pizza. He sank into his avocado green executive chair, tapped his fingers together, and thought for a while. Then he told me to lean back and get comfortable.

He led me through a series of deep relaxation exercises, instructing me to breathe deeply, to clench and release the muscles up and down my body, and to imagine my thoughts floating out the window. In no time at all I was surfing the clouds. Then the psychologist began telling me elaborate stories about the foods I'd listed. He started by describing the factory where the candy was made, where workers spat, dripped sweat, and blew their noses into large vats of syrupy concoctions. Rats climbed in and out of the cookie dough, leaving behind chocolate chip–sized turds. The long johns weren't really filled with cream, but were stuffed with rancid Crisco. It was Charlie and the Chocolate Factory in hell. My stomach was beginning to turn.

Then came the pièce de résistance: the pizza. The psychologist told me to imagine picking up a piece of hot, juicy, deep-dish pizza, covered with thick mozzarella that stretched away from my fingers in long, greasy strings. I took a big bite of the pizza, sank my teeth into a piece of sausage, and hit on something hard. I worked and worked at chewing the tough clump of meat, but it wouldn't give. I stuck my fingers into my mouth and pulled out a large, bony mass of gristle. Sticking out of the gristle were big tufts of slippery pig's hair.

"Pig," the psychologist intoned in his professionally soothing voice. "Pig, pig. Isn't that disgusting?" Later it would occur to me that hair probably doesn't grow on gristle. But at the time I was too grossed out to think clearly. Pig, I kept thinking to myself. That's what I was: A big, fat pig. After what seemed like hours, the fifty minutes were up, and the psychologist told me I was gradually going to become aware of my surroundings again, feel myself sitting in the chair, and finally open my eyes.

"How did you feel?" he asked eagerly. "Did you feel like throwing up?"

I nodded yes. I felt sick to my stomach. I felt terribly ashamed of myself. Fortunately, some tough part of my thirteen-year-old self felt like leaving and never coming back again. I suppose the psychologist's technique, which is called aversion therapy, was, to some degree, a success. I never did eat sausage again. I felt like a pig. And I would learn to throw up "bad" food.

And so my career as a dieter began in earnest. When I look back at photos of myself from that age, I'm surprised: I was plump, but hardly fat. Yet at the time it felt as if no one in the world was as fat as I was. Now it seems to me that if everyone hadn't paid so much attention to my weight, it wouldn't have been such a problem. I might have been a little heavy, since I come from sturdy stock on both sides of the family, but I probably wouldn't have been driven to overeat compulsively. I'll never be sure. All I know is that when I finally ended my dieting career a few years ago—prematurely, since most women continue well

the last century and particularly in the last two decades, are liv.
hectic lives, holding down two jobs: the traditional one of being a sexually desirable mother and wife, and the newer one of working to make
a living. The truth is that we hold down three jobs, and the third is, in
part, an expression of the uneasiness we feel about the tension
between the other two. The third job is being thin.

Most of us are convinced it's an important job. For one thing, our
efforts to control our weight give us the illusion that we have control
over at least one part of our chaotic lives. And it's the most visible
part: Being thin sends a visual message to the world that a woman is
competent at her other two jobs. She works hard at being attractive,
and is therefore good at her traditional job of being a desirable sexual
object, romantic partner, and consumer. By being lean, she also conveys the idea that she's disciplined, efficient, and in control of herself,
which makes her an ideal employee in today's competitive work world.
But the pursuit of thinness—which, unless you're born with the genes
of a jeans model, is time-consuming, stressful, and psychologically
debilitating—really prevents women from being successful at either
job. It keeps us from having real control over our own bodies, and our
own lives.

Very few American women I know are like some Italian friends of
mine, who take passionate interest in what they cook and eat. They
drizzle olive oil on vegetables with abandon, relish every bite of their
meals, and eat dessert or not as they please. Eating, for them, is a sensual experience, not a fearful one. They never feel guilty afterward.
Food isn't "good" or "bad" depending on the calories or fat grams it
contains, but according to how fresh it is and how lovingly prepared.
My Italian friends don't binge when they're upset, because food
doesn't have the power to overwhelm or hurt them. When they're finished eating, they're satisfied, and they don't think much about food
until the next meal; it's only one part of their full lives. They don't
worry about their weight and somehow they don't gain any.

Surely there are Italian women who have imported the American
bad habit of believing that food, fat, and their own bodies are the
enemy. There may even be Italian women who are afraid of olive oil.
But it's American women, and white American women in particular—
because women of color, who already deviate from the blonde ideal,
tend to have more respect for differences in size—who are especially
obsessed with their weight. American men are increasingly worried

about their weight, too, certainly, but the effects on women are much more penetrating and severe.

I was luckier in my diet career than many women. I was too young to have been given amphetamines, as many women were a decade earlier, with devastating consequences to their health. I was never fat enough to suffer the pain and discrimination that the truly obese endure. I never went on a liquid diet, shedding pounds rapidly only to see them boomerang back again. I didn't get my stomach stapled, my jaw wired, or my intestines shortened. I didn't suffer a stroke after taking over-the-counter diet pills, or die after ingesting herbal weight-loss remedies, as some women have. I wasn't like a very bright and talented college friend of mine, whose bulimia has consumed her life ever since, keeping her in miserable jobs, floating in and out of eating disorders treatment centers, lost and depressed.

I was more fortunate than that. I not only recovered from a serious eating disorder and weight obsession, I developed a healthy, positive, and downright pleasurable attitude about eating and my own body. But my awareness of the time and energy I lost, and of what so many other women continue to lose, haunted me. So I decided to take another look at the diet culture, this time not as a participant but as a journalist. I wanted to investigate the pressures that act on women to lose weight as well as the diet industry that exploits those pressures for a tremendous financial profit.

I set out to explore Dietland. I started with the same set of facts about dieting that most people already know: Nearly half of all American women, and a quarter of all men, diet, according to the Centers for Disease Control and Prevention (CDC). Most diets, several studies have shown, don't work for at least nine out of ten people, who will just regain the weight. (People who lose weight on their own and aren't counted in medical studies seem to do slightly better at keeping the pounds off.)[2] Still, we keep trying, and collectively we spend an estimated $34 billion to $50 billion a year on dieting—that's about the gross national product of Ireland—which comes down to roughly $500 a year per dieter.[3] Despite our efforts, we are still gaining weight: in the past decade, the average American adult has put on eight pounds.

Together, these facts suggest that we've invested a great deal in dieting—of money, not to mention of hope—and we're not getting much in return, except that we're getting fatter. What's going on? One widely held view is that we have no willpower. We fail at our diets, exercise less than our ancestors, eat too much, and sit around watching television, soaking up ads that encourage us to eat even more junk food. Our fat genes are running amuck in this saturated environment, say the obesity researchers, so we need more and more drastic diets and drugs to make us "normal."

There may be some truth to this view of why we're fat, but it puts far too much blame on the dieters. For one thing, a lot of research shows that some people are just born big and can't do much to change their basic body size. Other people may indeed have unhealthy habits, eating too much junk food or moving around too little, that make them fat. But there's something about the diet culture itself—the intense focus on unnatural slenderness, the cycles of deprivation and bingeing that wreak havoc on the body, the habit of thinking of food in terms of "good" and "bad," the depression that results from starvation and failure, and the notion that you need to have a great body to even begin to exercise—that encourages people to eat compulsively, shy away from movement, and gain weight. Our culture's efforts to make us thin, like my parents' attempts to get me to lose weight as a child, have backfired.

I began my research in the library, thumbing through old issues of *Ladies' Home Journal* and *Cosmopolitan*, looking for clues as to why our culture has become so obsessed with weight in the past hundred years. I wanted to know when slimness became an aesthetic preference in the United States, and more importantly, a sign of moral superiority. I became interested in looking at the changing images of ideal female bodies over the years, how we've gone from appreciating plump women to trying to emulate emaciated ones—and what those changes reveal about our culture.

Many of us today believe that it's those media images of thin women that are the main culprits in causing our weight obsessions and eating disorders. And no wonder. The current ideal body—the extreme is Kate Moss, so thin that New Yorkers spray-painted "Feed Me" on bus shelter ads with her image—is absurdly unattainable for most women. A model, on average, is five feet nine and a half inches tall, weighs 123 pounds (Moss is shorter and thinner), wears a size 6 or 8, and often has too little body fat to menstruate. Genetically speaking, she's something of a freak. The average American woman, on the other hand, is five feet four inches, weighs 144 pounds, and wears a size 12 (maybe 10 on top). But if fashion ads featuring skinny models were the only cultural pressures acting on us to be thin, we could resist them the way we can usually resist buying blue eyeshadow or wearing lime green this season. Ads with bony women reflect what sells in the culture; although they contribute to the mania for thinness, they didn't cause the problem in the first place.

The cultural pressures to be thin run much deeper than that. The drive to control our bodies—which is made up, in varying parts, of optimism, scientific zeal, morality, spirituality, and a good deal of entrepreneurship—is rooted in our peculiarly American character. But media images do tell the story about those deeper cultural values. Over the past century, changes in our culture's notion of what an ideal body looks like, and how much diversity is allowed in that ideal, tell us a great deal about our views of women and how women's roles have changed. Apart from that, these ideals also reveal shifts in the way we view our bodies as either natural and unchangeable, or completely malleable with the help of science, technology, and discipline.

After I explored the reasons why we're so interested in losing weight, I wanted to see how we do it. I investigated as many facets of the diet industry as I could. It's probably fair to say that I became as obsessed with the diet industry as I was, at one time, with dieting. I went to every guru, hypnotist, and weight-loss seminar I could find. I jotted down phone numbers from photocopied "Lose Weight Now, Ask Me How" flyers tacked up on telephone poles. I watched late-night TV diet infomercials, read the latest no-fat or high-protein weight-loss books, ate fake chocolate fat-free cookies, and sampled diet powder drinks. At health-food stores, I scoured the shelves for weight-loss products, deciphered their labels, and eventually talked with the families of women who had died taking those products. I rejoined Weight Watchers after many years, as well as Jenny Craig and several other commercial diet centers. I put ads in newspapers and interviewed numerous dieters and former weight-loss counselors about their long experiences with products and programs. In the end, I found that most of these diet programs were scams; they didn't help people lose weight, and many were even harmful.

Then I turned to science and medicine. No matter how much people can resist the cultural pressures to be thin, it's hard to argue with medical reasons to lose weight. Here, I expected to find a more sensible and ethical view of weight control, as well as some sort of consensus on the health risks of being fat. But what I discovered was a great deal of controversy and confusion in the field. Even the most basic questions about fatness—Is obesity really harmful? How fat do you have to be to be at risk? Is there any way to lose weight and keep it off? If not, why bother? Is yo-yo dieting itself harmful?—are hotly debated.

As a test, I asked several diet doctors and obesity researchers whether they thought I was overweight, and if so, what I should do about it. Some of them examined me: I've been weighed, measured, tested, and dunked naked in a water tank in a canvas sling to determine my body-fat percentage. I described myself to others on the phone: five feet six inches tall, 155 pounds. Some of the physicians lectured me, put me on a 500-calorie-a-day diet, and gave me big bottles of diet pills. Others recommended a 1,200-calorie-a-day diet, with a prescription for dexfenfluramine (Redux) later on if I wasn't "good." Still others asked me more detailed questions—Do I exercise much? What are my eating habits? Are my relatives large? How long have I maintained this weight? How big is my waist compared with my hips? What do my cholesterol numbers look like?—before deciding that my weight was probably fine. A few congratulated me for being in wonderful shape, eating a healthy diet, and maintaining my weight for so long—and asked me how I did it.

As it happens, the question of whether I'm overweight relates to many more people than just me. My Body Mass Index (BMI)—a fancy way physicians have of describing your weight according to your height (weight in kilos divided by height in meters squared)—is exactly the same as for the average five foot four inch, 144-pound American woman: 25. I'm like the typical client at commercial weight-loss programs who thinks she needs to lose twenty pounds. But physicians and researchers haven't figured out whether the average-sized American woman is at a health risk for her weight, or whether she's just fine as long as she gets some exercise. Nor have they determined at what point obesity definitely is a health risk (there's no question that extreme obesity *is* unhealthy), and what, if anything, can be done about it that will help in the long run.

In addition to asking physicians and researchers whether I was fat, I read hundreds of medical journal articles, attended scientific conferences on obesity and nutrition, spoke to patients, and interviewed many of the most prominent obesity researchers, dietitians, and eating disorders experts in the field. I tried to be as thorough and fair as a lay person could be in examining the available evidence and theories on the health risks of obesity, as well as the effectiveness of medical treatments for weight loss.

What I found is that many physicians and obesity researchers are as influenced by cultural ideals about weight as the rest of us. More disturbingly, many of them are as interested in making money off of diets and weight-loss plans as the commercial programs they disdain. In fact, many physicians were quick to sign up with commercial diet centers to dispense unproven and dangerous combinations of diet pills to just about anyone who walked through the door. When fenfluramine (Pondimin) and dexfenfluramine (Redux) were taken off the market in September 1997, some physicians, undeterred, continued to prescribe dicey combinations of phentermine and Prozac, or phen-Pro.

This is troubling, because when we listen to our doctors or read the results of a scientific study in the newspaper, we usually believe them. When a Harvard study concludes that we need to lose weight for our health even if we're just slightly over the ideal, we take it to heart. But I realized that we need to view the science about obesity with as much skepticism as we do other kinds of weight-loss hype.

For example, in September 1995, a study came out which convinced many women that being ten to twenty pounds over the ideal is dangerous to their health. This widely publicized study was based on data from the long-term Nurses' Health Study involving 115,195 female nurses over a period of sixteen years. The researchers, JoAnn Manson and her colleagues at Brigham and Women's Hospital and Harvard Medical School found that the leanest nurses in the group, most of whom were between the ages of thirty and fifty-five when the study began in 1976, were the ones who were most likely to live the longest. Those who had put on a few pounds had a greater chance of dying early. A five foot five inch woman, the researchers told the media, had no increased risk if she weighed less than 120 pounds. At 120 to 149 pounds, her risk went up 20 percent; from 150 to 160, it went up 30 percent; and from 161 to 175 pounds, the risk was 60 percent higher than for the lean women. "We can no longer afford to be complacent about the epidemic of obesity in America," Manson proclaimed in a press release. "Even mild to moderate overweight is associated with a substantial increase in risk of premature death."

It sounded alarming. The press repeated and exaggerated the

study's conclusions—"An extra twenty pounds can kill you," one local TV anchor put it—running color charts of ideal weights, hinting that those of us who are heavier than the ideal might as well start shopping for cemetery plots. But looking more closely at the details of the study, the gloomy picture of fatness and early death practically disappeared into meaninglessness.

First, the study was based on very few people, since only 4,726 of the nurses, or just over 4 percent, died. Of those, only 1,499 were women who had never smoked (cigarette smoking could account for many of the deaths). Of the nonsmokers, only 184 women died from cardiovascular disease, which was the sole disease clearly associated with weight. Of those deaths, plotted on a graph, the risk according to weight increased very slightly for that five foot five inch woman from 120 to 175 pounds, and only went soaring upward when she hit about 190 pounds (BMI 32). At 161 to 175 pounds (BMI of 27 to 29), the women did have a 60 percent increase in death rate, but the death rate was so low to begin with that 60 percent more than almost nothing was still almost nothing. In fact, when Manson warned of increased risks at a BMI of less than 27, she was actually talking about a statistical "trend," as she told me. In other words, when you draw a line on a graph showing how the risk of early death increases with weight, the line starts going up—just barely—at that point. But the increased risk was so small that statisticians say they're not confident it's even there. It's insignificant, which Manson admitted to me.[4]

Overall, the study didn't prove very much more than that middle-aged, relatively affluent, mainly white American women have very low death rates, and that only those who gain quite a large amount of weight stand much of an increased risk of dying early. The study also didn't examine how fitness may have affected the women's longevity and risk of disease. It made no distinction between heavy couch potatoes and heavy long-distance swimmers. It's quite possible that the tiny increase in risk of death had to do with getting too little exercise, which contributes to weight gain but may be the more important factor in health. Other studies that have added fitness to the equation of weight and early death have found that people who exercise live longer, regardless of their weight.[5]

Exercise is just one example of many factors that confound the question of how weight affects longevity. There's an enormous variation in human size, shape, and musculature, and it seems simpleminded to believe that everyone of a certain height should weigh the same amount. Nor can you make conclusions about individuals from a study that involves a large group of people. Weight is very individual—not something you can prescribe from a height-weight chart.

The results of this study, then, were essentially the opposite of what was reported: Being twenty or forty pounds over the ideal makes little difference to your health. Why were the results interpreted the way they were? Perhaps it was a matter of cultural bias and genuine concern about the increasing amount of obesity in the country. And maybe financial interests played a role. Manson, the leading author, was a paid consultant to Interneuron Pharmaceuticals, Inc., the company that developed the diet drug dexfenfluramine. In September 1995, at Food and Drug Administration (FDA) hearings on whether this drug should be approved, Manson used her study to testify about the health risks of obesity in order to justify the use of a drug that is rarely, but sometimes, quite harmful. Telling women who are mild to moderately overweight that they are at a substantially increased risk of dying early because of their size might well give their doctors a medical rationale for prescribing such a diet drug, which would, of course, boost sales considerably.[6]

After I studied diet doctors and obesity researchers, I turned to the anti-diet movement. I interviewed researchers, therapists, and activists who challenged the ideas that propel the diet culture. Some of them have shown how simply quitting dieting does a great deal toward enhancing self-esteem, and other have devised systems to help people develop healthier eating and exercise habits. Fat activists argue that most of the problems fat women experience are not due to their weight but to the culture that makes life miserable for them. I tried to approach these people and groups with the same skepticism with which I looked at other aspects of the diet industry. Here, too, I found cases where people made false promises, exaggerated their research, or ignored other scientific findings. But on the whole, their attitudes about women and weight were much more positive, productive, and realistic than those held by people who promote dieting.

Finally, I tried to gather sensible ideas from various researchers about improving weight problems from a different point of view, by developing healthy and sustainable eating and exercise habits, and by building a more positive body image. My hope, in writing this book, was not only to debunk the diet industry but to suggest that there are ways to get out of the vicious cycle of dieting and feeling bad about yourself, and truly to feel healthier and better about your body.

My other hope, at the end of this personal investigation, was to be done with my own dieting and weight obsession forever. That's hard to accomplish in this culture, but at least I can say that I no longer want to be skinny, and I can eat pizza without feeling the slightest bit like a pig. With any luck, this book may spare other women from having to endure a similar journey through Dietland, and encourage them toward some of the same pleasures at the end.

So, *buon appetito.*

Chapter 1

The Inner Corset

Once upon a time, a man with a thick gold watch swaying from a big, round paunch was the very picture of American prosperity and vigor. A hundred years ago, a beautiful woman had plump cheeks and arms, and she wore a corset and even a bustle to emphasize her full, substantial hips. Women were *sexy* if they were heavy. In those days, Americans knew that a layer of fat was a sign that you could afford to eat well, too, and that you stood a better chance of fighting off infectious diseases than most people. If you were a woman, having that extra adipose blanket also meant you were probably fertile, and warm to cuddle up next to on chilly nights.

Between the 1880s and 1920s, that pleasant image of fat thoroughly changed in this country. Some people began early on to hint that fat was a health risk. In 1894, Woods Hutchinson, a medical professor who wrote for women's magazines, defended fat against this new point of view. "Adipose," he wrote, "while often pictured as a veritable Frankenstein, born of and breeding disease, sure to ride its possessor to death sooner or later, is really a most harmless, healthful, innocent tissue." Hutchinson reassured his *Cosmopolitan* readers that fat was not only benign but attractive, and that if a poll of beautiful women were taken in any city, there would be at least three times as many plump ones as slender ones. He advised them that no amount of starving or exercise—both just becoming popular as means of weight control—would change more than 10 percent of a person's body size anyway. "The fat man tends to remain fat, the thin woman to stay thin—and both in perfect health—in spite of everything they can do."

But by 1926, Hutchinson, who was by then a past president of the American Academy of Medicine, was having to defend fat against fashion, too, and he was showing signs of strain. "In this present onslaught upon one of the most peaceable, useful and law-abiding of all our tissues," he told readers of *The Saturday Evening Post*, "fashion has apparently the backing of grave physicians, of food reformers and physical trainers, and even of great insurance companies, all chanting in unison the new commandment of fashion: 'Thou shalt be thin!' "

Hutchinson mourned this trend, and was dismayed that young girls were attempting to rid themselves of their roundness. He tried to understand the new view people took toward fat: "It is an outward and visible sign of an inward and spiritual disgrace, of laziness, of self-indulgence," he explained, but he remained unconvinced. Instead, he longed for a more cheerful period in the not-so-distant past when a little fat never hurt anyone, and he darkly warned that some physicians were deliberately underfeeding girls and young women solely for the purpose of giving them a more svelte figure. "The longed-for slender and boyish figure is becoming a menace," Hutchinson wrote, "not only to the present, but also the future generations."

And so it would. But why did the fashion for plumpness change so dramatically during those years? What happened that caused Americans to alter their tastes, not only to admire thinner figures for a time but for the next century, culminating in fin-de-siècle extremes of thinness, where women's magazines in the 1990s would print ads featuring gaunt models side by side with photo essays on anorexia?

Many things were happening at once, with dizzying speed. Foremost was a changing economy: in the late 1800s, for the first time, ample amounts of food were available to more and more people who had to do less and less work to eat. The agricultural economy, based on family farms and home workshops, shifted to an industrial one. A huge influx of immigrants—many of them genetically shorter and rounder than the earlier American settlers—fueled the industrial machine. People moved to cities to do factory work and service jobs, stopped growing their own food, and relied more on store-bought goods. Large companies began to process food products, distribute them via

s, and use refrigeration to keep perishables fresh. Food be-
nore accessible and convenient to all but the poorest families.
e who once had too little to eat now had plenty, and those who
tendency to put on weight began to do so. When it became possible for people of modest means to become plump, being fat no longer
was seen as a sign of prestige. Well-to-do Americans of Northern
European extraction wanted to be able to distinguish themselves,
physically and racially, from stockier immigrants. The status symbols flipped: It became chic to be thin and all too ordinary to be
overweight.[1]

In this new environment, older cultural undercurrents that were
suspicious of fat began to surface. Europeans had long considered
slenderness a sign of class distinction and finer sensibilities, and
Americans began to follow suit. In Europe, during the late eighteenth
and early nineteenth centuries, many writers and intellectuals—the
poets Keats and Shelley; Emily Brontë and Anton Chekhov—had
tuberculosis, which made them sickly thin. Members of the upper
classes believed that having tuberculosis, and being slender itself,
were signs that one possessed a delicate, intellectual, and superior
nature. "For snobs and parvenus and social climbers, TB was the one
index of being genteel, delicate, [and] sensitive," writes the essayist
Susan Sontag in *Illness as Metaphor.* "It was glamorous to look
sickly." So interested was the poet Lord Byron in looking as fashion-
ably ill as the other Romantic poets that he embarked on a series of
obsessive diets, consuming only biscuits and water, or vinegar and
potatoes, and succeeded in becoming quite thin. Byron, who at five feet
six and a half inches tall, with a clubfoot that prevented him from
walking much, weighed 202 pounds in his youth, disdained fat in
others. "A woman," he wrote, "should never be seen eating or
drinking, unless it be *lobster salad* and *champagne*, the only truly feminine and becoming viands."[2] Aristocratic European women, thrilled
with the romantic figure Byron cut, took his advice and despaired of
appearing fat. Aristocratic Americans, trying to imitate Europeans,
adopted their enthusiasm for champagne and slenderness.

Americans believed it was not only a sign of class to be thin but a
sign of morality. There was a long tradition in American culture which
suggested that indulging the body and its appetites was immoral, and
that denying the flesh was a sure way to become closer to God. Puritans such as the minister Cotton Mather frequently fasted to prove

their worthiness to God and to cleanse themselves of th[e]
jamin Franklin, in his *Poor Richard's Almanack*, chided [
eat lightly in order to please not only God but also a
Reason: "Wouldst thou enjoy a long life, a healthy Bod[y]
orous Mind, and be acquainted also with the wonderful works of God?
Labour in the first place to bring thy Appetite into Subjection to
Reason." Franklin's attitude toward food reveals a puritanical distrust
of appetite as overly sensual; it also presages diets that would attempt
to bring eating in line with rational, scientific calculations. "The Difficulty lies, in finding out an exact Measure"; he wrote, "but eat for
Necessity, not Pleasure, for Lust knows not where Necessity ends."
By the 1820s, even schoolboys were learning the lesson that it was
immoral to overeat: "Do not eat more than is necessary," says one
New York City grammar school reader. "Persons who eat too much
are called gluttons. They are stupid, and heavy, and idle; and, very
often, they have a sad pain in the head and stomach."[3]

At the end of the nineteenth century, as Woods Hutchinson
observed, science was also helping to shape the new slender ideal.
Physicians came to believe they were able to arrive at an exact measure of human beings; they could count calories, weigh people on
scales, calculate "ideal" weights, and advise those who deviated from
that ideal that they could change themselves. Physicians were both
following and encouraging the trend for thinness. In the 1870s, after
all, when plumpness was in vogue, physicians had encouraged people
to *gain* weight. Two of the most distinguished doctors of the age,
George Beard and S. Weir Mitchell, believed that excessive thinness
caused American women to succumb to a wide variety of nervous disorders, and that a large number of fat cells was absolutely necessary
to achieve a balanced personality.[4] But when the plump figure fell
from favor, physicians found new theories to support the new fashion.
They hastily developed treatments—such as thyroid, arsenic, and
strychnine—to prescribe to their increasing numbers of weight-loss
patients, many of whom were not exactly corpulent but more than
willing to part with their pennies along with their pounds.

As the twentieth century got under way, other cultural changes
made slenderness seem desirable. When many women ventured out of
their homes and away from their strict roles as mothers, they left
behind the plump and reproductive physique, which began to seem
old-fashioned next to a thinner, freer, more modern body. The new

consumer culture encouraged the trend toward thinness with fashion illustrations and ads featuring slim models; advertisers learned early to offer women an unattainable dream of thinness and beauty in order to sell more products. In short, a cultural obsession with weight became firmly established in the United States when several disparate factors that favored a desire for thinness—economic status symbols, morality, medicine, modernity, changing women's roles, and consumerism—all collided at once.

Thinness is, at its heart, a peculiarly American preoccupation. Europeans admire slenderness, but without our Puritanism, they have more relaxed and moderate attitudes about food, eating, and body size (the British are most like us in both being heavy and fixated on weight-loss schemes). In countries where people don't have quite enough to eat, and where women remain in traditional roles, plumpness is still widely admired. Other Westernized countries have developed a slender ideal, but for the most part, they have imported it from the United States. Russian women wouldn't dream of spending a month's salary on herbal weight-loss shakes if they didn't want to look like the women in American ads. Japanese girls wouldn't have soaring rates of eating disorders if they weren't exposed to so many Western images of skinny perfection (and high-fat Western snacks). The Chinese wouldn't be so successful in selling millions of bars of soft seaweed defatting soap in China and Japan (claiming to "discharge the underskin fat out of human bodies") if they hadn't taken the idea from us. No other culture suffers from the same wild anxieties about weight, dieting, and exercise as we do because they don't share our history.

The ideal of female thinness that developed in the United States from the 1880s to the 1920s wasn't just a momentary shift in fashion; it was a monumental turning point in the way women's bodies were appraised by men and experienced by women. The change can be traced through the evolution of three ideal types: the plump Victorian woman; the athletic but curvaceous Gibson Girl; and the boyishly straight-bodied flapper. By 1930, American women knew how very important it was for them to be thin. "How decisively even ten or fifteen extra pounds detract from one's appearance and make the most expensive gown dowdy!" proclaimed an ad for reducing salts in *Cosmopolitan* magazine. "A youthful slender figure means *everything* today." From then on, despite moments when voluptuousness was admired again, à la Marilyn Monroe, American women could never be too thin.

The Pleasingly Plump Victorian Ideal

Lillian Russell, a well-known actress and the most famous American beauty of the late nineteenth century, would be considered quite fat by today's standards. She would be the depressed-looking model in a "before" ad, pictured later, after a presumably quick weight loss, proudly showing off how far the waistband stretched in her old polyester fat pants. But to the late Victorians, Russell had all the attributes of face and figure that women coveted most: luminous white skin, soft dimpled cheeks, long golden hair, and a voluptuous body. Tall and stately, fairly bursting from her corset, she sometimes tipped the scales at over 200 pounds.

Russell was a singer and actress who charmed audiences with her sweet doll's face, open laugh, and generous spirit. She was a perfect icon of the plush era, when heady economic times loosened the corset strings—and strict morality—of the Victorians and made way for the Gay Nineties. Russell was a lady, but she knew how to have a good time; she frequently indulged her passion for rich food at New York's best restaurants with her companion Diamond Jim Brady. (During one gargantuan meal at Delmonico's, he offered her a large diamond ring if she could eat as much as he did. Russell discreetly slipped into the ladies' room to remove her corset, returned to the table, took a deep breath, and won her ring.)

In photographs, Russell hardly looks obese, though her voluminous skirts, flounces, and trains leave her proportions below the waist a mystery. Her arms and face have the appealing plumpness of a healthy baby. With her hair piled high, in elaborate costumes and feathered hats, she is a proud prima donna, a glory of a woman from a time when being feminine meant having a good deal of soft, female flesh.

Russell's hourglass body type was widely admired, but it wasn't an "ideal" in the sense that women everywhere believed they, too, had to have her proportions to be considered attractive. Corset ads from the late nineteenth century show a wide variety of body silhouettes—"For every ideal type!"—without any suggestion that a fashionable woman ought to be one particular shape. Dr. Warner's Coraline Corsets, for instance, were modeled in advertisements by four lovely women of very different sizes: "Made in twenty-five different patterns to fit every variety of figure—tall, short, slender, stout, either long, short or medium waisted." As long as a woman was cinched in at the waist, not nearly as much importance was placed on her actual body size as would be in later years.

A beautiful face was far more important then than a good figure. Victorians admired doll-like women who seemed as pampered, porcelain, and immobile as the genuine article. Several articles in *Cosmopolitan* magazine—then a general-interest magazine with rose-cheeked beauties on the cover instead of thin women with improbably large amounts of cleavage—muse at great length about feminine beauty but hardly mention the body. In 1890, one *Cosmopolitan* writer listed the attributes of the most admired American women: "Golden hair united to brown or hazel eyes, soft, smooth skin with faint olive shading, little color in the cheeks, features sharply defined (although relieved by a slight facial fullness), and the figure healthily rounded."

When pressed, a late Victorian man might admit he preferred a little meat on a woman's bones. It was considered impolite to comment on most women's bodies, but actresses were an exception. "There was nothing wraithlike about Lillian Russell; she was a voluptuous beauty, and there was plenty of her to see," wrote the critic Clarence Day in *The Saturday Evening Post*, recalling one of Russell's performances. "We liked that. Our tastes were not thin, or ethereal. We liked flesh in the Nineties. It didn't have to be bare, and it wasn't, but it had to be there."[5]

Slender actresses of the era held no candle to the likes of Lillian Russell. When the slim French actress Sarah Bernhardt visited the United States in the 1880s, she was openly mocked for her skinny body (which would seem rather large for an actress today), and was caricatured in cartoons as a broomstick, a boa constrictor, and a body made of water pipes.[6] Photographers of the era preferred plump women as models, too. One expert, advising would-be photographers in an 1896 *Cosmopolitan* article, wrote, "The model must be far from thin, with no suggestions of hollows in the face or of collar-bones, for the camera seems to accentuate such defects." Those are the kinds of "defects" that have made contemporary supermodels famous.

Personal ads from the late nineteenth century suggest that men seeking romantic partners preferred women who, if not fat, at least had plenty to love. In his social history of dieting, *Never Satisfied*, Hillel Schwartz describes how one prospective suitor, five foot ten and 160 pounds, looked for a woman who was shorter than him and weighed 130 to 160 pounds. Another specified he didn't want anyone "tall, lean, or lank-looking." These personal ads are quite different from ones today, where the adjectives "slim," "svelte," and "fit" are invariably listed long before "witty," "well-read," or "loves to fly-fish" are mentioned.

Women who would be considered twenty to forty pounds overweight today were just fine by the standards of the late Victorian age. For any woman today who has a body image problem, browsing through turn-of-the-century American magazines is excellent therapy. Page after musty page of *Cosmopolitan*, *Ladies' Home Journal*, *Vogue*, and *Harper's Bazaar* contains portraits of plump women. A woman who feels depressingly large and ungainly compared with the extremely slender ideal these days might well recognize her body type as the one celebrated in late Victorian drawings. Pin up the hair; don a corset, hoop-skirted dress, and button-up shoes: she, too, would draw admiring glances from men in handlebar mustaches.

Not that she'd want to have lived then. The late Victorians admired plumpness mainly because it emphasized a woman's traditional role as a homebound mother who was entirely dependent on her husband. Feminine identity then was based on an idealized image of motherhood and domesticity. The corseted body fairly shouted that a woman was not only built to reproduce—exaggerating the breasts and hips— but that, hampered by her clothing, she was only fit to stay at home. The picture of the ideal woman, painted in so many magazines of the era, was of a placid, blissful, childlike mother. One 1886 illustration in *Cosmopolitan*, titled "Maternal Felicity," depicts a plump, well-to-do woman darning, with a baby in the crib and another child at her side; her face has such a calm, vacant sweetness that she must either have a lot of household help or very little going on upstairs. In the Victorian imagination, both would be ideal. A Victorian woman couldn't forget that her main purpose in life was to bear children and then civilize them. At the time, the English biologist and novelist Grant Allen described women as "the sex sacrificed to reproductive necessities."[7]

During the Victorian era, the plump and corseted body not only emphasized a woman's maternal role but her economic status as well.

The leisure-class Victorian woman, ideally, was a trophy wife who was a visible sign of her husband's success. Being plump was a signal that a woman was free from menial drudgery and that her husband could afford to keep her well fed. The corset physically prevented her from doing any work. "The corset is, in economic theory, substantially a mutilation, undergone for the purpose of lowering the subject's vitality and rendering her permanently and obviously unfit for work," wrote Thorstein Veblen, the famous American economist of the age, in his *Theory of the Leisure Class* (1899).

Like Chinese foot-binding, corset lacing severely limited women's physical freedom and was considered essential for real femininity. Hoop skirts, bustles, and dresses that took yards and yards of fabric made it even more difficult to get around. Victorian corsets weren't like the lingerie we think of today, the stretchy little undergarments-as-outergarments that appeared on fashion runways in the early 1990s. They were extremely rigid contraptions with heavy stays which, when pulled tight, exerted some twenty to eighty pounds of pressure on the wearer.[8] The Victorians' justification for these horrendous garments was that women were such weak creatures that they needed help staying upright. Even girls learned that for health's sake they must wear corsets from an early age: "Beautiful children wear Good Sense," says one 1892 ad for the Good Sense Corset Waist (a "perfect health corset"). Corsets were touted as being necessary to support muscles, organs, and breasts that would, left alone, droop and collapse. Medical theories at the time held that women were so frail, they couldn't afford to waste their precious reproductive energies on mental or physical exertion.[9]

But the health justification for corset lacing was merely a way for the establishment to support a particular fashion in female body types and behavior, as the medical world would do a few years later, when physicians would advise women to go on crash diets to lose weight for the sake of "health." Corsets put so much force on women's bodies that they often constricted the lungs, squeezed the liver and small intestines, dislocated the stomach, and compressed the bladder. Some women's corsets were laced so tightly that, over time, their ribs grew into their livers or other organs.[10]

Corsets also prevented women from eating much, but ladies were considered too delicate to have any real appetite. Despite the fact that women were ideally supposed to be plump, it was considered unseemly for them to be caught in the indelicate act of eating. Women hardly ate at the dinner table—even though many binged in secret. Like Scarlett O'Hara, who was admonished to eat before a ball so she wouldn't appear to be hungry, women ate in private. Refraining from food was a sign that one was wealthy enough not to have to worry about when the next meal would come. It was also a sign of propriety: any appetite for food was equated with an unladylike appetite for sexuality. As an actress, Lillian Russell got away with eating more because it was a mild way of titillating her public. She publicized her huge meals in much the same way actresses today send out press releases about their latest sexual partners. But for most women, it was fashionable to refrain from eating long before it became fashionable to be slender. The long tradition of seeing food abstention as an essential character-istic of femininity and class would make it that much more important, later on, for women to diet.[11]

Corsets also interfered with women's appetites for change. They kept women literally tied to their roles as mothers and homebodies. A new suffragist movement was brewing—Lillian Russell's mother, Cynthia Van Names Leonard, who ran a shelter for prostitutes left homeless after the great Chicago fire, was one of the leading feminists of the time—and the more freedom beckoned, the tighter the corsets were laced. Without corsets, women might become like one of those suffragists who, as one *Cosmopolitan* writer warned, were "Brawling, noisy, homeless shriekers . . . always holding 'congresses' and de-nouncing the tyrant man." Corseted women couldn't very well leave the home, as a few renegade women were beginning to do, to enter the professions or do charity work.

That left little for leisured women to do. Unable to work, a woman's job was to be, as Veblen put it, the "chief ornament" in the home, as delicate, immobile, and perfectly decorative as a piece of fine china. They were at once objects of conspicuous consumption and con-sumers of objects. Sewing, shopping, and beautifying themselves were the only activities that gave well-to-do women any outlet for personal expression. Soon, those activities became a Victorian woman's primary occupation: to be a consumer. How much a woman bought, like how much time and money she spent on her appearance, showed off how much wealth her husband had. In Edith Wharton's classic novel *House of Mirth* (1905), the wealthy Rosedale, who wants to marry Lily Bart, puts a woman's value as a status object and consumer more succinctly:

"You need money and the right woman to spend it . . . I want my wife to make all the other women feel small."

Being a consumer, and buying things to look fashionable, became an essential part of a woman's identity. Her sense of well-being and usefulness depended on how well she decorated her home and represented herself as the lovely wife her husband would be proud to show off. Women became very susceptible to advertisements aimed at changing fashions, and changing themselves. They were extremely receptive to the helpful hints offered by advice magazines, which were proliferating at the time. When magazines began to give them intimate advice about their own body size—whether to be plump or thin, for example—they would take that advice.

It wouldn't be long before the pleasingly plump ideal would pass out of fancy. Fashions in corsets would pull the small waist, originally intended to enhance the plump appearance of the breasts and buttocks, tighter and tighter. The hourglass effect became so pronounced that many women, aware that they could use padding and bustles to create a plump appearance, began to try to reduce their body size by dieting in order to have an ever slimmer waist.

By the late 1890s, magazine ads were peddling patent diet remedies and rubber reducing garments. In 1896, Lillian Russell began the first of her many efforts to lose weight. Russell spent most of the rest of her career on highly publicized diet regimes, just as Elizabeth Taylor would do several decades later. The once great "American Beauty" would have to fend off reviews that compared her with a white elephant and criticized her for not being able to fit into the narrower, slinkier dresses being worn onstage by younger actresses. "Pounds and pounds were accumulating on her already stuffed figure," wrote her biographer, Parker Morell. "But what of it? she deluded herself by asking. The hour-glass figure would never go out of style. Yet there were indications that its sands were running low, and that a closing century might decree a new aesthetic for the feminine form."[12]

The Gibson Girl

In the early 1890s, an ambitious young illustrator dropped off a whimsical drawing of a dog barking at the moon at the offices of *Life* magazine. The art director liked the little sketch, agreed to publish it, and asked Charles Dana Gibson to try his hand at a few more. Gibson began to draw what he was interested in most: beautiful young women. The women in his illustrations were different, however, from the society beauties who had appeared in magazine pages before then. They were tall, slender, and had an air of freedom and vitality about them that was utterly fresh. The women, who were all variations on one type, had upswept hair, dainty facial features, rather broad shoulders, a tiny waist, and a vigorous build. They were the first women to appear in magazines who looked strong enough to swing a tennis racket. The Gibson Girl, as her type was called, was a wholesome, active, well-to-do young woman; she was as relaxed and lovely playing croquet or tennis as she was sitting in the parlors of society's best homes. She wasn't real, however; she was a pure fantasy, a perfect ideal that few women could hope to approach.[13]

From the 1890s until World War I, the Gibson Girl was a sensation. She was everywhere: in magazines, books, calendars, and on wallpaper. The Gibson Girl was more slender than the pleasingly plump ideal—though still quite large by today's standards—and full of a new physical vigor. She still had some of the characteristics of the late Victorian ideal, however; she had wide hips and a large, shelflike bust, and her cinched-in waist bore evidence of straitlacing (though illustrated women, of course, could achieve the effect without a painful corset). The Gibson Girl was a transitional figure between plump and slender beauty ideals. She was partly voluptuous and ornamental, but more slim, commanding, and independent-looking than the doll-like late Victorians. Her clothes were less fussy, confining, and elaborate than her predecessors', and so more of her natural body was revealed. In only a few years the Gibson Girl would bare her legs at the beach, making the lower half of a woman's body public for the first time. Before the Gibson Girl, a woman's lower body was merely a shapeless, massive pedestal on which the bust of a perfect, porcelain woman rested. The Gibson Girl's legs, exposed, were long and slim with dainty ankles. She would pave the way for a much more slender ideal: the flapper.

Charles Dana Gibson didn't create this new image of an ideal woman out of whole cloth. Rather, he was a young and fashionable man who was able to capture the spirit of the dawning era. The Gibson Girl was athletic because women in Gibson's social set, influenced by women abroad, had taken up croquet, tennis, and other genteel sports.

She wore simpler, less encumbering clothing to accommodate her active lifestyle. The Gibson Girl reflected the success of the early feminist movement's goals of freeing women from the strict confines of their clothing and their home. But she also represented how those feminist impulses had been safely harnessed in a new female ideal that was still corseted, demure, and hardly threatening. In illustrations, the Gibson Girl played sports and expanded her leisure activities, but she was never seen going to medical school, doing social work, organizing for the vote, or engaging in any other of the activities women's reformers were involved in at the time.

The Gibson Girl personified the new "natural woman" who came into vogue at the turn of the century. The first real woman of this type widely known in the United States was the British actress Lillie Langtry. This aristocratic woman—and one-time mistress of the Prince of Wales—had a body that was quite similar to the Gibson Girl. At five foot eight, she was tall, with a large bosom and hips, and a strong, broad-shouldered frame. She was known to exercise, as the upper classes in England had been doing for years. Americans, accustomed to plumper women who had delicate features, didn't like the looks of Langtry when she first toured the country in 1882. To them, she represented the worst of what could happen to a woman if she exercised: her arms and legs would become hard and stringy, with masculine-looking muscles showing through her formerly soft padded skin. The fear then, according to the historian Lois W. Banner, was that exercise burned an excessive amount of fat, and women would risk losing their bosom and hips, becoming appallingly thin.

Nevertheless, Langtry became more popular as elite Americans realized that exercise was the favorite pastime of the high-class British they tried to imitate. In 1896, *Cosmopolitan* society writer Ada Wentworth Sears, returning from a trip abroad, reported: "In England, especially, a stranger cannot help being forcibly impressed today, by the attention paid to women's athletics and to woman as an athlete." Sports (though no strenuous ones) were fast becoming necessary social graces. "If they wished to be numbered among the smart set of England or America," Sears decreed, women "must be adept at all kinds of outdoor sports." Sports were attractive to bored, leisure-class American women, who saw them as a welcome addition to the limited number of pursuits they could be involved in outside their homes.

By 1904, the Victorian ideal had become clearly outmoded. One writer for *Cosmopolitan*, Rafford Pyke, described the Gibson Girl look as the swing in the pendulum of fashion from the Victorian age, when the genteel young female had to be delicate in order to be admired. "And so she pinched her waist and shielded her complexion from the sun, and was ashamed of showing any appetite for food, and made herself interesting by having fainting-fits and hysterics whenever anything went wrong." In a few short years that look had entirely changed. "Nowadays that sort of young woman is extinct; and we have in her place the hail-fellow-well-met type, the cycling girl, the golfing girl, the yachting girl, the girl who eats like a coal-heaver, drinks 'highballs' and carries a cigarette-case in the pocket of her Norfolk jacket." Strength, not frailty, wrote Pyke, was the new watchword of contemporary femininity—though he feared that women would take things too far and begin to act like men.

Athletics really took hold because the aristocratic fancy for sports turned into a broader movement for physical fitness, whose advocates encouraged women's sports, particularly in colleges. Women's colleges were new, and critics still believed that intellectual work would sap away women's physical vigor. In response, a few of the more daring women's colleges organized physical education classes to prove to their antagonists that women had the capacity to develop strength in both areas. Calisthenics courses were offered, as well as rowing and tennis. At one college, a teacher hung wicker fruit baskets on the walls and devised a game whereby members of one team tried to keep the others from throwing the ball into the basket. (Eventually a few men tried playing "basketball" too, though it would be years before the slam-dunk was invented.) Women who participated in sports in college didn't relinquish them when they finished school; they joined gyms and country clubs, and, reform-minded, many of them lobbied for exercise classes for poor women in YWCAs and for immigrant women in settlement houses. Exercise was hailed as a health remedy for women who had been suffering from nervous disorders, hysteria, and a variety of other ailments.

It was also a remedy for a new health problem: corpulence. Beginning in 1901, insurance companies started to chart "ideal weights," and to show how being overweight was statistically linked with an early death. None of the early insurance charts was based on data about women; instead, the conclusions about women were made up from data about a rather narrow population group, men who were old and wealthy enough to get life insurance. But for the first time it seemed possible to measure the body like a machine to test its longevity. Scales became widespread, and people began to think of their bodies in terms of acceptable numbers. A pseudoscience developed which made it seem that all human beings, no matter what their build, shape, or genetic background, could be put on a single scale that could predict how long they would live and how healthy they might be. Manufacturers and entrepreneurs devised "scientific" systems for exercise, including baths, calisthenics, rolling around, and massage, to help people measure up to the ideal.

People began to believe that there was one perfect physical form that men and women could achieve if they worked hard enough at it. For women, that ideal was still rather fleshy. In the 1905 "Most Perfect Formed" contest, held in Madison Square Garden and produced by *Physical Culture* magazine, the woman who won first place had large hips and thighs, and though she appeared sturdy and strong—particularly compared with Victorian ladies—she was much, much softer than today's aerobicized ideal.

Of all the exercise regimes advocated by the new physical fitness buffs, the bicycle had the most lasting impact on women's health, clothing, and freedom. "To women, [the bicycle] is deliverance, revolution, and salvation," wrote Mrs. Reginald deKoven for *Cosmopolitan* in 1895. "It is well nigh impossible to overestimate the potentialities of this exercise in the curing of the common and characteristic ills of womankind, both physical and mental, or to calculate the far-reaching effects of its influence in the matters of dress and social reform."

For Lillian Russell, the bicycle would be the salvation of her career—or at least, her figure. Diamond Jim Brady ordered her a gold-plated bicycle, with her monogram set in diamonds and emeralds on the handlebars. The two of them wheeled around Central Park Reservoir every day. When guests visited their country house, they had to abide by the rules: Everyone had to be on time for meals and exercise at least an hour of each day of the visit. Russell lost a little weight; enough, at least, that newspapers printed some of the first "before" and "after" photos, one of which bore a caption speculating that Russell had had her fat surgically removed. (By 1912, like many fading celebrities today who make exercise videos to salvage their careers, Russell posed in a series of colored motion pictures that showed her engaged in calisthenics and other exercise routines. She ended up writing a syndicated beauty column for the *Chicago Tribune*.)

The bicycle changed women's fashions in body size, and led to some reform in women's dress. Some corsets eased up; the Good Sense Corset Waist advertised in 1897 that it was "yielding to every motion of the body, permitting full expansion of the lungs." Women couldn't very well ride a "scorcher," as the bicycle was called (because of its blinding speed), in tight corsets and voluminous skirts, either. Fashionable women began to wear "knickerbockers," a kind of split skirt that recalled the bloomer, though most wore a shirtwaist blouse and shortened skirts that, shockingly, displayed their ankles to the public.

The bicycle and the new dress it inspired gave women more freedom to move in public. But while the new physically fit ideal was liberating to women, it would lead to more self-consciousness about their bodies. A woman's body could be more easily discerned under a bicycling outfit than previous costumes. Soon, enough of the body would be revealed to make it subject to criticism. A consciousness of legs meant that legs, for the first time, had to adapt to beauty standards. And the standard was clear: the Gibson Girl.

The Gibson Girl's popularity cut across class lines, creating a single national ideal of womanhood. By 1900, the Gibson Girl's sporting outfit, a shirtwaist blouse and a simple skirt, had become fashionable everyday attire for women. The Gibson Girl was more than an admired type, as Lillian Russell was; her appearance coincided with the development of mass-circulation magazines and advertisements, and she was the first mass-marketed ideal image to appear in newspapers and advertisements everywhere. She was both an ideal look and an ideal attitude of womanhood—wholesome, demure, active, and carefree— "A Big American Girl," as Gibson put it, in dedicating his 1896 collection of drawings. Women were no longer content to be admired for their particular traits, whether thick dark hair, an inconspicuous nose, or lovely green eyes. Now they wanted to look just like the Gibson Girl, or despair of being beautiful or fashionable.

That goal, however, was nearly impossible to reach. Above all, the Gibson Girl was a fantasy: she was never a flesh-and-blood woman, but an artist's creation. "The Gibson Girl in America represents the American girl not as she really is but as she tries to be according to

Mr. Gibson's lesson to her," one writer of the day reflected. Like a Barbie Doll, the Gibson Girl wasn't real, and had impossible proportions. Ironically, though the Gibson Girl image was equated with freedom, her body type was extremely difficult to achieve in real life. Corsets that created a Gibson-like S-curved posture, with a thrust-forward bust and arched back, were particularly uncomfortable.[14]

It didn't take long for advertisers to capitalize on the Gibson Girl—and on the sense of inadequacy women felt before her. Advertisers who were now selling women's clothing, soaps, and other feminine products on a mass scale realized the rich possibilities of selling items by linking them to an ideal image. "The type Gibson created," wrote the advertising historian Frank Presbrey, "became a popular means of attracting attention to an advertisement."[15] Advertisers used Gibson-like illustrations to sell everything from women's clothing to trips to the seashore. Manufacturers advertised that their products created the "Gibson effect."

Women would buy products advertised by a Gibson Girl in the hope that some of her beauty, social position, and vitality would rub off on them. The Gibson Girl was so popular that any woman who could afford to was practically dutybound to buy a product that would make her look like her. No one could ever look quite as good as the fantasy Gibson Girl, yet magazines and advertisers would keep reminding women how important it was to go on trying. Eventually, the Gibson Girl would give way to an even more elusive ideal: extreme slenderness.

The Flapper

Just before World War I, there were hints that the tight-laced image of Victorian womanhood was beginning to unravel. The Gibson Girl, in her bicycling outfit, had loosened up that image a bit, but she was still a primly buttoned-up Victorian lady. The first sign that young women were ready for something much more daring may have come a few rainy spring days in the early teens, when groups of smartly styled working girls and co-eds began to wear their galoshes deliberately unbuckled. This silly fad went against every rule about how proper young ladies were supposed to wear their rain boots, which was what made it so much fun. Their loose galoshes flap-flap-flapped on the pavement as the young women—"flappers"—defiantly strode by.

There were other signs that women were changing, particularly in the world of fashion, and that the new image of womanhood would be much more liberated, sophisticated—and slender—than ever before. In 1908, a French designer named Paul Poiret completely changed the hourglass silhouette by creating a straight, slim, Empire-waisted dress that erased any signs of a woman's hips and breasts. Soon, society women were wearing slinky dresses that favored a more small-breasted, slender figure. For the first time, extremely fashionable women, like the vain Undine Spragg in Edith Wharton's *The Custom of the Country* (1913), despaired of being too curvaceous: "Only one fact disturbed her: there was a hint of too much fullness in the curves of her neck and in the spring of her hips.... Excessive slimness was the fashion, and she shuddered at the thought that she might some day deviate from the perpendicular."

By April 1914, when *Delineator* magazine asked its sophisticated readers, "Don't you want to be thin?" the answer was obvious. "This is the age of the figure," the magazine advised. "The face alone, no matter how pretty, counts for nothing unless the body is straight and yielding as every young girl's."[16] In the early 1920s, Gabrielle "Coco" Chanel, an athletic young French fashion designer, emphasized the youthful dress silhouette by dropping the waistline to the hips, raising the hemlines to mid-calf, and creating the uniform of the new young woman: the flapper.[17]

A flapper was an impulsive, flirtatious, jazz-dancing young woman who had utter disdain for anything old-fashioned. She was, as F. Scott Fitzgerald described her in 1920 in *This Side of Paradise* (the novel was a primer for flapperhood in its day), the "Popular Daughter" of a Victorian mother, who rebelled against primness and propriety at every turn. The Victorian mother was all gentility and manners; the daughter laughed at her morality, smoked cigarettes, and kissed on her first date. Where her mother treasured her long tresses, the flapper bobbed her hair in a saucy, carefree style. The mother, in her perfectly arranged house and clothing, barely moved; her daughter was lively, athletic, and constantly on the go. The Victorian mother was a still photograph and her daughter a motion picture.

The flapper rebelled not only against Victorian manners and morality but against the body that went with it. Instead of having an hourglass figure, whose curves suggested motherhood and domesticity, she was boyishly slim. Rather than wearing a confining corset that emphasized her breasts, hips, and waist, the flapper bound her breasts and dieted to appear even younger and thinner. She bared more of her body, in a sleeveless sheath that hit just below the knees. The flapper did everything she could to liberate herself from the delicate, claustrophobic life her mother led. She was modern, sharp, sexy, and energetic. Ultimately, however, she wanted to marry a rich man and settle down to a lifestyle that was, in some ways, as decorative and confining as her mother's. In a society where looks were becoming more and more important, she'd have to work even harder than her mother did, starving herself to keep up her "liberated" appearance. When the dancing stopped and the dust had cleared, the flapper would find she had traded the old Victorian corset for a new one: an inner corset.

Like the Gibson Girl, the flapper wasn't entirely real. She was a creation of the movies and literature, but she epitomized the spirit of the modern age. F. Scott Fitzgerald is credited with creating the flapper image based on his own wife, Zelda, who was slim and petite, with short, slicked-back hair. Fitzgerald's female characters were shocking for the age, but rather harmless. They smoked and drank and kissed with abandon; they wore rouge and eye pencil, ran with a fast crowd, and spoke knowingly about Freud. They were invariably beautiful, and beautiful, as in the case of Rosalind in *This Side of Paradise*, meant being slim, young, and springy: "She was slender and athletic, without underdevelopment, and it was a delight to watch her move about a room, walk along a street, swing a golf club, or turn a 'cartwheel.'"

Fitzgerald's women had traded Victorian tradition and morality for a new kind of narcissism. The flapper's self-absorption had a materialistic side to it, too; money bought fun, new clothes, and allowed her to stay out late at clubs with the smart set. "I like sunshine and pretty things and cheerfulness—and I dread responsibility," says Rosalind, explaining why she can't marry a man she loves because he isn't rich. "I don't want to think about pots and kitchens and brooms. I want to worry whether my legs will get slick and brown when I swim in the summer." Ultimately, though, the heady, self-centered lifestyle was an empty one for a smart young girl, who, once her youth and beauty wore off, would be left with as few options as her mother had. "Here am I with the brains to do everything, yet tied to the sinking ship of future matrimony," says Fitzgerald's sophisticated, bob-haired Eleanor. "If I were born a hundred years from now, well and good, but now what's in store for me—I have to marry, that goes without saying."

But for the moment, the flapper celebrated her new freedoms—smoking, drinking, dancing—with abandon. In the years just after World War I, the emphasis was on living in the present, with the knowledge that the future was fast upon them. The genteel Victorian culture had been shattered by the horrors of the first modern war, and a sense of hedonism and cynicism prevailed. "The girls I wrote about were not a type—they were a generation," Fitzgerald reflected in an interview several years later. "Free spirits—evolved through the war chaos and a final inevitable escape from restraint and inhibitions."[18]

Several other social forces contributed to the free-spiritedness of the flappers, and to the physical symbol of their freedom, slenderness. Women had won the right to vote, and demonstrated their new sense of equality with men by cutting off their hair and doing away with other obvious symbols of sexual difference, such as the corset and the maternal body. But flappers didn't really care much about voting. They preferred the other masculine freedoms that went along with the new equality, such as staying out late and drinking gin fizzes. Unlike their feminist foremothers, social housekeepers who wanted to clean up vice and squalor and mother the whole world, flappers weren't very interested in "feminine" social reform. The turn-of-the-century feminists who won the vote had done so by claiming that women would have a purifying influence at the voting booth because as mothers, they were morally superior to men. By the 1920s—not unlike the 1990s—the term "feminism" had begun to smack of Victorian morality among young women. The flappers weren't interested in that kind of morality. They were much more interested in their freedom to be as immoral as men.[19]

Even more than the right to vote, birth control gave women a new sense of freedom. Contraceptives had made it possible, for the first time, for women to choose whether or not they wanted to be mothers, and to limit the size of their families, which decreased sharply in the United States between 1890 and 1910.[20] Many women were able to delay marriage and instead go to college, secretarial jobs, and even professions. More than anything, though, the availability of contraceptives meant a change in attitude. No longer like the pure, chaste Victorians who couldn't have sex without having children, women in the twenties had a new freedom to explore sexuality for its own sake. Though most women clearly drew the line at sex before marriage, kissing and petting no longer meant ruin. Women began to have power over their own sexuality; a flapper could flirt and tease and begin to demand something for herself.

The flapper's sexuality was still young and innocent, and expressed itself in a young and innocent body. A flapper had the body of an adolescent boy, not a grown-up woman. Her androgynous look made her appear less overtly sexual than a full-bodied, hourglass-figured woman would have looked in the same slinky clothing. Roberta Seid, in her book *Never Too Thin*, suggests that the Victorian woman was able to show off her sexual characteristics—her large breasts and hips—because there was no danger she would act on her sexuality: "The suggestiveness of her clothing and shape were simultaneously denied by her demureness and presumably unsexual nature." But in the 1920s, when women actually began to exercise some freedom, sexual and otherwise, their overtly sexual characteristics had to be repressed. "When women became more overtly sexual and exposed more of their bodies, this kind of amplitude might seem, in a sense, too blatant," Seid says.[21] In the same way, a fashion advertisement of a nude boyish model doesn't seem pornographic to us today; but put a fleshier model in an underwear ad, and it might not look quite so much like art. Without obvious curves and sexual characteristics, women's sexuality still appears to be under control. Beneath the twenties' message of sexual freedom was the symbol of female restraint: the slender female body.

The flapper's body, to put things in perspective, was slender only in relation to the plumper figures that went before. It is some measure of how extremely slim the ideal has become today that Clara Bow or Louise Brooks, both actresses who were considered quite slim for their time, would look very meaty next to most contemporary ingenues. Mary Campbell, who was crowned Miss America in 1922 and again in 1923, and had a typical flapper's body, was five foot seven and weighed 140 pounds.[22] Annette Kellerman, a champion swimmer and actress who advertised her 1926 book, *The Body Beautiful*, in the pages of the *Ladies' Home Journal*, was just shy of five foot four and weighed 137 pounds.[23] But the flapper defined a new silhouette that was straight and modern, and would only get thinner.

The slender body befitted the new aesthetic of the modern consumer age, also light and streamlined. This aesthetic was reflected in the speed of automobiles, the angles of abstract art, the design of new products, and the images of mass media. Everything was straight, quick, and lean. Movie actresses had to be thinner than those on stage or in still photographs, because a body in motion appears to be larger than one standing still.[24] Fashion drawings, following the lead of modern art, became elongated stick figures that only suggested a body. The long, elegant figures focused attention on the neat lines of the clothing, rather than on the curves of the human body. At first, fashion drawings and models, viewed together in the pages of women's magazines, were oddly different; the real-life models looked plump and squat compared with the illustrations. But models became thinner and thinner to compete with the stick-figure illustrations, and women reading the magazines became thinner and thinner to compete with the models.

A woman's appearance became much more important to her than it had been to her mother. In this new, fast-paced culture, all the things that used to make up a person's identity—family, church, and community—became less important than her looks. "In mass culture, the old roadblocks to social mobility came down," writes Robert Sklar about the twenties. "You could change your name, ignore your religion, leave your background a thousand miles behind. But you could never afford to neglect your appearance."[25]

A woman's appearance was much more than skin deep: it was a measure of who she was. The flapper's role as an object was even more important than it was for her Victorian mother. The flapper had to be a good consumer, keeping up with fashion and buying the latest in beauty products. With the speed of invention and fads, she had a more difficult time keeping up-to-date than did her mother, but she loved the challenge. The ultimate freedom to the self-absorbed flapper was not political equality, as her feminist forebears might have hoped, but the freedom to buy whatever she pleased.

Advertisers were quick to tap into this new sense of "freedom." Piggly Wiggly grocery stores ran an ad campaign in the twenties featuring a woman in a shopping market in a stylish cloche hat: "Here she is free—to reach her own decisions." Advertisers offered women the power and freedom to choose between products. "They promised fake liberation through consumption," writes the social historian T. J. Jackson Lears.[26] The most blatant example of advertisers subverting the real impulse toward women's political freedom into the false freedom to buy products came with smoking campaigns. In 1929, Edward Bernays, advertising man for a tobacco company, organized a march of cigarette-puffing women down Fifth Avenue, led by the feminist Ruth Hale, to demonstrate women's newfound freedom to smoke.[27] They'd already come a long way, baby.

This new "freedom" to buy was hardly liberating. Women became bound to buying products that would make them more attractive, and better sexual objects. They couldn't easily resist the onslaught of advertisements that the new consumer culture had to offer, because many of the ads deliberately spoke to their deep-seated fears and desires. For women whose grandmothers had been trained that their role in life, as the turn-of-the-century feminist economist Charlotte Perkins Gilman put it, was to "consume, consume, consume," it was difficult to turn their back on ads that told them essentially that their human worth depended on how well they kept up with fashion and popular standards of attractiveness—including slenderness.

The narcissism of the flapper turned into a kind of masochism as advertisers pointed out, over and over again, all the things that needed to be corrected with new products. Women in the twenties had problems their mothers never dreamed of, or at least would never mention in polite company. The makers of Lysol disinfectant, for instance, marketed their product as a feminine hygiene deodorant with the assurance that women who used it would achieve "immaculate cleanliness," and the satisfaction that comes "When you know you are meticulously groomed." Pond's Cream warned of "The little flaws that make one homely." Odorono deodorant featured a woman relating "the most humiliating moment in my life: When I overheard the cause of my unpopularity among men." Listerine depicted the bad-breathed woman who was "Often a Bridesmaid but never a Bride." The message was clear: Women could never reach emotional fulfillment or be attractive to men unless they bought products that would improve themselves.

It was during the 1920s that advertisers hit on a problem that was visible enough for women to be embarrassed about, difficult enough to require buying lots of products, and best of all, would never go away: fat. Advertisers made women feel humiliated that they weren't as slim as the beautiful women in their illustrations. They sold bath salts, laxatives, reducing brushes, stimulating belts, scales, mail-away diets, and scores of other obesity cures. Every advertisement chided women for being overweight. "Overweight these days is a woman's own fault," proclaimed one ad for a musical reducing record. And every advertisement promised that a woman would not only lose weight with the product, but her life would be better afterward.

With all these pressures from advertisements, fashion, movies, stylish friends, and even doctors who were starting to warn of the dangers of being overweight, women began to do anything to be slim. They starved themselves and chewed gum laced with laxatives to lose weight. Told to "Reach for a Lucky instead of a sweet," they took up smoking to lose weight; it was, as the ad said, "the modern way to diet." They followed a number of wild fad diets recommended by physicians and pseudophysicians, many of which involved fasting, purgatives, and odd combinations of foods.

Carl Malmberg, author of *Diet and Die*, wrote in 1935 that the craze for slimness that swept the United States after World War I led many physicians to try to rationalize the fad—"Scientists and health authorities have set out to prove that it is healthy as well as fashionable to be thin." Some of those diets were the result of a mutually beneficial alliance between physicians and food producers. The United Fruit Company, for instance, was happy to advertise Johns Hopkins University physician George Harrop's banana and skimmed milk diet with the AMA seal of approval. The Hollywood Eighteen-Day Diet (585 calories a day) was promoted by citrus growers—grapefruit was a centerpiece of the regime—as being the product of careful research on the part of French and American physicians.

Despite being medically approved, the results of these diets were sometimes disastrous. "There are many people who were never intended by nature to have the appearance of slimness," Malmberg observed. "Many of these people nevertheless set out to achieve this ideal, and in doing so too often ruin their health in what is, for them, an impossible task." Crash dieting, he reported, was responsible for the deaths of several Hollywood celebrities in the thirties. Louis Wolheim, who lost 25 pounds in less than a month for a role in the movie *The Front Page*, was so weakened by dieting that he failed to recover from an attack of appendicitis. Renée Adoree, a boyish-figured movie star renowned for her strenuous dieting efforts, collapsed and died in Hollywood in 1930, weighing only 85 pounds.[28]

The cultural pressures to be thin in the 1920s were already so extreme that some women resorted to vomiting, as they would again in a later era that made slenderness the price of women's freedom. In 1926, when a group of physicians gathered for an Adult Weight Conference, one prominent physician had a disturbing report about his patients' very modern form of dieting. "I discovered," he said, "that many of our flappers have mastered the art of eating their cake and yet not having it, inducing regurgitation, after a plentiful meal, either by drugs or mechanical means."[29]

Barbie and Beyond

By the 1920s, the inner corset was squeezing women, and for the most part, it would not let up for the rest of the century. From then on, women would be under pressure to be thinner and thinner, even though the average woman in the United States grew taller, with bigger bones and a larger frame. Film stars and fashion models became more slender because their angles photographed better on screen and in magazines. Louis B. Mayer, upon signing Greta Garbo to MGM, grumbled, "In America, men don't like fat women."[30]

In the movies, being thin was a sign of an aristocratic background and swanky style, in imitation of Europeans. Immigrants who made money often tried to slim down to appear to be longtime members of the aristocracy. In his book *The Kennedy Women*, Laurence Leamer describes how the four-generation-old obsession with food and diet that haunts the Kennedy women—who were always chided as children not to gain weight—began as a way to distinguish early members of the family from lesser immigrants. "The obsession with fat came originally from Joe (their father), whose parents in their later years had grown as portly as prosperous peasants, their Irish roots painfully evident," writes Leamer. "Joe wanted his wife and children sleek and lean."[31] Losing weight in the first few decades of the century was mainly an upper-crust concern. During the Depression, when some people had so little to eat that advertisers were even beginning to sell cures to put on weight, only the well-off, perversely, starved themselves on diets of grapefruit or caviar.

During World War II, many women were too busy worrying about their new jobs and the fate of their families to be concerned about their body size. Ideal body sizes stayed almost the same as they were in the flapper period, though they became somewhat more sturdy and curvaceous. In the 1920s, the bust-waist-hip measurements of Miss America winners averaged 32-25-35 (with bound breasts). In the 1930s, the contestants' measurements grew to 34-25-35; in the 1940s, they were 35-25-35.

But after the war, with women back at home, there was renewed emphasis on fitting an ideal shape. Two competing ideal female body types developed: the buxom blonde and the elegant brunette. The blonde was the direct descendant of light-haired Lillian Russell; she had large breasts, erotic appeal, and working-class sensibilities. The ideal buxom blonde—Marilyn Monroe, Jayne Mansfield, or any *Playboy* bunny—was curvy, with an emphasis on torpedo breasts; in the 1950s, the average Miss America now measured 36-23-36.[32]

The voluptuous body became more popular in the fifties because America had a new romance with peaceful suburban domesticity after World War II. The ideal fifties woman had the maternal, turn-of-the-century hourglass figure of her Victorian great-grandmother, though she wasn't quite so plump. Marilyn Monroe in *Some Like It Hot* (1959) seems absolutely fat by today's standards. The camera feasted on Monroe's backside when she bent over, showing off the full expanse of her derriere; nowadays, that shot could only be a visual joke. When she turned around in her tight dress, she revealed a rounded tummy.

This chubby woman was the unabashed object of sexual attraction in a movie. But she wasn't exactly the center of intellectual interest, whipping off the kind of sharp comebacks that Bette Davis and Myrna Loy always had ready. "Guess I'm not too bright," Monroe tells the saxophone player she falls in love with, and that's the deepest line she gets. Marilyn Monroe, and blondes like her, were unthreatening because though they were maternal-bodied and oozed sexuality, they were also childlike, innocent, and a little dim. Monroe herself, of course, was a smart cookie, but she knew enough to play dumb. The annoying association between blondes, breasts, body fat, and brainlessness continues even today.

The elegant brunette was thinner, longer, and more sophisticated. She had a lot more brains and class than the buxom blondes, and was the strong, smart, independent heroine in movies. Katharine Hepburn, Audrey Hepburn, and others of their type came to dominate women's magazines. Thin women—designers would argue—were the perfect clothes hangers. After reading a copy of *Vogue* magazine in 1946, the British writer George Orwell commented rather disparagingly on the increasingly slender body type found in its pages. "Nearly all these women are immensely elongated," he said. "A thin-boned, ancient Egypt type of face seems to predominate: the narrow hips are general, and slender, non-prehensile hands like those of a lizard are quite universal."[33]

In 1947, when the French designer Christian Dior unveiled his New Look designs, dresses with full skirts nipped narrowly at the waist, fashionable women everywhere had to become thinner to squeeze into them. Muriel Maxwell, who was a cover girl in the late forties, later recalled how the new fashion shook the modeling world. "We wondered where in the world we were going to get models who could get into them," she said. "Then out of the woods came these nymphs with no lungs and very little of the flesh that keeps you alive. These new kids really don't eat."[34] By the end of the fifties, when dieting was becoming more and more prominent in women's magazines, the slender Suzy Parker was the typical model, not Marilyn Monroe.

In 1959, a body type was born that was a combination of the buxom blonde and the elegant brunette. She had large, erotic breasts, a tiny waist, relatively narrow hips, and long legs. Like the Gibson Girl, she wasn't real, and her proportions were impossible for ordinary women to attain. Her name was Barbie. At eleven and a half inches tall, Barbie became the ideal that little girls everywhere could measure themselves against. Blown up to life-size, Barbie's measurements would be 38-18-34, and she wouldn't have enough body fat to menstruate.[35] This impossible but ubiquitous ideal—90 percent of American girls ages three to eleven own one or more Barbies—would keep women dissatisfied with their own proportions.[36] In their attempts to become like the plastic Barbie, many grown-up women would resort to starving themselves to skinniness, and then get plastic implants to replace the fat they lost in their breasts. (In 1997 Mattel released a new Barbie, less busty with smaller hips—in other words, more like a supermodel.)

From the time of Barbie on, both the buxom *Playboy* types and the brunette model types got thinner and thinner. When one group of researchers compared the height, weight, and body measurements of *Playboy* centerfolds from 1959 to 1978, they found that while the height increased by 20 percent, the body size decreased significantly. In 1959, the playmates weighed 91 percent as much as the average women; but by 1978, the figure was only 85 percent of the ave-rage weight (other studies have shown that playmates have become thinner and thinner every year since). When the researchers looked at Miss America Pageant contestants during that same period, they found that their average weight declined even more than the play-mates'. Before 1970, the contestants weighed 87 percent of what an average woman weighed, and after, 84.5 percent of average. The win-ners, it turned out, weighed even less than the rest of the contestants. The researchers noted that only 5 percent of women aged twenty to twenty-nine were as thin as the Miss America winners.[37] The same trend toward thinness was happening in Europe; in 1951, Miss Sweden was five foot seven and 151 pounds; in 1983, she was five foot nine and 109 pounds. Beauty queens were now not only the fairest but the thinnest of them all.

In the sixties, the fascination with youth culture and freedom gave way to flapperlike images that were even more boyish and slender than their predecessors. In 1966, the ultimate clothes hanger ap-peared: Twiggy. Lesley Hornby (now Lawson), known as "Twiggy," the seventeen-year-old model from England, weighed between 92 and 97 pounds and measured 31-22-32. A few models and hip sophisticates, such as Edie Sedgwick, imitated her style, but Twiggy's extreme slen-derness only made a major splash in fashion spreads. Today, super-models have celebrity status, and are more influential style-setters than are actresses, but Twiggy didn't have that kind of clout. Young women didn't seriously expect they could look like Twiggy the way they believe they can—and should—look like Kate Moss, who is about the same size. Twiggy did contribute to a more general slender trend, though, as the bikini-clad actresses and models who were the seven-ties ideals—Cheryl Tiegs and Farrah Fawcett—became thinner and thinner.

In the seventies, the thin ideal coincided with another wave of feminism; the androgynous, dress-for-success look became popular, along with a physique that didn't look too overtly female in the work-place. The main mission for many women was to gain power in a male-dominated world, and they found that they could fit in to that world more easily if they were thin. Like the flappers, they wanted to cast off the traditional maternal and domestic female role—and the body that went with it. Many feminists of that era, therefore, have ignored the backlash social forces that work extra hard to control women's bodies precisely at the times when they're seeking to have more control over their own lives.

During the eighties and early nineties, women's bodies became leaner and stronger. There were varying ideals—super-thin waif models, more curvaceous Cindy Crawford types—yet not one of them had a suspicion of fat on their bodies. Jane Fonda kicked off the fit look in 1981 with her *Workout Book*, initially shaping the fitness revolution as a feminist response to a damaging ideal. "In pursuit of the 'feminine ideal'—exemplified by voluptuous film stars and skinny fashion models—women, it seemed, were even prepared to do violence to themselves," wrote Fonda. She described her own history of addiction to diet pills and diuretics, and her bout with bulimia, as evidence of how debilitating these ideals can be. Fonda found that exercise was the answer, allowing her to cope with both the social demands to be attractive and to be a strong and effective working woman. "I could create for myself a new approach to health and beauty which would not only make me look better, but would enable me to handle the intense, multifaceted life I live with more clarity and balance, to say nothing of more energy and endurance."[38]

As it was for the Gibson Girl, exercise became both a vehicle for liberation and further oppression when it was tied to an ideal body. Despite her good intentions, Fonda succeeded in creating a new feminine ideal that has proven, in its way, just as damaging as the old one. The super-fit body has become another image to which most women can't measure up. The goal of exercise, for many women, isn't to achieve good health, but a perfectly disciplined, slender body. Exercise companies use this new ideal to sell products the way diet companies always have, promising a fantasy body. Soloflex weight machines, for instance, have an ad featuring a lean, buffed-out, headless woman's torso in a bikini. "You don't have to be a model to have a body like this," the ad reads. "All you need is just $39 a month."

Most people can't attain that kind of sculpted physique without devoting huge chunks of their lives to the goal. Madonna is a good example of someone who started out with a subversive, rebellious, sexy body and tamed it through exercise into a disciplined and—disappointingly—more socially acceptable ideal. She reportedly works out four hours a day, six days a week. At five foot four and 100 pounds, she is 12 percent body fat; for a time, every morsel of food she ate was entered into a computer.[39] Oprah Winfrey is another woman who once presented an alternative image to the world; she was a role model for those who didn't believe that a large African American woman could be a serious success. But she, too, felt compelled to whip herself into the dominant feminine ideal.

Winfrey's dieting tribulations, first losing weight on Optifast, and then, after regaining her 67 pounds plus more, going on exercise and a low-fat diet, have been public events. Dropping from 222 pounds in 1993 to 135 pounds in 1994 consumed a great deal of her time. Every day, Winfrey reportedly undergoes at least two bouts of exercise; she runs up to eight miles, works out on the StairMaster for 45 minutes, and does 350 sit-ups. She also has a personal chef who monitors her 20 grams of fat a day. Winfrey didn't stop losing weight when she became healthy; she stuck with it until she became a model of obsession which few real-life women have the time or resources to follow.[40]

In her book *Moving Beyond Words* (1994), Gloria Steinem describes how working out and building muscles may be "revolutionary" for women, since it is a way out of society's "thin vs. fat dichotomy." She uses bodybuilder Bev Francis as a positive example of someone who is pushing the cultural ideals of femininity in a radical way. But bodybuilding, the extreme of the aerobicized ideal, creates another ideal that abhors fat, and practically banishes femininity completely in its imitation of a male physique as a source of "female power."

In 1995, at the world women's bodybuilding championship, the Ms. Olympia contest held in Atlanta, I saw what this ideal looks like. When I first walked into a party before the event, packed with fans and contestants showing off their stuff, I was startled. There were thick bulbous calf muscles teetering on stiletto heels. There were meaty, veined forearms, and knuckly fingers that ended in long, painted nails. Thigh muscles bulged through black Lycra skirts. The hair was big, but the biceps were bigger. One competitor told me she got involved in bodybuilding in college because she disliked her "too-soft" body. Her efforts to control it at all costs reminded me of someone with an eating disorder—as did the way she eats, consuming only skinless chicken breasts and oatmeal for weeks before competition. Another, five foot nine and 161 pounds, with an upper body like armor, said she wanted to redefine the feminine ideal. "I could never achieve a petite, dainty look, and muscularity is a look that women should be able to choose," she said.

It's refreshing to meet a woman who likes being big, but in this culture you can only be big if you're also hard; you can't be strong *and* soft. Many of the women, I found out later that weekend, take steroids containing testosterone to build their muscles, with obvious masculin- izing side effects—husky voices, male pattern baldness, chin stubble. The women who are trying to achieve the ultimate in feminine physical perfection, ironically, look surprisingly like men.

Not all women in our culture, of course, strive for this hard-body ideal. Exercise, for them, is just one way to control fat. The fear of fat, after one hundred years, has become extreme. We believe—and in this culture it is true to a great extent—that we must be slender to be suc- cessful. We can't get away from that message, particularly if we read magazines: Nine West shoe ads feature near-anorexic models in mini- skirts telling us, "We all need diversions, we all need clever friends, we all need to lose 5 pounds (OK, maybe 10)." *Redbook* describes how we—like Oprah, Demi, and Cher—can lose weight easily, even if we don't have our own personal trainers and chefs. A *Mirabella* cover proclaims "Waif Goodbye: Return of the Real Woman," with a photo of a new voluptuary who weighs about five pounds more than the gaunt starvelings of the year before. In *Vogue*, supermodel Christy Turling- ton, whose ribs are visible in Calvin Klein underwear ads, complains to a magazine writer that she has a beer belly. In my local newspaper, fashion designer Bill Blass gives advice on how to be well dressed, saying, "Forget it, unless you are skinny! Don't even attempt it unless you are. It doesn't work otherwise."[41] It only makes sense that two- thirds of all American women, including many who are average-sized or thin, believe they're overweight.

In this culture, even women who are only slightly over the ideal weight—who can't squeeze into those size 8 jeans—are scrutinized and penalized for their size. Women who are only 10 or 20 pounds over the ideal are often passed over for jobs or promotions. "There's a glass ceiling for overweight people," says University of Vermont Professor of Psychology Esther Rothblum, "and it's a lot lower for women than men." Consider that flight attendants at United Airlines are sus- pended from duty and subject to dismissal if they're only 11 pounds over the ideal weight chart, even though at that size, their weight doesn't hamper their performance. That kind of bias is hardly unusual in image-conscious jobs. An editor I know at a fashion magazine who was looking for a new assistant recently told me, "If the most perfect person in the world for the job walked in today, and she was over-weight, there's no way we'd hire her." A corporate headhunter put it even more plainly: "All things being equal, the thinnest person always wins."

That's true: one recent study of more than 10,000 young people aged sixteen to twenty-four found that overweight women are 20 percent less likely to get married than slimmer women. The study pointed to a second dismal consequence of being fat in this culture, which is economic: the heavy women had household incomes averaging $6,710 a year less, and were 10 percent more likely to be poor.[42] In another study, when one group of college students was asked what type of person they'd be least inclined to wed, they said they'd sooner tie the knot with an embezzler, cocaine user, ex-mental patient, shoplifter, nymphomaniac, communist, blind person, atheist, or marijuana user than a fat person.[43] Some people think it would be better if fat people were never born: one survey of parents found that 11 percent of them would abort a child they knew had a genetic tendency to be fat.[44]

Even kids know how bad it is for them to be heavier than other kids. A hearty four-year-old I know is worried about whether she has a "fat butt" and already believes she should only eat fat-free cookies. Surveys have shown that by fourth grade, 60 percent of all girls want to be thinner. From kindergarten on, if you show kids drawings of children with different body types and ask them what kind of people they are, they'll say that the thin children are cuter, more popular, nicer, neater, and smarter than those with an average or chubby body. When reporters on one television magazine show recently asked kids what would be the worst thing that could ever happen to them, most had a quick reply: "Getting fat."[45]

It's no wonder that when *Esquire* magazine polled 1,000 women in 1994, more than half of them said they'd rather get run over by a truck than gain 150 pounds. Most women can't make it through a day without getting disgusted with themselves for not having a better—meaning thinner—body. We expect the impossible from ourselves. Women who are naturally large-boned and robust damn themselves for not being delicate and slim. Women whose bodies have just under-gone the astonishing job of childbirth burst into tears when they can't fit into their jeans, or get mad at themselves when they realize they're in no shape to pose on the cover of *Vanity Fair* wearing only body paint, as actress Demi Moore did two months after she had a baby. We

ourselves and cripple ourselves by constantly obsessing
weight. As one psychologist and body image expert, Marcia
_ninson, says, "If you talked to your friends the way you talk to
your body, you'd have no friends left at all."

Given the obvious debilitating effects of weight obsession on
women, it's surprising that many feminists continue to ignore this
obsession as a political issue, and personally buckle under to the
expectation that we should all try to become thin. There are excep-
tions, of course. Among lesbian feminists, where the issue of living up
to a male-defined sexual ideal rarely registers on the radar screen,
there is more tolerance for fat. There's also a group of feminist writers
and therapists who have devoted themselves to women's problems
with weight and eating, including Susie Orbach, Kim Chernin, Susan
Bordo, Geneen Roth, Susan Kano, Carol Munter, Jane Hirschmann,
and many others. These women have recognized that their personal
battles with weight are rooted in a culture that tries to control
women's size as a way of controlling their power. Although their work
has influenced many intellectuals and therapists, their concerns
haven't made it very far into popular culture. Naomi Wolf, who wrote
The Beauty Myth (1991), is one of the few highly visible feminists who
has drawn attention to weight obsession as a serious women's issue;
she, too, knows from firsthand experience with anorexia how debilitating the problem can be. It's telling that Wolf's book was most
strongly attacked by "new feminists" for putting too much emphasis
on the gravity of eating disorders as a social problem.

A few feminists are achingly aware of both their personal desires
to be thin and the social cost of those desires. In her book *Femininity*,
(1984), Susan Brownmiller describes how she can hardly pass a group
of construction workers in New York City without sucking in her
stomach, adding, "I expect I will continue to be obsessed with weight
until . . . I am past the age of sexual judgment and no longer concerned
with what a man might think."[46] But she knows that this self-
conscious, insecure drive for a perfect appearance is debilitating for
us; it is, in her words, "the ultimate restriction on freedom of mind."
The feminist philosopher Susan Bordo, whose book *Unbearable
Weight* (1993) dissects the oppressive meanings of the thin female
body in Western culture,[47] is herself a bit anxious about her weight;
she joined Nutri/System, she told me, to lose 25 pounds before she
wrote her book. But her desire to be thin, she says, illustrates how

enmeshed we are in the diet culture, how conflicted we feel about weight issues, and how we contribute to perpetuating the pressures to be thin. "We almost can't help wanting to be thinner," Bordo says. "We live in a culture where there are very real rewards for being thin."

As a society, we have yet to develop an image of femininity that conveys women's real power. This, I imagine, is one that might have the curves and body fat of a mother as well as the strength and stride of a person who is as intellectually and physically capable as a man. We have yet to acknowledge how different women's bodies are from men's, and how diverse we all are, size-wise, from each other. We're stuck, as the Victorians were, molding women, molding ourselves, with painful and debilitating stays.

Chapter 2

The Truth That Will Change Your Life (Only $39.95): Diet Gurus

She startles you in the midst of your sleepy late-night channel-surfing. "Stop the Insanity!" shrieks the almost bald-headed woman on the infomercial. "Discover the Truth!"

Frightening. *Now* you're awake. The truth this woman prancing around in *Flashdance* exercise wear seems to be talking about is how to lose weight. "Eat! Breathe! Move!" she tells the audience. Just buy her product, the ad promises, and you'll not only trim down but your whole life will be better.

Susan Powter, the star of this infomercial, is a real motormouth, a fitness queen who sounds like a cross between Camille Paglia and Phyllis Diller. She alternately jokes about her ex-husband, rages about the lies told by the diet and fitness industries, exhorts women to take control of their lives by eating less fat, and shows off "before" and "after" photos of herself. All you can imagine is that the sad-looking fat woman in the first snapshot transformed herself into the lean machine in the second after she discovered amphetamines. She will not shut up.

"Change the way you look and feel *forever*, says Powter, with the fervor of an evangelist. She describes, over and over, how she transformed her life by shrinking herself from a 260-pound housewife to someone who can jump up and down in a size 2 thong bikini without wiggling. In the process, she got revenge on her ex-husband and became rich, famous, and happy. And she did it, she assures us, without dieting.

"This program is easy and it works," Powter insists. "No more starvation, deprivation, or dieting. It's over." Just send four "easy" payments of $19.95. Whoa! Find the Visa card—pick up the phone!

Plenty of people have. Powter is one of the latest, and most successful, in a long line of American diet gurus whose fortunes have risen and fallen while selling their followers a vision of personal transformation through weight loss. Like Sylvester Graham, Jack La-Lanne, Robert Atkins, Judy Mazel, Nathan Pritikin, Richard Simmons, Stephen Gullo, and countless others before her, Powter took her personal experience with weight loss, turned it into a package of nutrition, exercise, and feel-good philosophy, and marketed it to the entire nation.

At the core of every diet guru's philosophy is the belief that losing weight will not only make you a smaller person—at least, temporarily—but a *better* person. Becoming thin, they profess, will change your life, put you in control, open your heart, solve your emotional problems, or put you on the path toward spiritual enlightenment. Diet gurus promise that if you follow them, and buy their product, this dream of success will happen to you. And if it doesn't, it's not because you were never destined to fit into a size 2 bikini. It's because you don't have the strength and commitment to stick it through—you're a failure, a bad person.

Diet gurus are popular because in a society that is increasingly image-conscious, we judge each other more and more by our bodies. Whether or not we're good people has less to do with our background—families, education, church, accomplishments, or relationships to others in our community—and is communicated more by how we look. Our bodies have to convey the message that we're disciplined, in control, and effective. "People used to try to develop a better self, and act out all the projects of transcendence, transformation, and purification, in the context of community or religious work," says Susan Bordo. "Now they go to seminars with diet gurus."

Diet gurus, we think, will help us become thinner, better people. They begin their pitch by emphasizing how terrible it is to be fat. They know; they've been there. They've been obese and sloppy and unable to fit into their size 18s anymore. They've been embarrassed at the beach, abandoned by their husbands, and confined to their houses for fear of running into anyone they know. They've dieted and fasted, lost their hair, and come close to dying. They paint a miserable picture of life as a fat person, which contrasts nicely with the vision they're selling of living, as they do, as glamorous and exciting slender people. Susan Powter accomplishes this by mocking fat people; Richard Simmons sheds tears over them. By exaggerating the psychological, physical, and moral problems associated with being fat—there are, after all, successful, happy, well-adjusted fat people out there in the world—gurus are that much more likely to make a sale.

Diet gurus offer their followers many different paths to lightness, though each believes that theirs is the only true way. Their particular diet and exercise plan isn't very important, though; it's the motivating force behind it that matters, the personality that enlightens, inspires, entertains, or flogs followers into an almost religious devotion. The dieters believe it is the guru himself, or herself, who will transform them; the diet itself is just the daily practice that reinforces their devotion. In his crusade to save Americans from fatness, for instance, Richard Simmons touches as many people as he can, whether by hugging them, calling them, or looking into their eyes with his own gaze of conviction: "I know you can do it!" Many fat people believe that just *meeting* Richard Simmons in person is enough to motivate them enough to become thin.

The danger of putting so much faith and power in the guru, however charismatic and motivating he or she may be, is that it takes an equal measure of power away from the followers. Rather than figuring out for themselves what exercise and eating habits might give them the most pleasure and health for the rest of their lives, they believe that they have to follow the guru, go to his classes, buy his tapes and books, and that without him, they are helpless. Instead of imagining that they deserve to live positive and productive lives even while they're fat, the followers feel ashamed, and put everything on hold until that magic day when they're thin. Then, when the guru's diet doesn't work as promised, and their lives don't change, they end up feeling like more of a failure than ever before.

as weighing his feces to see what was being digested. Like other diet practitioners who have no medical credentials themselves—such as weight-loss counselors at Jenny Craig—he took to wearing white jackets to give himself a look of authority. Fletcher wrote a best-selling diet book, *The AB–Z of Our Own Nutrition*, and performed feats of strength to publicize his health claims.[2]

It became fashionable to "fletcherize." At dinner parties, people were so busy chewing there was scarcely time for conversation. Henry James told Edith Wharton he had not only taken up the new method, but that he was "a fanatic." John Harvey Kellogg, soon to be a cereal magnate, advocated fletcherizing at his Battle Creek, Michigan, health sanitarium (along with his other quackish obesity cures, which included cold rain douches, cold dripping sheets, sweatpacks, and plunge baths). At Yale, one professor did a study and concluded that people who fletcherized regularly experienced an increase of 50 percent in muscular endurance (and not just of the jaw muscle), had a greater immunity from common sicknesses, and were cured of the desire for drinking excessive alcoholic stimulants. To Fletcher, this proved once again that following his diet, as he put it, would result in "a higher general morality."

Fletcherism passed out of fashion in the early 1900s, mainly because younger scientists were putting forth the theory that it was what you ate, and how much, that mattered more than the way you chewed it. In the 1890s, the chemist Wilbur O. Atwater had broken food down into its nutritional components—protein, fat, and carbohydrates—and discovered that gram for gram, fat had the most calories. In the early 1900s, a chemist at Yale University, Russell Chittenden, took Atwater's idea of measuring food as calories—the amount of heat required to raise the temperature of 1 gram of water 1 degree centigrade—and applied it not only to energy taken in but energy burned in exercise. Calorie counting was born: Americans now had a simple and scientific way to calculate how much they needed to eat and exercise to lose weight. It would be decades before anyone challenged calorie counting with the idea that the body uses some types of food differently from others, and that everyone burns calories at a different rate. For now, everything and everybody was reduced to a simple in-and-out equation.

Dr. Lulu Hunt Peters was the first diet guru to popularize calories, in 1917, with her best-selling book, *Diet and Health, with Key to the*

Calories. Peters, who had shed some 50 pounds by counting calories, offered her readers a diet regime that is as depressingly familiar as Weight Watchers. The dieter would start with a fast, then work up to 1,200 calories a day. Once she lost the weight, she would go on a maintenance diet. Two million copies of her book were sold, an astonishing number for the time.

Peters drummed calorie counting into the heads of her readers. "Hereafter you are going to eat calories of food," she wrote. "Instead of saying one slice of bread or a piece of pie, you will say 100 calories of bread, 350 calories of pie." Peters compared the body to a machine, and told her readers they needed constant vigilance to keep it functioning properly; the scale, she said, was the most important piece of furniture in the house. Although Peters based her diet on what she viewed as strict science, the moral lesson was clear. If you could control your calories, you could control your weight. Being fat meant you had no discipline or control; it was a sign of moral weakness.[3]

For the next several decades, calorie counting was the practice almost all dieters engaged in, making businesslike accounts of their food intake, checking daily totals against the weekly numbers on the scale. Diets came and went—the Hollywood Diet, the Hays Diet, the grapefruit diet—but all relied on calories. From the time of the Depression to World War II, calorie counting faded into the background of America's consciousness—it became much more important to count up pennies for the day's food, or the numbers of young men missing in war—but it returned again in the 1950s. Then, women's magazines picked up the task of giving their readers a moral education in weight loss. Mass-circulation magazines had a larger pulpit than any meeting-hall diet guru ever dreamed.

Writers who wrote for women's magazines became the new diet gurus, every month preaching the same message of how life gets better with weight loss, and printing new diets, varying the methods and menus that ultimately added up to the same dismal calorie counts. From 1951 to 1953, the number of articles on dieting listed in the *Reader's Guide to Periodical Literature* increased fivefold. Women's magazines had found that diets were one of the best ways to boost their circulation figures. "Next to fashions," wrote Helen Woodward, a women's magazine executive in the fifties, "the most important subject in all these magazines has been reducing. Each new diet . . . is treated as a miraculous new discovery. Then, in a little while there is a totally different diet, again a miracle."[4]

The magazines ran gushingly inspirational stories of dieters, illustrated with "before" and "after" photos, which emphasized the magical transformation that occurs when people lose weight. During the fifties *Ladies' Home Journal*, for instance, featured one of these fairy-tale stories nearly every month: "From forlorn fatty—to fashion model," "The no-willpower diet," "I dieted during my second pregnancy," "I was a two-ton Annie." Failing on these diets was rarely covered, but one story—"I gained back 110!"—described a woman who, having reduced from "a monstrous 295 pounds," gained it back, to her shame and disgust. The magazine assured its readers, however—without actually resorting to real data—that 80 percent of dieters had kept their weight off for five years; those who had discipline and self-restraint could avoid such a miserable fate.

By 1960, dieting and slenderness, once signs that indicated a deeper religious nature or sensitive temperament, had practically become a religion in themselves. "Weight control is emerging as the new morality; fat, one of the deadlier sins," wrote Lesley Blanch, in *Vogue*. "The bathroom scales are a shrine to which believers turn daily. Converts are marked by the usual unctuous zeal. Doctors become father confessors to whom grievous sins are whispered." Blanch noted that Americans were practically wallowing in sin, in their marshmallow-salad cuisine, and that reformation seemed to be in the air. "Perhaps we are witnessing the first stirrings of a gigantic puritan revival, destined to lead the nation along a stony path of self-denial." Such a movement, she said, could only take place in a land of prosperity and health, where people could afford to look sickly. "Today skeletal bodies, pallid lips, and sunken, black-rimmed eyes are admired; any natural glow of health is carefully painted out with cosmetics."[5] The writer was making fun of dieters, but it was clear, with thinner and thinner models in the magazine's pages, that the editors, at least, were taking this new religion dead seriously.

Eventually, the flock of dieters became too large to be guided only by impersonal beauty editors at women's magazines. There was too much potential for someone to lead these masses of fervent dieters; too big a market to ignore. Diet gurus also had a much better way to reach masses of people than they had at the turn of the century, in churches and meeting halls, or later, in women's magazines: television.

Jack LaLanne

Halfway through his TV exercise show, Jack LaLanne's German shepherd Happy would trot across stage with a sign in his mouth: "It's Glamour Stretcher Time!" All over America, housewives watching the show in their living rooms would go fetch their mail-order elastic ropes, grasp the handles on the ends, and exercise in time with Jack LaLanne. "A-one, and a-two," he said brightly, looking them straight in the eye while they pulled the elastic across their chests. "That's right! Feel the stretch."

Women in the early 1960s who dreamed of looking as glamorous as slender Jackie Kennedy tuned in to LaLanne every day for exercise and inspiration. LaLanne promised not only to make these women trim, but with the help of his Glamour Stretcher, he'd give them a more "youthful bustline," and take a little padding off the "old back porch" as well. He led them in kicks, twists, bicycle movements in the air, and a full half hour of "fun-nastics." By 1960, he had the biggest national daytime show on television, and by 1964 (the year after Betty Friedan wrote *The Feminine Mystique*), 8 million housewives tuned in to his show each weekday morning after breakfast.[6]

Like most diet and exercise gurus, Jack LaLanne started out as a pathetic physical specimen, but transformed his body after he had an experience in which he saw what was, for him, the light of Truth. That moment came to LaLanne, a San Francisco youth who was the son of a telephone installer, when he went to a standing-room-only health lecture at a hall in Oakland. The lecturer, Paul Bragg, was an evangelical, Sylvester Graham type, who exhorted the packed crowd to give up the evils of sugar, soft drinks, and processed foods, and turn instead to carrot juice, green vegetables, and clean living. LaLanne's mother had taken her sickly son up to talk with the man personally; from that moment on, LaLanne's mind was changed, and his body would soon follow.

LaLanne began exercising and eating health foods: unprocessed foods, raw milk, vegetables, and vitamins. When he was nineteen, his father died, and LaLanne was convinced the cause was overeating and underexercising. That gave him reason to turn his personal devotion to a healthy body into a crusade. He opened his own gym in San Francisco, which soon turned into a string of gyms. In 1951, he started his own calisthenics program on a local TV station. There, he was able to reach more viewers with his health message than any other diet guru ever dreamed before; eventually seventy-three stations carried his program. He was also able to sell more products than other diet gurus. He started by peddling his five-dollar Glamour Stretcher—"a whole gym in a rubber cord"—on his show, then extended his line into a huge mail-order business that included diet drinks, vitamins, protein wafers, and inspirational diet books: "Be slimmer and trimmer! Lose ugly pounds systematically! Enjoy fat-free cooking." (LaLanne was way ahead of his time with the low-fat diet.) By 1965, LaLanne, Inc. exceeded $4 million a year in sales.

LaLanne wasn't just in it for the money, though (although the Hollywood mansion was nice). He was on a crusade, and no one doubted his sincerity. When one San Francisco columnist called him "the Billy Graham of muscles," LaLanne—who always told his viewers about being sure they have plenty of "vitamins F in G, Faith in God"— was flattered. But he told Peter Wyden, who profiled LaLanne in 1965 in his book *The Overweight Society*, that there was a difference between himself and Billy Graham. "He puts people in shape for the hereafter," LaLanne said. "I get them fit for the here and now."

People swore that LaLanne had indeed transformed them. Bette Davis, Merle Oberon, and Mrs. Gary Cooper reported exercising in front of their televisions every morning. "Every man, woman and child should learn to follow his philosophy of living," Oberon said. LaLanne not only cured people's "pooped-out-itis," as he called it; viewers testified to other miraculous cures: they were finally able to get pregnant, their arthritis disappeared, their "home lives" improved. At fifty, with a perfect 48-28-35 physique, LaLanne himself was a remarkable testimonial to the power of his energy foods and exercise. Like Horace Fletcher, he performed feats of strength to publicize his program; each year, to celebrate his birthday, he put on another show. One year, he swam handcuffed from Alcatraz prison across San Francisco Bay in less than an hour; when he arrived at Fisherman's Wharf, he did thirty push-ups to boot. Another time, he performed a thousand push-ups in under half an hour for TV's *You Asked for It* program.

Despite his popularity, the U.S. government thought LaLanne's marketing was a little too eager. In 1962, the FDA seized thousands of bottles of LaLanne Protein Wafers and cans of LaLanne Instant Breakfast, saying that the health claims on the labels had been overstated. LaLanne's star faded as other celebrities, such as Debbie Drake, took over the TV limelight; later, a string of diet and exercise gurus patterned after Jack LaLanne would appear, most notably Jane Fonda, Richard Simmons, and Susan Powter.

LaLanne had added a new dimension to the diet gurus' puritanical quest for spiritual salvation through the body: exercise. After LaLanne, dieting wasn't enough to prove you were truly devoted to self-improvement; you had to have muscles, too. LaLanne never gave up his crusade to make America fit. Even in 1995, at the age of eighty, he was promoting a health care company and doing physical feats— lifting his wife for an audience.

Paperback Diet Gurus

From Brooklyn to Beverly Hills, the seventies and early eighties were a heyday for diet gurus, especially for the best-selling ones. Americans were hungry for an alternative to calorie counting, desperate to fit into bikinis, and happy to buy a paperback at the checkout stand that would tell them what to do. By this time, the idea that you could change your life by losing weight seemed evident to most people; the question was how to do it.

In 1980, *Consumer Guide* published *Rating the Diets*, which listed more than a hundred paperback diets—the wine diet, the lollipop diet, the astronaut diet, the desperate housewife diet, the born-again diet. Most were named after a diet doctor (Dr. Atkins' Superenergy Diet, Dr. Blackburn's Balanced Deficit Diet, Dr. Kremer's No-Breakfast Diet, Dr. Stillman's Quick Weight Loss Diet, Dr. Solomon's Easy, No-Risk Diet), a celebrity (Eileen Ford, Helena Rubenstein), or a nice address (the Hollywood Emergency Diet, the San Francisco Weight Loss Method, the Scarsdale Diet, the La Costa Spa Diet). They all made more or less the same promise: to lose weight fast.

One of the most imaginative of these best-selling diet books was *The Beverly Hills Diet* (1981), written by Judy Mazel in tropical prose. "A La Jolla housewife is popping grapes at her bridge luncheon . . . a New York book editor is packing papayas in her briefcase. What is going on?" It was, she claimed, the diet phenomenon of the eighties. "The diet embraced by everyone from 'Dallas' star Linda Gray, actress Sally Kellerman, and singer Englebert Humperdinck to hundreds of skinnies shouting the praises of the Beverly Hills Diet—a way of eating that has turned slimhood into a reality." Who could resist?

Mazel was inspired to go into the diet-counseling business when, at the age of thirty, a disembodied voice commanded her to exit off the L.A. Freeway and buy cashews. It was a spiritual quest. She drove up to a health-food store where she found a book on food combinations which became the basis for her diet. She'd already tried Stillman, Atkins, carbohydrate counting, and everything else. "All were rigid prescriptions for failure," she said. Mazel, one step past Horace Fletcher, realized that the key to weight loss is *digestion*. As long as everything you eat is fully digested, you can't gain weight. It's the enzymes in food, Mazel claimed, that help it get digested, but only in certain foods and combinations. In her book she reveals those combinations, explains her theory about the four stages of the digestive process, and describes the best source of enzymes of all: tropical fruit. Mangos, papayas, and pineapples, in large quantities, she found, *really* got digested. "If you have loose bowel movements, hooray!" she wrote. "The more time you spend on the toilet, the better."

The Beverly Hills Diet, in other words, is a step-by-step outline of how to binge and purge, with natural laxatives. The "have-it-all" theme was one of the most popular in diet books; people love to hear that they can eat all they want without gaining weight. "I still eat a triple order of potato pancakes without choking, an entire roast beef without blinking an eye, a whole, extra-rich cheesecake without a single gasp," she confesses, sounding a lot like an experienced bulimic. On her diet, however, you don't get to eat those foods every day. Day one involves pineapple in the morning, and bananas at night. (One woman I know who tried the diet said her mouth was so sore from eating just pineapple that she couldn't eat anything else for days.) Days two and three are mainly papaya, and day four is watermelon. After endless days of fruit, on day eleven you finally get the big binge: three and a half bagels for breakfast, and three ears of corn for dinner. Then it's back to fruit again.[7]

Throughout her book, Mazel chronicles her obsession with her weight, fixating on her "wonderfully lean hipbones," as she described them. In an article in the *International Journal of Eating Disorders*, which appeared not long after *The Beverly Hills Diet* was published, two eating disorders researchers, Orland W. Wooley and Susan Wooley, picked apart Mazel's book—and her psychology. "The Beverly Hills Diet marks the first time an eating disorder—anorexia nervosa—has been marketed as a cure for obesity," they wrote. Mazel's binges, her obsession with her 102-pound weight, her belief that you can never be too skinny, and her periods of starvation, they said, had all the hallmarks of anorexic psychopathology.[8] Her vision of how to achieve a glamorous, Beverly Hills lifestyle (and hipbones) made her book a big seller for years, and no doubt contributed to more than one eating disorder.

The paperback diet books that were most influential in the seventies and eighties were the ones written by diet doctors. Medical researchers were becoming more interested in studying obesity, and people were starting to listen more to what doctors had to say about losing weight. Now the moral directive to lose weight had the authority of medicine behind it. The scientific understanding of fatness was still uncertain enough, though, that any doctor who wanted to could test his or her personal theories about dieting on the paperback-buying public. Often—since they were, after all, trying to sell books—these doctors told the public what they wanted to hear.

"You can eat luxuriously—heavy cream, butter, mayonnaise, cheeses, meats, fish, fowl," promised Dr. Robert Atkins, a cardiologist. "I don't recommend [exercise] for anybody 40 years of age or over," said Dr. Herman Tarnower.[9] These men were the new experts on weight loss, authorities who looked out from their book jacket photos fully clad in lab coats and stethoscopes, surrounded by a library of medical texts. They were no longer dispensing the forgiving, big-sister diet advice of the fifties' women's magazines; they were sternly and inflexibly telling women what to do, with the full weight of their professional paternalism.

Dr. Herman Taller was the first doctor guru to become a huge best-selling author, with *Calories Don't Count* in 1961. His high-fat, high-protein, low-carbohydrate diet was a modern version of Banting's *Letter on Corpulence*. This diet had surfaced again in the 1940s, when a physician named Alfred Pennington studied overweight employees at duPont and came up with the idea that people needed to eat fat to get thin. He had the curious theory that people could metabolize fat completely, but not carbohydrates, so it was the carbohydrate leftovers that were making people fat. In 1961, Taller, a Brooklyn obstetrician-gynecologist who had a weight problem, read both Banting's and Pennington's diets, and, converted, published his own diet. He claimed that by eating fats, you stimulate the body's fat-burning system, which makes the stuff burn more efficiently. He thought vegetable fats were especially good for weight loss, since he believed they softened other body fats and flushed them out of the body. In 1967, after selling more than 1 million copies, Taller was found guilty of six counts of mail fraud for using the book to promote a particular brand of safflower capsules, which the court called a "worthless scheme foisted on a gullible public."[10]

That year, Dr. Irwin Stillman published another low-carbohydrate diet, *The Doctor's Quick Weight Loss Diet*, written with Samm Sinclair Baker (who later co-wrote the *Complete Scarsdale Diet* with Herman Tarnower and, barely credited, Jean Harris). Stillman was a strict carnivore, allowing his patients to eat only lean meat, poultry, eggs, and low-fat cheeses. His personal weight-loss theory held that the protein molecule is so big and complex it takes the body more energy to digest it, so you can eat as much as you want of protein without gaining weight. The authors advertised that patients would lose between 7 and 15 pounds the first week, and 5 pounds thereafter. These large amounts of protein, however, put people in a state of ketosis, where, without enough carbohydrates, the body breaks down fats for fuel faster than the body can eliminate the ashy protein leftovers. These leftovers, the ketones, not only cause bad breath but constipation, nausea, and weakness as well. The high-protein content of the diet also spiked the dieters' cholesterol levels to all-new highs. Stillman himself died of a heart attack in 1975—after some 20 million people had been on his diet.

The next "diet revolution"—as he called it—came from Robert Atkins, the cardiologist, who also advocated a protein diet. After reports of his diet appeared in *Harper's Bazaar* in 1966, and *Vogue* in 1970, he began treating celebrities, and soon became a celebrity himself. Atkins's diet is based on meat, with plenty of fats allowed. Dieters could add tiny amounts of carbohydrates to their diets, but only as long as urine test sticks showed that there were ketones in the urine; he believed that these protein byproducts helped control the appetite. As with the Stillman diet, eating only animal meat and saturated fats elevated cholesterol levels, strained the kidneys, and denied the body the necessary vitamins, minerals, and fibers found abundantly in fruits and vegetables. Doctors at the time criticized the hugely popular diet;

Frederick Stare, a Harvard obesity specialist, said it bordered on malpractice to recommend such large proportions of saturated fats and cholesterol when the hazards to the heart were well known. The American Medical Association (AMA) called it a "bizarre regimen" that is "without scientific merit."

But Atkins fought back, calling, in the language of the times, for a "diet revolution." He was lit with a kind of moral zeal. "Political action and protest on your part can help revolutionize the food industry, by forcing it to decarbohydrate many foods—just as it has de-calorized some foods—*but with a federal law to back this change!*" he told his readers. "Martin Luther King had a dream. I, too, have one. I dream of a world where no one has to diet. A world where the fattening refined carbohydrates have been excluded from the diet."[11] Atkins resurfaced again in 1992, with the hardly changed *Dr. Atkins' New Diet Revolution.*

A more sober protein doctor was the cardiologist Herman Tarnower. He was also perhaps the most paternalistic of the bunch. His *Complete Scarsdale Diet* (1978), a high-protein diet that added up to about 700 calories a day, specified exactly what the reader could eat and not eat. Tarnower's diet was an exercise in following doctor's orders: the dieter was supposed never to make substitutions; to give up all alcohol, butter, and oil; and to have nothing between meals but carrots and celery. And when Tarnower said celery, he didn't mean green peppers or zucchini. "I think it is important to *follow the diet as written,*" he wrote. "Your *attitude* toward a diet is an important ingredient in the success or failure of that diet for you. When you start playing fast and loose with it, you're on your way off the Diet."[12] Breakfast every day on the Scarsdale Diet was invariable: one half a grapefruit, one slice toasted protein bread, and black coffee or tea. Period.

Tarnower not only had rigid ideas about what women should eat but how they should act. Like other doctor gurus, he was giving women prescriptions in feminine morality, from a distinctly male point of view. When one reader wrote to him, "When I diet, I get cranky, and my husband says, 'I like you better fat than cranky'; have you any suggestions?" Tarnower responded, "You should be able to diet without getting cranky. Your husband, I am sure, would like to have you attractive, lean, and pleasant." His attitude makes one sympathize with his lover Jean Harris, the former school headmistress who later did prison time for his murder.

Doctor gurus are still with us today. Some of them rely on the same old protein diet. A flurry of protein-based diet books came out in 1995 as a response to the low-fat, high-carbohydrate diets of the preceding few years, including Michael and Mary Dan Eades's *Protein Power*, Barry Sears's *The Zone*, and Adele Puhn's *The 5 Day Miracle Diet*. Though these diets add enough carbohydrates to the mix that people don't go into ketosis, and don't rely as much on animal proteins, they are nearly as nutritionally immoderate and scientifically suspect as the original protein diets. Sears talks about "good" carbohydrates and "bad" carbohydrates, seemingly randomly distinguishing between different types of vegetables, fruits, and grains. It's rather astonishing, after so many recent studies have demonstrated the importance of vegetables and fiber in preventing disease, that people would still recommend a high-protein diet as "healthy." (Like Taller, some of these new protein diet authors promote products in their books, often making unproven claims about their effectiveness. Among others, according to the *New York Times* writer Marian Burros, Barry Sears makes money off the nutrition bars he mentions in his book, and Cliff Sheats, who wrote *Lean Bodies Total Fitness*, promotes dietary supplements and even his own brand of longhorn beef.)[13]

Others rely more on their personality than on their diet gimmick. Stephen Gullo, a Manhattan celebrity diet shrink who is quoted everywhere in women's magazines (*Self* uses him as an author one week and an expert the next), charges his patients $500 a session to give them stern admonishments. "It's better to wear Italian than eat Italian," he tells them. "Eat white and green!" His diet book, *Thin Tastes Better: Control Your Food Triggers and Lose Weight Without Feeling Deprived* (1995), emphasizes little psychological tricks—identifying "trigger foods"—and is fairly high in protein and low in carbohydrates, especially grains. Like many doctor gurus, Gullo has done no new studies to back up his diet. He just has a new shtick, and a marketing strategy. He preaches one-on-one to celebrities and wealthy people, and lets his advice trickle down to the rest of us via popular magazines and gossip columns. His advice to women, like that of all paternalistic gurus, sounds like advice to children: Never eat when you're hungry ... Don't use slips as excuses to eat more ... Exercise won't bail you out. As one client told the *New York Times*, "The tapes are made for idiots. The diet was too restrictive. He's outrageously expensive."[14]

Dean Ornish

On the West Coast, Dr. Dean Ornish, a physician based in Sausalito, California, whose book *Eat More, Weigh Less* was a bestseller in 1993, is less overtly authoritarian and sounds more spiritual. But like Taller or Stillman, Ornish recommends that dieters stop eating an entire food group. In his case, he campaigns against fat, not carbohydrates. Nutritionally, his diet is just the opposite of Taller's or Stillman's—and it is healthier, no doubt about it, but in some ways just as extreme. Ornish recommends that everyone get their fat level down to less than 10 percent of their diet. That doesn't mean just cutting back on cheeseburgers and fries; that means no fat, period, except what naturally occurs in vegetables, grains, beans, and fruits.

Ornish follows in the footsteps of Nathan Pritikin, a Southern California diet guru who wrote the best-selling *Pritikin Program for Diet and Exercise* in 1979, and believed that exercise and very-low-fat eating could reverse cardiovascular disease. Pritikin, who started the enormously successful Pritikin Longevity Center in Santa Monica, thought his strict regimen was not only the best way to lose weight but the best way to live, and he preached his message widely. "It is possible," Calvin Trillin wrote about Pritikin in *The New Yorker* in 1981, "that when the Deity finally decides to reveal the Truth to the human race He may choose as His messenger a Southern California health guru who has a how-to book in the top ten and has managed to recruit both John Travolta and Barbra Streisand as disciples."[15] But many critics have wondered whether people who don't have cardiovascular disease or other health problems need to devote themselves to such a Spartan practice.

Ornish, who started out as a cardiologist trying to reverse heart disease, took the Pritikin low-fat, low-cholesterol, high-fiber diet, along with the exercise, added meditation, and group support, and tested it. He proved that it is indeed possible to reverse coronary heart disease in unhealthy middle-aged people. Most importantly, he forced the medical establishment, which for the most part had relied on drugs and surgery to treat heart disease, and pooh-poohed alternative approaches, to take another look at prevention and holistic methods of healing for cardiovascular patients.

Then, like Pritikin, Ornish extended his valuable but limited observations to the general population. No one had studied the effects of such a diet on a normal female population of dieters. Nor did Ornish separate the effects of meditation, community, and exercise from the effects of diet. He based his initial recommendations to the general public on studies involving only forty-eight middle-aged people with coronary heart disease, with only five women among them. There may be no reason for normal people to go to such extremes. Why give up fat entirely if there's nothing wrong with you? It isn't necessarily true that if less fat is good, then drastically less is better. A super-low-fat diet may even cause a deficiency in fat-soluble vitamins in some people, and for others who are susceptible to diabetes, a high-carbohydrate diet could be harmful. But Ornish says abstinence from fat is less complicated than trying to figure out how to cut down. "It's easier to make big changes than small changes," he says.

Like other diet gurus, Ornish writes with a slightly religious tone. His diet, he seems to believe, will not only change your body but your higher self. "This is a book as much about transformation as on weight loss. If you are overweight, then you know what it means to be in emotional pain. When you're suffering, your distress can be a catalyst, a doorway to real healing." Later, he writes of what happens when his diet pushes you through that doorway. "Many people find that eating a low-fat vegetarian diet—that is, the Life Choice [Ornish] diet—makes them feel more open, aware, and connected." He includes a testimonial from a devotee who went from overeating and numbing his pain, "living half a life," to learning to connect with people, having more control over his own fate, and achieving more insight. "I feel like I'm waking up after being asleep for a long, long time," the man said.[16]

Ornish's followers can develop an almost cultlike devotion to his principles. In 1995, at a conference of diet doctors, I met a young physician who was interested in starting a weight-loss and preventive health care practice (he'd failed his board exams in psychiatry, so decided to become a diet doc instead). He was in his mid-thirties and wiry-lean. He had changed his diet completely, and vowed never to eat fat again, so he wouldn't end up like the overweight members of his family. I wanted to find out more about why he was becoming a diet doctor, so we decided to discuss things over dinner. We were in San

Antonio, right downtown, where tables for outdoor restaurants stretch along both sides of the river. I had already scouted out the menus earlier in the afternoon, spotted some blackened tuna, tequila-marinated grilled prawns, and other healthy Southwestern dishes, and was looking forward to my dinner. The Ornish acolyte, however, insisted we drive to a vegetarian restaurant he had found in the phonebook instead. We spent half an hour driving to the other side of town, where we sat down in a nearly empty mall café that was trying to project something like a hippie spirit. The physician ordered plain pinto beans—"Those are made with no fat, right?"—and plain baked potatoes, no sour cream or butter. I ordered sautéed spinach and mashed potatoes (with butter), and had a cookie for dessert.

I had the cookie to torment him. The physician had spent almost all the time, energy, and conversation that evening getting his eating situation just right, perfectly no-fat. Yet he was so thin he practically needed reverse liposuction. Then, after he dropped me at my hotel, he went to find a twenty-four-hour gym where he could work off dinner. I have seen eating obsessions up close before, but never one with such a strong sense of righteous healthiness.

I called up Dean Ornish to find out why an otherwise healthy person would want to follow his program—which, he insists, is for everyone, not just those who want to lose weight. What's wrong with just cutting back on fat and eating lots of fruits, vegetables, and whole grains, without going to extremes? I told him that I have been a fish-eating vegetarian for fifteen years, I eat mainly nonfat dairy products, and use only a little olive oil to sauté garlic and vegetables.

"Olive oil?" he asked. I had said an evil word. "All oil is a hundred percent fat."

Chastened, I went on. I told him my height and weight, said I exercise nearly every day, have a low-waist-to-hip ratio (a better sign of health than is weight), and a rock-bottom cholesterol count. "Why should I eat less fat than I do?"

Ornish estimated that I probably already eat 15–20 percent fat (after his reaction to the olive oil, I was afraid to confess the occasional brownie or scone I eat to keep life interesting, but my fat intake is still pretty low). "If you want to lose weight, that might be one reason to eat less fat," he said.

"Why should I lose weight?" I asked. "How could I be in better health?"

He conceded there was no health reason for someone like me to lose weight; later, in a letter, he said it would cut my risk of breast cancer (the evidence on that point is actually very mixed). At bottom, Ornish's reason to tell normal, healthy people like me to lose weight and eat no fat is moral, cosmetic, and self-promotional. *"Eat More, Weigh Less* is a doorway to get people to eat this way," he told me. "That motivates people. If I wrote a book called *How to Help Heart Disease, Cancer, and Osteoporosis*, it wouldn't be number one on the bestseller list."

Nevertheless, I tried to eat out à la Ornish one evening. I went to Square One, the recently closed San Francisco restaurant that was the home of chef Joyce Goldstein, who contributed to Ornish's low-fat cookbook. "What would Dean Ornish eat?" I asked the waiter. He pointed me to the seared tuna *all'abruzzese* with wine, hot pepper, rosemary, and garlic, served with a pan ragout of white beans, broccoli, greens, and fennel. He added, however, that Ornish would not eat the sauce on the fish—I guess there was a drop or two of olive oil in it. I spent half the meal glowering at my companion because he got the sauce. Other than that it was delicious—proof that if I could eat at restaurants like Square One all the time, I could stay on the diet.

Other restaurants proved more difficult. At one, I ordered the Caesar salad with no dressing or cheese. "Let me get this straight," the waiter said. "You just want plain Romaine lettuce?" I meekly asked him to sprinkle a few anchovies on top, but then, after realizing that they, too, are packed in oil, I changed my order a couple more times. The waiter hated me. At a traditional Italian restaurant, it was easy to get balsamic vinegar for the salad, but I embarrassed my friend when I asked if the marinara sauce had any oil in it. "Only a little," replied Fabio, the waiter. "It's very light." I asked if it was possible to make it with *no* oil. Fabio was dismayed. "Maybe it is possible, signorina, but I don't think you would like the taste." When I refused his offer of grated cheese for the pasta, Fabio only shook his head. At dessert, he lovingly described the *tiramisu* and hazelnut chocolate torte. I ordered an espresso and a glass of port (thank God there's no fat in alcohol), but I still felt deprived.

If I had heart disease, diabetes, dangerous cholesterol numbers, high blood pressure, and smoked cigarettes all my life, I might go running to Dean Ornish. His holistic approach to treating serious diseases that are caused or encouraged by unhealthy lifestyles makes a lot more sense than drugs and surgery. But for those of us who are already healthy? Sure, you can spend your life counting the fat percentage in everything you eat. You can swear you'll never eat another olive, avocado, cashew, scone, marinated vegetable, hazelnut chocolate torte, taste of Gorgonzola cheese, or drop of olive oil. You may live longer if you eat a super-low-fat diet. Or it may just seem that way.

Richard Simmons

Richard Simmons, a curly-headed dynamo who has been in the diet business for more than a decade, is America's favorite diet guru. He has inexhaustible energy; he runs an exercise studio in Beverly Hills, produces his own fitness videos, sells his Deal-A-Meal diet plan on infomercials, checks in regularly on daytime TV talk shows, makes three hundred personal appearances at malls and conventions a year, and calls hundreds of fat people a week. Like Jack LaLanne, Simmons is on a personal crusade to transform every fat person in America, and he truly believes that if there were only enough hours in the day, he could do it.

For millions of Americans, Simmons, who was once a 260-pound teenager, has become an emblem of the hope that they can lose weight and change their lives. They feel that he personally can help them lose weight, and they write to him as a last-ditch diet effort. "I'd say every overweight person has written to me at least once," Simmons tells me. "I'm the last hotel on Weight Loss Boulevard. You have to have been living under a rock not have seen me on a talk show or infomercial."

Indeed. With his frantic schedule, Simmons almost succeeds in keeping pace with the growing number of fat people in the country. "Every day, CNN or somebody is telling us how many more fat people there are," he says, breaking into a TV anchorman voice. "Four out of five people are short and fat! Five out of eight have had a divorce and are fat!" He laughs, but humor is his way of dispelling the pain he believes comes with being fat. He laughs with fat people, and cries with them; he opens his arms to them in order to save them. "I want to take care of these people. I don't judge them because they're fat, I love them unconditionally. I just want them to come to class."

Like so many of his fans, Simmons has been fat, he's dieted, he's starved, and he's thrown up. He understands: even though he has succeeded in losing weight, he still has the desire every day, he says, to lick his finger and get the remaining greasy potato chip crumbs at the bottom of the bag. To overcome that desire, he has transformed his compulsion to eat into a compulsion to help others. "I'm Richard O. Simmons!" he chirps. "The O is for 'obsession.'"

Like Jack LaLanne, Simmons started out with an exercise studio, and it's in his studio that he really shines. His exercise class at his shiny pink and white "Slimmons" Studio in Beverly Hills is high-energy fun for people who might otherwise feel out of place in an aerobics class. Simmons prances up to the front of the room, his fuchsia tank top and nylon shorts sparkling in the mirror. "The disco's open all night!" he yells, throwing a record onto the stereo. Most of the people in the room are women in the 200-pound range, wearing bright makeup, neon leggings, and oversized T-shirts. A few people are larger; a man and a woman in the back of the room, discreetly furnished with ample chairs, are closer to 500 pounds. Simmons leads the group in slow stretching warm-ups before heating things up with grapevine steps, shuffles, and *Saturday Night Fever* moves. Soon, everyone is not only moving but panting and sweating. Between routines, Simmons keeps up a comedy patter on the theme of weight loss. "If you have a problem, a baloney sandwich is not going to solve it," he says. "Anyone here starving themselves?" he asks. "If so, you have to do the class naked. Those are the rules."

By providing an atmosphere where people of all sizes and shapes can exercise comfortably and have a great time, Simmons gives them an opportunity to transform themselves in the present, instead of in the distant after-picture future when they might become thin. Exercise lifts people's moods right now, and gives them the sense that their bodies are not just a source of shame but of pleasure. "I see people blossom," says Simmons.

But that isn't enough for Simmons—or for many of his students. They're here, primarily, to get thin. If they didn't think exercise helped them lose weight faster, they might not show up for class. At Slimmons, thinness is the fantasy, the motivation, and the ultimate goal. "Debbie lost sixty-seven pounds," Simmons tells the group, pointing to a blonde in her forties. "She had her belly button redone. She picked Cher's."

Simmons promises fat people they'll *really* start living when they lose weight. No matter how much fun you have jumping around an exercise studio, feeling good about your body for a change, life really won't be exciting unless you become thin. Until then, he feels sorry for you. He doesn't think it's possible to come to class, exercise, and be fit if you don't lose the weight—even though he acknowledges that most people, in the end, don't keep the pounds off.

"Fat kills," he tells me later, sitting on the lavender carpet of his *Gone With the Wind*–style mansion up in the hills above the studio. "You go from being chubby to fat, to obese, to morbidly obese. And then there's death." Simmons likes to tell Cinderella stories of people he's saved from that fate, who have lost 100 pounds or more on his program and gone on to lead glamorous lives. But he can't help everyone. His brown eyes redden. "I've lost so many people."

Simmons, to his credit, doesn't sell faddish diet products to help people lose weight. "I've never jumped on the bandwagon for the liquid diets—and I could've made a lot of money—or for the pills, or for the little frozen foods that don't look like much." Instead, he advocates a moderate low-calorie, low-fat, semi-starvation diet (about the same as most commercial weight-loss programs), along with exercise, and relies on his charm and willpower to inspire people to stick with it. He's well aware of the formula for his success: "Being approachable, being my TV persona, and looking the same—as long as I can fit into these Dolphin shorts, my weight's okay," he says. He isn't a stickler about getting super-thin; with a little potbelly himself, he's more realistic. "And I eyeball 400,000 people a year like this." He stares into my eyes with his liquid brown ones, in a well-practiced gaze that registers compassion, love, and heartfelt sympathy. "I don't know why I keep it up. I just keep going, I love it. I have a passion for what I do."

Leaning back against a large, lime sherbet–colored armchair, Simmons tells me he doesn't think of himself as a guru. "I'm a struggling guy who's lost some weight, and through humor is helping a lot of people. People think of me as a cousin they grew up with who made them laugh." If people look to him for inspiration and motivation, though, he's happy. "They do write to me and say, without you, I couldn't have done this, I never could've lost this two hundred pounds. And I figure, that's great. I'm glad I was there to help." His eyes redden again for a moment, and he looks away, surveying the living room with its many ornate dolls perched on display shelves and marble pedestals. "I never put myself on a pedestal with these people," he says. "They've followed me like a Pied Piper, but I've never led them down the wrong path."

It's not surprising that people follow Richard Simmons; he's honest, direct, sensitive, and a lot of fun to be around. I wanted to stay all afternoon, chatting away, and it seemed like he might have let me. He gave me a tour of his doll collection, his blown-glass plates, his cow-patterned kitchen (the stools had udders), and his Victorian Easter egg collection. He introduced me to his six Dalmatians, and showed me the dogs' future memorial park, complete with cypress trees, cala lilies, and marble walkways, which he had built right outside the house so that when the dogs need a final place to rest, they can be near him. He broke out alternately into tears and Broadway songs as we talked, and his humor was quick, spontaneous, and never mean. Before I left, he introduced me to his family of household assistants and a friend, telling them how I'd attended his exercise class that day. "She took the class, and she was the thinnest one there," he said. That actually wasn't true, but to Richard Simmons, it was the highest form of flattery.

Simmons doesn't believe that it's possible to be heavy and still feel fine about yourself. "I don't find fat pretty," he says. "I don't look at a fat woman and say, 'Oh my gosh, she's beautiful the way she is!'" He is adamant that fat people need help, and those who think they're all right—a view encouraged by fat activists, such as members of the National Association to Advance Fat Acceptance (NAAFA)—are just fooling themselves. "I get a lot of letters saying, 'I belonged to this fat organization, and they told me they were happy and fat, and they had a career and a man who loved them, but I couldn't buy it. I got out of it, and Richard, I need some help.'" He says he's puzzled why people at NAAFA don't like him. He wishes they did, he says; he'd like to help them lose weight, too.

Simmons is a frequent guest on daytime TV talk shows, where the story always involves a depressed fat person who—surprise!—gets to meet Richard Simmons, and is inspired to start on that diet and lose the weight once and for all. They are chubby Cinderellas, and he is the fairy godmother who swoops down and, with a wave of the wand, gives them the inspiration and willpower they need. "It's a great story, the Cinderella syndrome," Simmons tells me. "She's scrubbing the floor, can't go to the ball, and the fairy godmother comes. She gets the dress, the Tiffany jewelry, she goes to the party. We're raised on these stories. We all have this thing about happy endings. So, if Sally has a story about a fat woman, those get big ratings, because we want this big transformation. It's still hot, and it will never change. Never."

In his book *Richard Simmons' Never Give Up* (1993), every story is a story of miracles that happen when someone meets Richard Simmons and loses weight. Nancy dropped 112 pounds and saved her marriage. Charmi met Simmons and achieved the goal of her life, to become an aerobics instructor. One man was so fat it drove him to drug abuse and theft; he went to Simmons's class, lost 110 pounds, turned himself in to the police, and was sentenced to continue the class. A woman whose daughter got run over by a car ate to deal with her grief; she got Simmons's Deal-A-Meal, lost weight, and was able to adopt a new baby.

In real life, though, losing weight doesn't have much to do with adopting a baby, rehabilitating a criminal life, finding love, or saving your marriage. Losing weight is not likely to solve all your problems, heal the emotional scars of your childhood, or make you rich (unless you become a diet guru). Many people, in fact, have found the opposite to be true: Giving up the dream that dieting will transform them has let them get on with their lives, rather than putting everything off until that fantasy day when they're finally thin.

But for those who follow Richard Simmons, hope springs eternal. In spite of the many people who have failed repeatedly on his—like every—diet, Simmons is always there with an encouraging word. Michael Hebranko, who once lost 700 pounds and became a 200-pound television spokesman for Simmons, made the news in May 1996, when, at about 1,000 pounds, unable to stand for more than half a minute or breathe on his own, he was removed from his home with a forklift and transported to a hospital. Simmons, though saddened and worried about Hebranko, nevertheless told reporters he was sure that with his help, the man would get back on his diet and lose the weight again.

Susan Powter

Unlike Richard Simmons, Susan Powter isn't about to give you a big hug or cry with you over your mournful fatness. She'll yell at you to eat, breathe, and move, and scorn you if you don't follow her commands. She's more like a diet dominatrix than a diet guru. Powter, standing in the lobby of the Ritz-Carlton Hotel in a blond buzz-cut, executive-tailored pantsuit, and large square black glasses, is the picture of cold, hard-bodied, nineties-style femininity. She offers me a limp hand to shake, then strides several paces ahead to the restaurant, where she hollers at the host before he can scurry up to the podium with the menu. "We need a table! Breakfast!"

Powter orders with enthusiasm—Japanese breakfast, with an egg, salmon, rice, miso soup, and fruit—and eats with real gusto, which is a rare quality in a woman, one that I admire. She starts by telling me she isn't peddling a diet, but—like all diet gurus—enlightening people about the one true way they can lose weight and transform their lives forever. "I'm not a nutritionist, I'm not a doctor, I'm not a dietitian," she tells me, picking up her salmon with her long red nails. "I'm a housewife that figured it out. All I do is tell people the truth. It's attainable, it's simple, it works, and it's the truth."

She launches into her spiel promoting her talk show, her book, her program, her million projects, all the while talking through bites of seaweed and egg. Her first "Stop the Insanity!" TV infomercial, she says, topped the charts, selling 80,000 units of her product—a "no-diet" package—per month. Her confessional 1993 diet book, *Stop the Insanity!*, and its companions, *The Pocket Powter* and *Food*, hit the bestseller lists. She has a TV talk show, a series of exercise videos, a line of fitness wear, and an audio newsletter. A huge and devoted group of followers pay $39 a head to attend her motivational hotel seminars. This high school dropout, mother of two, and former topless dancer made about $1 million for every one of the 133 pounds she claims she lost on her "wellness" program (only to file for bankruptcy later).

You might think that Powter had something rather extraordinary up her sleeve. I not only had breakfast with her, I bought her books, called the toll-free number for her products, listened to her tapes, and went to one of her seminars. What's her secret? Contrary to what she says about being anti-diet, she mainly promotes a low-fat diet. Fat calipers, motivation tapes, an exercise video, and some recipes pad out her product. What really sells, though, is her personality. Angry and rebellious, Powter taps into the rage many women feel over having tried and tried again to lose weight, spending ridiculous sums on diet gimmicks and ending up fatter and feeling worse about themselves than before. Like them, she has experienced the pain of being fat, and can even joke about it. Unlike them, however, she has overcome her weight, been transformed, and wants to share her secret with everyone—for a price. Susan Powter ends up exploiting women's anger and frustration about dieting to sell them yet another diet.

Powter offers women an irresistible combination of promises. If they follow her simple low-fat eating and exercise plan, they will transform their lives. They, too, will melt from a size 22 to a 2. They'll show their ex-husband's girlfriends who's the thinnest of them all. They'll get revenge on all their friends and foes who have put them down for being fat, and they'll find new energy, exciting relationships, self-respect, and success. "Lose a little weight, gain some strength, and your whole life will change," Powter says.

Perhaps what makes Powter most appealing is her way to lose weight, which is very binge-oriented. At her hotel seminar, she tells the audience that you can eat all the food you want, as long as it's low-fat, and the pounds will still melt away. "You can eat popcorn until you throw up." she says. For the amount of fat in a fast-food burger, she points out, you can swim in a bathtub of noodles or eat 452 cups of grains. "You can eat truckloads of grain!"

She wheels out grocery carts of vegetables on stage, bottles and bottles of salsa, and bags of potatoes to illustrate how much you can eat for the amount of fat in a piece of cheese (which she calls "doody," borrowing the vocabulary of her elementary school–aged sons). One of the keys to Powter's success is how well she taps into the American binge-purge mentality. "Susan Powter's message," says Susan Bordo, the feminist philosopher, "appeals to our desires to consume as well as to the puritan element that says we've got to have willpower and control."

But the truth is that nothing short of actual bulimia will allow you to eat as much as Powter says you can and lose weight. Carbohydrates do have fewer calories, gram for gram, than fat, but eat enough carbohydrates and they turn to fat, too. Powter's "fat formula"—basically checking the label and making sure nothing you put in your mouth exceeds 10 or 15 percent fat—is also too simple. She doesn't take into account anything as confusing as the idea that one could eat a high-fat olive or a chocolate chip cookie now and then and still stay well within a low daily limit of fat. In her view, a dribble of olive oil in a pan is the same as deep-fat frying. "Where did we get the idea that if you wipe something with olive oil, it's any different than pouring it on?" she asks. "All oil is one hundred percent fat," she says, sounding a lot like Dean Ornish. "Fat makes you fat! Fat is disgusting! Eeech!"

Another appealing—but often false—promise she makes is that everyone can get thin on her program. Just eat, breathe, and move. It's true that exercise and eating less fat may make you healthier, but it isn't necessarily going to make you thin, unless, like Susan Powter or Oprah Winfrey, you spend several hours a day working out and lifting weights. For the ordinary woman who has a job and kids, her program is as much a setup for failure as any diet. Powter's message that it's simple and takes no time to lose weight is a myth, in a world full of myths that women should have more time to work, be at home, work out, and fit an ideal standard of attractiveness.

Some people are just big, and are never going to be thin, no matter how much Powter promises them. "You'll be floored at how quickly your body starts to shrink," she tells the audience. "You'll put on a pair of pants and they'll be hanging." Even if she did lose 133 pounds, as she claims—members of her family say she was never that fat— that doesn't mean other fat women can do it using her method. "Susan Powter does not look like a genetically fat person who's lost weight," observes C. Wayne Callaway, a George Washington University endocrinologist and obesity expert who sees a lot of fat people in his practice. "She had one event in her life where she gained a lot of weight; those people lose it more easily. Someone is two hundred sixty at eighteen years of age is not going to get down to her weight. It's grossly misleading."

I asked Powter over breakfast whether indeed she had been fat as a child, which is a good way to find out whether it's in the genes. "I wasn't morbidly obese as a child," she said, picking at her salmon. She went off on a rant about yo-yo dieting, gaining and losing 20 or 40 pounds, eating lettuce for four months . . .

"When you were five or six, were you fat?" I interrupted.

"I was a normal kid," she replied.

At the hotel seminar the next day, in front of hundreds of people, she used our interview, which I did for *Vogue* magazine, for stand-up material. "Yesterday," she said, swaggering around the stage like a model on a runway, "I was interviewed by *Voooooogue*." She paused to let the middle-class audience have a laugh at New York magazines and models, even though she is offering them the same impossible image of thinness.

"This journalist accused me of being mean to fat people," she said. (Not exactly: I'd asked her whether she was holding out false hopes to people who don't have it in the cards to lose a lot of weight.) "I'm always getting these assaults from the right-to-fat groups," she said. " 'I'm genetically fat, I'm from a big-boned tribe,' " she mimicked, then went back to her sergeant tone. "This is ridiculous. There are very few people with medically justified fat. Ninety-nine-point-nine percent of us are fat because we are eating too much high-fat food and we're not moving." She didn't cite the source of her statistics. "When you have three to nine inches of fat on top of Grandma's thighs? You can't even see what you've been given genetically." She pointed to her life-size "before" photo. "My stomach hung down to my knees."

Later, after a break, she came back on the stage. "You know that woman from *Vogue* I was telling you about?" she asked the audience. "Well, my manager said I had to say something nice about her." She made a big fake smile. "Well, she was lovely, she really was. And she was smart. She understood every word I said."

Actually, Powter, like many diet companies, doesn't pay that much attention to fat people. She's interested in a more lucrative market: helping normal-sized women who *think* they're fat get really thin, feeding their obsessions. Most of the people at her hotel seminar were about fifteen to forty pounds heavier than the ideal. On one of her tapes, describing how to use fat calipers to pinch and measure fat percentages, her volunteer weighs 133 pounds and has 21 percent body fat. By all standards, that's entirely healthy. "She's not obese," says Powter. "But she's a big girl. She could lose some body fat."

The woman mumbles her assurances that yes, she will lose that dreadful body fat. Powter, who constantly reminds everyone she went from 43 percent body fat to 14 percent body fat, says women can go as low as 8 percent body fat. "When you look emaciated and you're not getting your period anymore, you've gone too low," she advises. Most scientists, however, call 14 percent body fat "essential" fat required for women to menstruate and reproduce. Eight percent body fat is hovering around anorexia.

Finally, Susan Powter insists that her program is going to do women a world of good, and calls herself a feminist. "Everybody should be a feminist," she told me. "Who the hell shouldn't be a feminist?" But feminism, to her, is about giving women physical strength, thinness, and the illusion of control over their lives through diet and exercise. It's not about defying a culture that places impossible demands on women—including the expectation that we be thin. It's just gaining power and success. " 'Stop the Insanity!' is not weight loss, it's power," she told me. "You regain control and power in your life."

Power to Powter, too, means sexual power, which comes from losing weight. "My motivation was not, and still isn't, health," she said. "I wanted to look good. My motivation was to look better than my husband's girlfriend. Absolutely the truth. And you know what?" She laughed. "I do."

Powter's version of feminism comes down to women achieving power, as usual, through their bodies. "This is a strange version of feminism," says Bordo. "Her feminism has to do with making yourself the most attractive, invulnerable, compelling object that you can. And the degree you're in control of that, then you're in power."

For all her energy, anger, humor, and talk about "empowering women," Powter is selling women an old diet and an even older message: Focus on becoming thin and attractive, and your whole life will change for the better. It isn't surprising that after so many women bought her message—and failed to get down to her size, 2—Susan Powter's popularity, like that of so many gurus, is already waning. She's just the name of another diet that didn't work.

Chapter 3

Ten Pounds in Ten Days: Diet Scams

The phone rang in the middle of a Tuesday afternoon. "Hello," said the woman on the line. "Are you interested in losing weight?"

How did she know? Alarmed, I wondered whether "overweight" was somehow noted in my credit profile, a part of my computerized identity, available to telephone marketers everywhere.

"Well . . . yes," I confessed. It didn't occur to me that nearly every woman listed in the phone book is interested in losing weight, and this was just a random call.

"That's just great," the woman cooed, introducing herself as Darlene. I could tell right away by the warm, sympathetic tone in Darlene's voice that she'd be there for me if I decided, here in the middle of my work day, to finally do something about those terrible excess pounds.

Darlene gave me the pitch. Thermojetics, she explained, an Herbalife product, is the best new way to lose weight. "It's really phenomenal," she said. "It's scientific, and it doesn't involve any dieting, because everyone *knows* diets don't work. You don't even have to exercise."

Apparently, all I had to do to lose as much weight as I wanted, as she put it, was take two tablets a day, and my body would immediately start burning fat more quickly. My metabolism would increase and I wouldn't feel hungry. Between meals, I would automatically reach for celery sticks and cauliflower florets instead of handfuls of granola and hunks of Gruyère cheese. "Kind of like willpower for the body," Darlene said. She confided that she herself had lost five inches after only seven days of taking these tablets. "My boyfriend can't believe it!"

Amazing. Why hadn't I read about this stuff in the *New York Times*? "What's in them?" I asked her.

"Just herbs," Darlene said, matter-of-factly. "It's all natural." She seemed to mean that since it's all natural, it couldn't possibly hurt me. Then came the environmental part of the pitch: "You can heal your body and help save the planet, too," she explained. "You'll help save the rain forest where these herbs come from."

Lose weight *and* save the rain forest. Hmmm. "Exactly which rain forest herbs are they?"

"Organic herbs," she replied, as if that explained everything.

I asked her if she might have a list of ingredients. "I don't really know...." She trailed off. Then she found the list, and started reeling off names of herbs: "Chinese ma huang, yerba mate, bladderwrack, valerian root, purple willow, Hawthorne berry, uva ursi, alfalfa, cornsilk, parsely, marshmallow root, magnolia bark, pau d'arco, astragalus, fennel seed, goldenrod, and licorice."

I was surprised to hear you could get cornsilk and magnolia bark in the rain forest. And bladderwrack, it seemed to me, was what I'd end up with if I took all those ingredients at once. "Can you tell me how these work?" I asked Darlene.

She launched into more well-rehearsed territory. "This product regulates the metabolism, increases the body's ability to burn fat, and controls the appetite," she said. Whoever wrote the pitch was certainly up on the latest diet promises. "The whole point is that you don't deprive yourself, and you don't diet. You just add these pills to what you normally eat." Then she went into the pseudoscience. "The tablets help you retrain your body's ability to convert fat to energy," she began. "There are two systems in fat cells—storage and release. A lot of overweight is caused by an imbalance between these. So these herbs correct the balance. Your energy comes from the release of fat."

"Have there been any studies to prove this?" I asked her. "The product was three years in the making," she said. "I'm *sure* there are studies. It's thirty-five dollars for a month's supply. Will that be Visa or MasterCard?"

Every year Americans spend between 5 and 6 billion dollars on over-the-counter pills, herbal formulas, and teas that promise to make us thin. The Internet is crowded with ads for herbal supplements that promise miraculous weight-loss results, and salespeople at health food stores say these diet aids are flying off the shelves. In the fall of 1997, after the popular prescription diet pills dexfenfluramine and fenfluramine were pulled off the market, sales of copycat herbal diet remedies soared. Twinlab, which makes Herbal Phen Fuel (a combination of citrus aurantium, a mild stimulant, and St. John's wort, an herbal remedy for depression that is supposed to increase serotonin levels, as the banned diet drugs did) said it expected to sell $25 million in the nutritional supplements by the year's end.[1] HPF, which makes Herbal Phen-Fen, a combination of the stimulant ephedrine and St. John's wort, would only disclose that it was the "hottest-selling diet aid ever." And while the FDA issued a consumer warning against products that masquerade as prescription diet pills in November 1997, there is little the agency can do to stanch the flow of untested, ineffective, and sometimes dangerous herbal diet products.

Whatever the ingredient list of herbal diet aids—ephedrine, garcinia, 5-hydroxy-tryptophan, guarana, chromium picolinate, pyruvate, chickweed—all make the same promises to burn fat and raise the metabolism, and all back their claims up with scientific-sounding terms and lists of studies. But most of those studies are either fake or too small and poorly done to be accepted in medical journals. In fact, there is very little evidence that anything you can buy in a bottle at a health food store or drugstore will help you lose weight, unless you burn up a lot of calories walking to the store.

"There's no herb at the present time that can be taken safely that has been proven to induce weight loss," says Varro Tyler, professor emeritus at Purdue University who is an expert in medicinal herbs.

Even when the FDA knows that a product is ineffective, or indeed unsafe, there's very little the agency can do to protect consumers. There's a free-for-all in herbal supplements in this country, even though several people have died taking herbal diet pills or teas. In 1994 the Dietary Supplements Health and Education Act, championed by Republican Senator Orrin Hatch of Utah (a state where, not coincidentally, many herbal supplements are manufactured), took the teeth out of the FDA when it comes to regulating these products. In the past, if the FDA had a health or safety question about a food product, the burden of proof was on manufacturers to show that it was safe. Now it's up to the FDA to prove, in a lengthy and expensive investigation, that a product is dangerous before it can be pulled from the shelves. And despite its increased burden, the FDA has received no additional resources to conduct investigations of potentially harmful products.

The FDA doesn't allow herbal diet-aid manufacturers to make direct drug claims about their products. But manufacturers are adept at skirting the regulations. Rather than making direct weight-loss claims, they use product names—Mini Thins, Trim-Maxx, Super Fat Burners—that do more than hint. The Dietary Supplements Act also allows manufacturers to display "scientific literature" about the products alongside the bottles on the shelves. These booklets are often confusing, throwing around scientific terms that seem to suggest, without actually saying so, that a product will help you lose weight. One pamphlet for Garcinia-Max Diet System, for instance, states: "The search for safe means of supporting weight management without stimulants has now borne fruit. . . . Since 1965, Garcinia has been the focus of exciting new research examining lipogenesis—the metabolic processes by which fat and cholesterol are produced and stored in the body. The tart rind of its fruit is uniquely rich in hydroxycitrate—a nutritional factor that is especially relevant for people whose calorie consumption exceeds healthful levels." These claims are worded so that a consumer who reads that a product is "relevant" to overeating will come to the quick conclusion that it will make them lose weight.

The Federal Trade Commission is trying to crack down on the blatant weight-loss promises that many of these herbal diet products advertise. In March 1997 the FTC launched an "Operation Waistline" project to warn consumers that the billions a year we spend on "miracle" diet products is a complete waste of money. Most of these products, according to Richard Cleland, director of the FTC's weight-loss fraud division, contain herbs that are untested and unproven. Fraudulent diet companies typically promise to help consumers "blast off fat" and "lose thirty pounds in thirty days without dieting or exercise." In 1996, for instance, a Florida company called Slim America sold quantities of its Super Formula by mail, a product containing herbs that promised to "quickly evaporate virtually every ounce of visible fat from your waist, hips, thighs, and rear end so *lightning-bolt fast* you'll want to dash to the mirror every fifteen minutes to watch those ugly pounds magically disappear." Despite these rather flagrantly false promises, the company sold $10 million of its product before it was recently forced out of business by the FTC.

Joanne Ikeda, a University of California at Berkeley nutrition expert who testified in the case against Slim America, says such products are not only a scam but, more worrisome, they detract consumers from healthier ways of controlling their weight—making them that much fatter. "People figure a magic pill will take care of their problem, so they don't have to get outside and get some exercise," she says.

It's easy to blame the public for being gullible enough to buy diet products, forever willing to shell out money for a quick and easy cure in order to avoid the reality that losing weight is either impossible or requires major lifestyle changes. And it is true that several of the women who experienced serious side effects or died after taking these diet aids should have known the products were producing obvious negative side effects and stopped taking them. In most cases, people who have died taking these products have taken more than the amount recommended on the box. But with diet products, that goes with the territory. "Dieters think that if one pill or tea bag is going to make them thin, then ten will make them thinner," says Berg. In a weight-obsessed culture, where companies market diet products aggressively to exploit women's dissatisfaction with their looks, common sense sometimes loses out.

To complicate matters further, more physicians, including well-known obesity experts, have been willing to sell their credibility to back questionable diet products with promises that they'll work. At eleven o'clock at night, when you're home alone, miserable, and scraping the bottom of the ice-cream box, those medical promises, emotional appeals, and scientific claims can be difficult to resist—especially when help is only an 800 number away.

The media, rather than protecting their audience from diet scams by giving them well-researched information, sometimes end up promoting these frauds. Editors at fitness and women's magazines are constantly under pressure to come up with "news" about dieting to feed their readers' presumably insatiable appetites for weight-loss advice. Though some of these magazines are cautious and thorough in their approach to diet stories, others are quick to publicize any new diet remedy, no matter how questionable. A "diet breakthrough" is just too hard to resist, whether or not the diet aid du jour—chromium, amino acids, protein diets, herbs—has actually been tested by anyone but the promoter.

Some writers are paid by the product companies to place promotional articles in magazines. Some magazines will excerpt articles from books written by diet product promoters; the authors, who may be physicians or Ph.D.'s, are described as "experts" on dieting or nutrition, rather than as people who have a business interest in selling more of their product. More often, writers and editors resort to press-release journalism, relying only on the information and experts described in a publicity sheet to write a story. The press release may sound scientific, or even come from a university; the "experts," however, may have some financial interest at stake or may be exaggerating the importance of their study or discovery in order to inflate their reputations in the scientific community.

Even magazines that have the reputation—and resources—for doing decent health reporting occasionally engage in lazy promotional pieces about diet products. *Self* magazine, for instance, trumpeted a "Diet and Fitness Breakthrough!" on its cover in October 1994, proclaiming: "New protein superdrinks let you lose weight and add muscle." Inside, the writer Harry Hurt III allowed Dr. A. Scott Connelly, the inventor of "MET-Rx," which generated some $90 million in sales that year, to make exaggerated promises about his product for several pages. MET-Rx is one of many meal-replacement drinks that contain vitamins and amino acids (the building blocks of protein in the body) and claim to burn fat. The company typically places full-page ads in newspapers with headlines such as "Amazing Weight-Loss Story!! Medical Doctor's New 'Miracle' Engineered Food Transforms Colorado Man from 327 Pound Doughboy—Into Lean Powerful Athlete!"

Self's article was nearly as promotional as this breathless ad copy. "It is the brainchild of an honest-to-God physician, whose scientific research dates back some 20 years." We never get to look at any of Connelly's research up close, however, nor do we encounter any studies by anyone else—least of all someone who has published something in a respected medical journal—that might back up his claims. Hurt passes along Connelly's confusedly pseudo-scientific explanation that MET-Rx helps you lose fat and add lean muscle mass through something called "nutrient partitioning." How does that work? one wonders. "Exactly how this partitioning takes place, it turns out, is a trade secret," Hurt says, "but it has something to do with specifically engineered amino acids that are added to the mix." Ah-ha.

After three-quarters of the article (illustrated with photos of celebrities, including Clint Eastwood, Cher, and Sylvester Stallone, who apparently swear by the stuff), Hurt throws in a few obligatory nay-saying quotes to add "balance." But we get no dietitians who might wonder about the physical and psychological effects of abstaining from real food. We get nobody from the FDA or FTC to comment on the advertising claims. We get no researchers who have studied amino acids but have no financial interest in the product. (One physiologist I called who has studied supplements and metabolism, Hank Lukaski at the U.S. Department of Agriculture Human Nutrition Research Center, told me, "There is no evidence that amino acid supplements have any beneficial effect on weight loss.")

In the conclusion, all we get is Connelly telling us, once again, that his stuff works and is safe. "Will it actually produce the kinds of results it claims, and is it worth your trouble to give it a try? The answer depends in part on the strength of your commitment and your capacity to handle the costs." As with most diet products, the writer is telling us, if it fails, it's the fault of the buyer's "commitment," or, just as humiliating, their inadequate funds. Finally, Hunt sums up this publicityfest with words from a "satisfied MET-Rx user": "It's 'a whole lot less expensive than buying a whole bunch of food and vitamins.' " Talk about empty calories.

It's hard to go through a week without being assaulted with a barrage of bad information about diet aids. But if any of these products really worked, wouldn't we have read about them in, say, the *Journal of the American Medical Association*? Wouldn't we know friends who had lost weight that way? Yet people keep buying these products, and blaming themselves when they fail to help them lose weight. Bogus diet-product companies are making millions exploiting women's poor body images with empty promises that they'll look and feel better.

When the remedies fail, consumers invariably end up feeling worse about themselves.

But it's difficult to get consumers to stop buying these products—even when they suspect they won't work. "You're buying a fantasy," says Jeffrey Sobal, a nutritional sociologist at Cornell University. "I might buy a lottery ticket for the daydreams about being a millionaire, and others buy diet products to dream of being thin." Consumers may also be tempted by the products in order to prove they're at least doing something about their extra pounds. "You're telling the world you want to lose weight and you're trying," Sobal says. "It may be worth $39.95 to get somebody off your back."

Pink Lemonade, Poison, and Liquid Protein

Diet fraud has a long history in the United States, full of colorful American character types: confidence men, hucksters, shady doctors, and fly-by-night entrepreneurs. People have been peddling phony weight-loss elixirs since before the turn of the century. No sooner had fashion declared that women should be thin than advertisements appeared in magazines proclaiming quick weight-loss cures. "Weigh what you should weigh!" advised one 1896 ad for a diet remedy. "Get Rid of Fat!" Some of the early promoters, uncertain whether losing weight was necessarily going to be very popular for long, hedged their bets by advertising that their products would either help you add weight or reduce, depending on what you needed.

A few of the early diet preparations were quite dangerous, especially Marmola, Corpulin, and Kellogg's "Safe Fat Reducer," which contained thyroid. Physicians, too, prescribed thyroid, a drug derived from animal glands that can stoke the body's furnace so high it starts to burn up vital organs. Woods Hutchinson wrote in 1894 that doctors didn't have any idea how thyroid, often prescribed with potassium (and sometimes aresenic), worked. "Both cause, in some curious manner which we do not as yet understand, such an interference with the normal metabolism of the body as to cause the burning up and elimination of considerable amounts of body fat." But, he noted, if patients lost more than 10 percent of their body weight—the "movable ten percent," he called it—the results would be injurious. "The appetite becomes impaired, the sleep broken, and the heart's action irregular." If prolonged, the drug would set up a "serious and obstinate disturbance of the nervous system, and particularly of the nerves controlling the heart, accompanied by palpitation, sweating, weakness, and intense nervousness."[2]

Other early diet preparations contained strong laxatives or purgatives, or arsenic and strychnine. Most, however, consisted of simple washing soda, Epsom salts, or other innocuous ingredients. By 1914, *Good Housekeeping* printed an exposé on obesity cures entitled "Swindled Getting Slim," by Harvey Wiley and Anne Lewis Pierce, which could have been written today. "As the rage for slimness grows apace, with apparently no limit in sight, the number, audacity, and unadulterated foolishness of the alleged obesity-cures and flesh-reducers keeps step with the demand," they wrote. "Some are merely picturesque and amusing; some are dangerous; all are misleading, and no little ingenuity is shown in presenting simple old-time frauds under new names and new auspices, with marvelous scientific explanations as to how they work, and new assurances of harmlessness and effectiveness."[3]

Wiley and Pierce described the techniques—some of which are still used today—that diet hucksters used to sell their products and to escape the scrutiny of regulatory agencies. A few products, such as Manhattanite Jean Downs's "Get Slim," which contained pink lemonade, were outright fraud. Others, such as Berledet tablets, claimed their product "makes you thin without dieting," with the caveat in small print that the user should avoid all fatty foods and take long walks every day. Others again took a multifaceted approach to weight loss, such as Marjorie Hamilton's "Quadruple Combination," which combined recommendations for enemas, long walks, exercise, no liquids at meals, and no white bread, pastry, or potatoes with instructions on daily use of the diet powder, which turned out to be ordinary bath powder (you bathed in it, rather than ate it).

A few diet remedies contained some of the same herbs used in contemporary herbal formulas such as Herbalife. In 1921, for instance, the American Medical Association's compendium *Nostrums and Quackery* listed bladderwrack, kelp, and pokeberry as common ingredients in obesity cures. "There seems to be no explanation for the popularity of this species of seaweed as a remedy for obesity," the authors wrote of bladderwrack. "In fact, it is said that this particular seaweed is used in some localities as a food for hogs in the belief that it makes the animals fat!"[4]

Diet quacks used the mail to sell obesity cures, moving from state to state after being indicted for fraud, or simply changing the name of their cure to launch a new ad campaign. One particularly enterprising man, Walter Cunningham, purveyor of Marjorie Hamilton's Obesity Cure, frequently changed his state, obesity remedy, and wives. After having been jailed in Minneapolis for fraudulent real estate deals in 1906, Cunningham moved to New York, where he sold mail-order beauty creams under his wife's name. In 1909, he transferred to Chicago, sold the Evelyn Cunningham bust-developer and wrinkle-eradicator, then, after some legal trouble, changed the name of the products to "Della Carson." In 1911, he divorced his wife, married Marjorie Hamilton, and sold the Marjorie Hamilton mail-order fat reducer. When that received bad publicity, he promoted the Texas Guinan fat reducer. In the testimonial ads, Texas Guinan distinguished her product from previous "frauds," which the public never knew were sold by the same company. "It is not like the Marjorie Hamilton treatment—as absolutely different as day from night," Guinan proclaimed.

As they do today, turn-of-the-century diet aid promoters took advantage of the frustration people felt toward the medical establishment for failing to come up with an effective treatment for obesity. Actress-turned-diet promoter Texas Guinan ("I was a sight in tights at 204 pounds!") and others ridiculed physicians' treatments in order to sell more of their own products. Guinan—whose cure, for $20, consisted of a solution of water, alcohol, and alum, along with the advice to take a hot tub twice a day, and avoid bread, potatoes, sweets, and starchy foods—described how she squandered her money "trying the various fat-reducing treatments so heavily advertised by charlatans of the American Medical Association." Like diet guru Susan Powter today, who rails against "the boys at the AMA" for conspiring to harm women, Guinan didn't mince words about doctors to would-be weight reducers. "Tell the quack AMA doctors and specialists to go hang," she advised her followers.

Many of those quack doctors were busy selling their own, often more dangerous diet cures. One of the early ones was dinitrophenol, the first synthetic drug used for weight reduction. During World

War I, observers noted that fat men who worked in munitions plants and came into contact with the chemical lost a substantial amount of weight. After the war, physicians lost no time in prescribing it to dieters. Dinitrophenol, which is still used as a powerful insecticide and herbicide, is a metabolic poison that is toxic to all forms of higher life.[5] In humans, it speeds up the metabolic rate until eventually the body burns itself up.[6] By 1935, over 100,000 Americans had taken this drug, advertised in newspapers and magazines as a "new and safe way to lose weight." It wasn't long before severe side effects and fatalities were reported. Twelve women in the San Francisco Bay Area had been temporarily blinded by the drug, prompting the dean of Stanford University's Medical School to condemn its use. One physician who experimented with a large dose of dinitrophenol was, as Carl Malmberg put it, "literally cooked to death." By 1938, dinitrophenol had largely been discarded because of its ill effects, and the AMA announced it would withhold its approval of the drug.[7]

Another strange obesity cure that was popular among physicians for a time was human chorionic gonadotropin (HCG), a type of growth hormone that was injected into patients. This treatment became popular in 1957, when *Harper's Bazaar* printed a diet—"Slimming: A Roman Doctor's Treatment"—that consisted of five hundred calories a day for up to forty days, plus daily hormone injections. In the article, A. T. W. Simeons, a British endocrinologist, claimed his patients weren't hungry as long as they took shots of HCG, which is produced by the placenta and derived from the urine of pregnant women (variations on this treatment used the urine of pregnant rabbits and mares). It's the very hormone, in fact, that turns the stick blue on a home pregnancy test.

Human chorionic gonadotropin was legitimately used at the time to treat a condition called Fröhlich's syndrome, a hormonal imbalance that affects young boys, disturbing their sexual development, appetite, and sleep, and causing them to accumulate fat on the hips, buttocks, and thighs. Simeons reasoned that if the drug worked to melt away the fat on those boys with a rare genetic disorder, then, hey, it ought to do the same thing on normal, healthy women. The hormone, he wrote, would cause a "normal distribution" of fat on the body and would correct a "basic disorder in the brain." His diet book—*Pounds and Inches: A New Approach to Obesity*—included other gems of pseudo-medical advice, warning readers to eat no breakfast whatsoever, except for coffee, and to abstain from using any cosmetics or lotion on the body because it will be absorbed and added to the existing fat deposits *in* the body.

Simeons's treatment became all the rage; for a time, it was the most widespread medication given in the United States to lose weight, and was the main treatment used in eighty Weight Reduction Medical Clinics in California. Unfortunately, it didn't work: none of the mainly female patients seeking treatment, it turned out, was suffering from Fröhlich's syndrome. The medical establishment only started to become suspicious of the drug when reports surfaced that part-time doctors were being offered as much as $100,000 a year by weight-loss clinics to spend one afternoon a week sitting and writing pads of prescriptions for the drug.[8]

In 1962, the *Journal of the American Medical Association* warned against the Simeons diet, saying, "continued adherence to such a drastic regimen is potentially more hazardous to the patient's health than continued obesity." In 1974, the Food and Drug Administration required producers of HCG to label the drug with a warning against using it for weight loss or fat redistribution. The Task Force on the Treatment of Obesity in Canada warned that use of the hormone "touches on possible malpractice." Nevertheless, a few diet doctors continued with the treatment—it is legal, after all, for physicians to prescribe medications for purposes that are not approved by the FDA—often handing the patients the drugs and injection equipment so they could administer it themselves.[9]

In 1981, a physician and an entrepreneur joined forces for one of the most dangerous diet schemes ever: the Cambridge Diet. Jack Feather, who originated the idea, was a Walter Cunningham type who built a fortune in the 1960s with his wife Elaine selling women the bodies they wanted to have. They peddled figure salons, Mark Eden bust-developers, Trim-Jeans, the Sauna Belt, and then in the 1980s, the Cambridge Diet. In the 1960s and 1970s, romance and true story magazines were filled with Feather's fabulous promises for his products: "Astro-Trimmer—the most astounding waist and tummy reducer of all time!" Many featured lovely young women with enormous breasts, who swore their bustlines were the result not of nature or silicone, but a handheld exercise contraption. "The very first time I used Mark II I saw my bust line become rounder and fuller and actually grow three full inches right before my eyes!" one testified. For fifteen years, while the Feathers increased the size and fullness of their bank accounts, the U.S. Postal Service battled with them to stop making outlandish claims. Finally, in 1981, they were indicted on thirteen counts of mail fraud, and made a deal with the government to pay $1.1 million and stop selling bust-developers, Astro-Trimmers, and other diet aids. But by that time, they were ready to move on to their biggest scam.

In 1979, Feather had come across a copy of the *International Journal of Obesity*, which described University of Cambridge nutrition researcher Alan Howard's work putting patients on very low, 320-calorie-a-day diets. Feather decided he wanted to add a diet to his line of figure-enhancing products, and made a deal with Howard to put the diet on the market.[10] By this time, the very-low-calorie diet had already proven itself to be disastrous, since fifty-eight people had died after being put on the commercial liquid diets that were popular in 1976 and 1977.[11] The amount of protein in these drinks was insufficient to keep the body from feeding on its own stores of protein, including lean muscle tissue and vital organs. The Cambridge Diet, however, advertised that it was "the perfect food," and "provides you with scientifically balanced nutrition"; these claims were backed by assurances from Dr. Howard, who was hardly an unbiased scientific observer but continued to defend the product in scientific journals without revealing he'd been paid for his services.[12] It took journal articles by other well-known obesity researchers to bring to light the fact that even Howard's own research showed that the extreme diet burned up the body's muscles and organs.

After two months, the U.S. Postal Service and the FDA forced Feather to stop mail-order sales from ads that claimed that the Cambridge Diet would produce "no harmful side effects," was "metabolically balanced," and that people could stay on the formula for an "unlimited amount of time." Feather stopped selling the product through the mail, and instead created the kind of wildly profitable multilevel marketing plan used today by Herbalife. The diet sold by word-of-mouth, with counselors who served as cheerleaders and spiritual advisers for their clients. The diet counselor who sold the liquid formula not only got a profit from each can sold to his own customers but a percentage of the sales of each counselor he recruited into the Cambridge "family."

This pyramid scheme was so successful that some counselors were earning more than $150,000 a month. Successful counselors-turned-executives were rewarded with BMWs, Mercedes-Benzes, solid gold pens, and glitzy, celebrity-ridden hotel extravaganzas. Eventually, more than 3 million people had tried the diet, which Feather marketed as "an Ultimate Truth." For some, it was the ultimate diet: thirty people died from heart attacks before the FDA forced the company to stop selling the nutritionally inadequate diet drinks.

The Cambridge Diet debacle shows just how dangerous weight-loss marketing schemes can be. The problem with most weight-loss products sold over the years is they don't work, except to make the promoter wealthy. The problem with the rest is that they *do* work, temporarily, by promoting unhealthy weight loss through starvation, as in the case of the Cambridge Diet, or by stimulating the nervous system, as in the cases of ephedrine and over-the-counter diet pills containing phenylpropanolamine (PPA), which causes unpleasant side effects such as dizziness and irritability, and can even lead to strokes and heart attacks. If money were the only thing people lost in diet scams, it would be serious enough. But many people have lost their good health or their lives. No matter what the claims, no obesity cures to date really work to help people lose weight permanently. At best, they only make your wallet thinner.

Disturbingly, even after many of these schemes have been proven ineffective or dangerous, they persist. Even the poisonous dinitrophenol made a comeback. In 1987, the Texas State Board of Medical Examiners tried to revoke the license of Dr. Nicholas Bachynsky, who owned a $10-million-a-year chain of diet and smoking-cessation clinics, for using dinitrophenol in his weight-loss treatments. Sold under the name "Mitcal," and advertised with the promise, "Never Be Fat Again," patients were charged $1,000 per treatment for the poison.

Bachynsky testified in a 1986 trial that he'd prescribed the drug to some fourteen thousand Texans. Jurors found Bachynsky guilty of using the toxic chemical on his patients, he was fined $86,000, and his medical license was revoked. State District Judge Juan Gallardo overturned that order, finding that the medical board's claim that dinitrophenol is "a chemical compound with no proven therapeutic value and usually has a number of harmful and dangerous side effects upon persons who take it" was "not supported by substantial evidence." Bachynsky went back to practicing medicine.

It wasn't until 1990 that the Texas State Board of Medical Examiners was successful in taking away the diet doctor's license, after he pleaded guilty to a $60 million insurance scam that put him in federal prison for a ten-year term. He's no longer injecting weedkiller into weight-loss patients, but only because he got caught for another reason—falsifying his patients' insurance claims.[13]

And human chorionic gonadotropin is still being peddled at conventions of diet doctors. In the exhibit hall at the American Society of Bariatric Physicians' Conference, I picked up a bottle of HCG and read the package insert. "HCG," it said, "has not been demonstrated to be effective adjunctive therapy in the treatment of obesity. There is no substantial evidence that it increases weight loss beyond that resulting from caloric restriction." I asked the vendor whether the physicians buy this for weight loss. He shrugged. "They buy it," he said. "It's up to them what they use it for."

Herbal Ephedrine

Pamela Bradley, a hazel-eyed Wisconsin woman who worked at a cheese factory, had been struggling for years to lose weight. In 1994, at five foot four and about 160 pounds, she wasn't obese, but her weight was still a constant source of concern to her. Her husband, she told her mother, frequently criticized her for being fat. She was worried about the marriage: If she just lost some weight, she thought, things might go more smoothly between them. Pamela dieted, and because she felt run-down from dieting, she took over-the-counter herbal diet pills to perk herself up.

On the morning of November 18, 1994, Pamela awoke complaining to her husband that she had chest pains and a gassy feeling in her stomach. She said she thought she'd be all right, and he went outside to work on the car. Pamela got up to take her morning shower, went into the bathroom, and turned on the faucets. Several minutes later, her husband noticed that the water had been running for what seemed like a long time. When he came inside, he found his thirty-year-old wife dead on the bathroom floor.

At first, newspapers reported that Pamela Bradley's death was mysterious. An autopsy revealed that she had died of heart failure. It wasn't until January 1995 that the toxicology report came back: "The deceased died from an overdose of diet pills containing ephedrine," the coroner concluded, "causing the heart to go into cardiac arrhythmia that would then go into cardiac arrest." Pamela Bradley had taken about six times the recommended dose of diet pills containing the herb ephedra. The herb contains an active ingredient, ephedra, which can, in large doses, cause the heart to go galloping out of rhythm. "Her heart," says Bradley's mother, June Joas, recalling how the coroner described the effects of ephedrine, "was wiggling like a bunch of worms."

Despite the fact that it is a potentially dangerous drug, ephedrine is the main active ingredient in many herbal diet remedies, including Herbal Phen-Fen, Herbalife's Thermojetics, Nature's Nutrition Formula One, Diet Max, and many others. Ephedrine comes from the Chinese herb *ma huang*, and is an amphetamine-like chemical that acts as a stimulant, particularly in combination with caffeine. It has been approved for use by the FDA as an asthma drug and a decongestant, and is used in prescription drugs for those conditions. It has also been sold over the counter as herbal recreational drugs, with names like "Herbal Ecstasy." In low doses ephedrine speeds up the body, causing restlessness, insomnia, and nervousness. In larger quantities it can drive up blood pressure, increase heart rate, and even cause seizures and strokes.

The FDA reports that there have been at least 18 deaths caused by ephedrine since 1994, and more than 800 complaints of adverse reactions to the drug, ranging from nervousness and headaches to myocardial infarction, cardiac arrhythmia, psychosis and seizures. "Deaths have occurred in first-time users," says one senior FDA official. "These were otherwise healthy people."

In 1997 the FDA issued proposed guidelines to limit the amount of the drug per capsule to eight milligrams, and to limit the maximum recommended intake to 24 milligrams per day. The guidelines were, in fact, the FDA's first regulatory initiative under the 1994 Dietary Supplements Act. The agency also proposed barring ephedrine from being combined with other stimulants, such as guarana and other sources of caffeine. The regulations would prohibit manufacturers from promoting the use of ephedrine for more than a week, meaning they effectively couldn't make promises that the drug would, in such a short time, help people shed pounds and build muscles. Despite the modesty of these proposals—and the stacks of evidence the FDA amassed about the adverse effects of the drug—the agency received over 30,000 responses to the initiative, mostly from herbal manufacturers who wanted the drug to continue to be completely unregulated.

Even if the regulations pass, ephedrine will still be available over the counter to anyone who wants it, and the likelihood is that there will continue to be many adverse effects. The irony is that while ephedrine may help people lose a little weight in the short term, as with every other diet drug, the weight comes right back in the long run. "The only way ephedrine might work is by causing your hand to become so jittery you can't get food to your mouth," says Varro Tyler.

At least, if the new regulations pass, consumers will have been warned that the drug can have serious side effects, instead of assuming that anything they buy in a health food store is perfectly healthy. In 1995, for instance, Vivien Harrison, a 52-year-old elementary school teacher, took three tablets of an herbal product called Stim and Trim, which was supposed to give her a little extra energy for a better work-out and help her lose a few pounds. An active and average-sized woman, Harrison had been taking the product for less than a month—and she took fewer than the number of pills recommended on the label. She went out to run errands with a friend, and began feeling headachy and woozy, as if she were coming down with a cold or flu, then felt an intensely tight constriction in her chest.

In the emergency room, doctors told Harrison that her blood pressure—which had always been normal—was soaring dangerously high. In fact, they found, Harrison had suffered a heart attack. The doctors were puzzled: An angiogram revealed that Harrison's arteries not only weren't blocked, they were slick as Teflon. She was in excellent physical condition. Only one thing explained why her blood pressure had shot up to the point that her heart went into a spasm: The herbal weight-loss pills she'd taken, which contained ephedra.

Harrison, who bought the product in a regular drugstore, had no idea it was anything but perfectly safe. "There was no warning on the bottle that would make a healthy person cautious," she says. "You don't think that something on the shelf, available to all ages, could be so dangerous. But what I've found out is that in the supplements industry, there's absolutely no regulation." Two years later, Harrison was back to being active, but her heart is permanently damaged.

These days she never knows how hard she can push herself physically, and is always afraid that she may be on the verge of another attack. "It puts you in a state of constant fear."

Dieter's Tea

Christopher Grell, a San Francisco lawyer, remembers everything about that quiet evening at home in July 1991. His wife June, a thirty-seven-year-old blond woman with a big smile, had put their twenty-one-month-old son to bed and sat down for her usual cup of tea. Grell noticed that she drank her tea strong that evening, using two bags of Laci Le Beau Super Dieter's Tea that she'd bought at the health-food store. After reading for a while, they went upstairs, turned out the lights, and kissed each other good-night.

In the morning, Grell got up early, played outside with his son, and then went upstairs to wake June for breakfast. Grell called her, then nudged her, then shook her hard. June didn't move. In a daze, he put his son in the crib and called 911. By the time the paramedics arrived, he knew his wife was dead.

The coroner had no explanation for why June Grell's heart had suddenly stopped; she was a healthy woman with no history of cardiac problems. Grell asked him if June's death could have had something to do with the tea she drank that evening. He said he didn't know.

For more than a year, anguished and depressed, Grell did nothing. Then he wrote to the manufacturer of the dieter's tea—Nutrition Products in Fresno, California—to find out whether it might have contained any ingredients that could have contributed to his wife's death. A lawyer wrote back: "Laci Le Beau Super Dieter's Tea is not a drug, it is a food beverage . . . none of the herbs in the tea are known to be deleterious to health."

Grell wasn't so sure. He read the list of herbs printed on the box, consulted several books about herbal remedies, and found out that the tea contained senna, a potent laxative, along with uva ursi, a diuretic. He wrote to the Food and Drug Administration to find out whether anyone else had experienced problems with herbal dieter's teas, which are made by several companies. He eventually received a stack of complaints about adverse reactions, including cramps, nausea, heart palpitations, and severe diarrhea. There was also one other death.

Grell, a products liability attorney, is now convinced that overuse of Laci Le Beau Super Dieter's Tea caused his wife's death, as well as the heart-rhythm disturbances that led to the deaths of three other young women since then. He is suing the manufacturer and distributors of the tea, and is on a campaign to warn consumers against other herbal diet products. "People believe that whatever they buy in a health store is going to be healthy," Grell says. "As long as it says 'natural,' they think it's fine to take."

The box of lemon mint Super Dieter's Tea June Grell bought, for instance, said only that it contained "all natural herbs," based on an "ancient Chinese formula." The directions suggested that users "start with a small amount . . . and gradually increase the amount to fit your needs. . . . If the tea is too strong, dilute with a little more water until you feel comfortable with it." While the label cautioned users, "for best tasting tea, never over-steep," there is no indication that the tea contains a laxative that can cause diarrhea, cramping, and with long-term use, problems with the colon and even the heart.

Even very careful label readers can't tell what's in the product. "I read labels from top to bottom," says Randi Fine, an Owings Mills, Maryland, mother of two who quit using a dieter's tea after she experienced heart palpitations. "I even picked up an herb book at the health-food store to try to figure out what was in that tea." But on the box she purchased, the laxative senna was identified by its lesser-known names, locust plant and Cassia, neither of which Fine could find in her sourcebook. "Unless you know what a product has in it, how can you be sure you're using it safely?" she asks.

Dieters are particularly vulnerable to the side effects of laxatives like senna. Used for long periods, senna can flush important minerals called electrolytes out of the body; among these is potassium, which sends electrical signals to the heart and keeps it beating normally. It's easy to get enough potassium in your diet—the mineral is found in abundance in potatoes, winter squash, bananas, and orange juice, for instance. But laxatives prevent potassium from being absorbed by the body. And when a person is on a strict diet or has bulimia and is losing fluids through purging, consuming senna can make an already unhealthy situation much worse. "Dieters don't always know how badly they've put their body out of whack," says Olga Woo, a pharmacist and poison-control expert in San Francisco. "Senna is a very strong laxative. In a small percentage of people, it pushes them over the edge. They can get depleted of potassium, and that causes the heart to beat irregularly. Sometimes the messages to the heart get confused and the heart stops."

People who use senna can also become addicted to its laxative effects. George Triadafilopoulos, a gastroenterologist at Stanford University, has several female patients who used dieter's teas and who now have chronic constipation. "No one should take this on a regular basis," he says. "It should be clear on the label that this can cause long-term problems."

Frederick Stine, the chief executive officer of Nutrition Products, which makes Laci Le Beau Super Dieter's Tea, denies that the company's product is dangerous in any way. Stine points out that senna is approved by the FDA as a food flavoring at levels below 12 milligrams per serving. "We make sure our levels are far below the levels that constitute a laxative effect," he says. "It's just a flavor."

But internal reports of tests conducted by the California Food and Drug Branch of the Department of Health and Human Services (DHS)—which has been investigating complaints against the tea for the past ten years—show that the senna in any given cup of dieter's tea can be much higher than the FDA-approved level, depending on how the drink is prepared. When testers allowed dieter's tea to steep for two minutes, the drink contained as much senna as an over-the-counter laxative. Labels on over-the-counter laxatives warn buyers not to use the product for more than a week, but, notes the California DHS memo, "Consumers have no way of knowing that long-term ingestion of sennosides in the quantities found in [dieter's tea] may put them at increased risk of life-threatening cardiac arrhythmias and loss of normal bowel function."

Because of the deaths in the dieter's tea cases, an FDA advisory committee recommended in August 1995 that a number of herbal diet aids—including Super Dieter's Tea, Trim-Maxx, 24-Hour Diet Tea, and Ultra Slim Tea—and others carry a warning cautioning consumers that the products contain laxatives; can cause adverse effects; do not significantly reduce the absorption of food calories; and can lead, in chronic cases, to serious injury or death.

Regulatory officials say consumers must share some blame; they note that people with eating disorders typically abuse these products and keep their behavior secret. "The point of view of many people in the agencies is that if a woman taking an herbal product starts to experience a laxative effect, why does she continue?" says Stuart Richardson, chief of the California Food and Drug Branch. "There are all kinds of products out there that are being abused," he adds. "You can't eliminate them all." At the FDA, a senior official says, "The women who died after taking herbal diet aids were young and very concerned about their weight. The pressures to get thin, and to do it by shortcuts, may be a major factor in these deaths. We can't regulate that issue."

But dieter's teas and herbal diet pills are marketed, by their names, to dieters—the very people who may have obsessions with weight, as well as dangerously low electrolyte levels. The companies are targeting the very people who are most vulnerable to overusing the product.

Betty Helphrey wishes that her daughter, Debbie, had known more about the risks posed by herbal products. The twenty-year-old Florida college sophomore died suddenly after drinking a dieter's tea every night for several months. Her mother still sees the tea on sale at her neighborhood mall. "If you're twenty years old, and you buy something in the health-food store," Helphrey asks, "how are you supposed to know it's going to hurt you?"

Over-the-Counter Diet Pills: PPA

Phenylpropanolamine, or PPA, is the most widely used—and abused—diet pill available without a prescription. The drug, a stimulant and appetite suppressant that is a close chemical cousin to amphetamines, can raise the blood pressure and cause anxiety, nervousness, and other jittery side effects. In rare cases, even with only one dose, PPA can send the blood pressure soaring dangerously high, and cause a stroke. Because of its speedy side effects and potential risks—and because it has not been proven to have long-term effects in helping people lose weight—95 percent of the developed nations in the world have banned PPA as a diet aid.

In the United States, PPA can be found in nearly every supermarket and drugstore under such names as "Dexatrim," "Acutrim,"

"Thinz," and "Appedrine." PPA is also a common ingredient in cold medications, including Contac and Dimetapp. If you've ever stayed wide awake at night after taking medicine for the sniffles, it's probably because what you took had PPA in it. The companies that sell PPA as a diet pill—the giant of the bunch is Thompson Medical, which also makes Slim-Fast—spend $40 million a year advertising their products, and bring in at least $200 million a year from sales.[14] American consumers take 6 billion doses of products containing PPA per year. And nearly every year, a few of them have severe reactions to the drug.

Unlike dieter's tea, packages of diet pills do contain warnings. In small type, the consumer is warned not to take more than one caplet per day, and not to take the pills at all if you are being treated for depression, an eating disorder, or have heart disease, thyroid, high blood pressure, or any other medical problems. In much larger type, however, there's a more compelling message, especially to women who might be depressed or have eating disorders: "You and Dexatrim . . . A Successful Team for a Slim and Trim Figure." The Dexatrim label tells consumers "How to lose weight fast and keep it off," and suggests that once you've reached your goal, you should weigh yourself every day, and if you gain a pound or two, just go back to taking Dexatrim.

The FDA began investigating PPA in 1972. Despite many reports of adverse reactions and deaths, particularly among young women who were obsessed with losing weight, the agency has yet to reach a decision on whether the product is safe. Ron Wyden, the senator from Oregon, has been trying to get the FDA to regulate PPA for several years. "What you have is a situation where young women will pop into some pharmacy or store, buy a fistful of these products, and suffer some serious health consequences," he says. Wyden has asked the FDA to at least put the pills behind the counter, where they'd have to be requested and pharmacists could describe the dangers, and to stop selling them to minors. But he's gotten nowhere with his efforts, and sounds exasperated. "There's tremendous lobbying by the pharmaceutical industry," he says.

Wyden began his efforts to get PPA regulated in 1990, when he first held congressional hearings on diet pills. During those hearings, one expert after another stepped up to testify to the potential dangers of PPA. Thaddeus Prout, M.D., an associate professor of medicine at

Johns Hopkins University School of Medicine who had been on a committee that evaluated diet drugs for the FDA in 1970, said, "I defy anyone to find another medication that has had so many misadventures so often reported." Prout said that there was no reason the drug shouldn't be put behind the counter, if not taken off the market. He pointed out that the diet pills don't even work: like other appetite suppressants, they can stop people from feeling hungry for a few weeks, but long-term studies prove they have no lasting effect in keeping weight off. Most of the studies presented to the FDA that showed that PPA was safe and effective, he said, were poorly done and paid for by the diet industry.

Another witness, who is a physician and public health specialist, Paul Raford, testified that records from the American Association of Poison Control Centers showed that pill for pill, more adverse reactions were reported from people who had used PPA than any other over-the-counter drug. In 1989, 47,000 people called their poison-control centers to complain that they had experienced side effects to diet pills that were serious enough to require a hospital stay or medical care. Several studies on the drug, said Dr. Raford, show that in 10 to 27 percent of users, their blood pressure rises 20 to 40 points.

Vivian Meehan, the president and founder of the National Association of Anorexia Nervosa and Associated Disorders, told the subcommittee that teenaged dieters and girls with eating disorders frequently abuse diet pills, sometimes taking three to five times the recommended dose. In the previous six years, she reported, there had been eleven cases of young patients who had suffered cerebral hemorrhage and inflammation of the blood vessels after taking PPA. The medical journal *Pediatrics* had listed numerous other side effects reported in young people, including seizures, hallucinations, headaches, confusion, mental disturbances, hypertension, cardiac irregularities, anxiety, paranoia, and mania. Meehan asked the committee to put PPA drugs behind the counter, and make them available only by prescription to minors.

University of Michigan researcher Lawrence Krupka described a study he conducted of 2,400 undergraduates, in which he found that 45 percent of the women and 6 percent of the men had tried diet pills. Nearly one-fifth of them started using the products before they were sixteen, and none had talked to a physician before taking the pills.

A twenty-year-old college junior, Jessica McDonald, told the subcommittee how she had taken diet pills when she suffered from anorexia nervosa and bulimia between the ages of twelve and seventeen. "I wanted to lose weight, and I wanted to lose weight fast," she said. "If I could lose weight with one pill, I could lose weight by taking more pills. I would take the whole bottle—eighteen to twenty at a time." The pills made her feel terrible, she said. "I would get weak, dizzy, nauseous, and, on more than one occasion, I even passed out." She asked the subcommittee to regulate the sale of diet pills to minors, the way alcohol or cigarettes are regulated. "Having diet pills open and so easily available just adds focus to the obsessions many Americans already have with dieting," she said.

Tony and Diana Smith told the committee how their daughter Noelle, who had been struggling with eating disorders since the age of fourteen, had died of cardiac arrest in 1989 at twenty. Noelle, a swimmer and gymnast who had worried about being fat since she was ten years old, used diet pills, laxatives, and diuretics, as well as obsessive exercise and self-induced vomiting to lose weight. The Smiths read out portions of a letter that a friend of Noelle's, whom she had met at an eating disorders hospital, had sent them. "She once told me that her use of diet pills had accelerated to as many as eight to ten boxes a week," the young woman wrote. She described how Noelle had complained of not being able to concentrate, and of feeling nervous and irritable. "I believe that the availability and the easy access to diet pills, laxatives, diuretics, and Ipecac was a major contributing factor to her eating disorder which led to her tragic and untimely death."[15]

Despite this testimony, the FDA refused to change the status of the over-the-counter pills, even to make them unavailable to minors. For the next few years, Ron Wyden made repeated requests to the FDA to speed its investigation. In May 1993, Donna Shalala, Secretary of Health and Human Services, wrote Wyden a letter to say that "FDA has not side-stepped a final determination regarding the status of this drug." The agency had determined that PPA is effective as a weight-control agent, but only, she said, "when used in conjunction with exercise, behavior modification, and an appropriate weight loss diet." Under those conditions, in other words, it is just as effective a weight-control agent as pink lemonade. As to the potential safety problem of increased risk of stroke, Shalala said that "remains to be resolved." In the meantime, nothing would change. "The agency does not believe ... that there is a basis for removing PPA from the marketplace while this additional information is being collected." Apparently, the industry, and its lobbyists, don't think so, either.

In 1994, the FDA issued a statement that it was working with the Nonprescription Drug Manufacturers' Association—an organization of pharmaceutical companies, including ones that manufacture PPA, and hardly an unbiased group on this matter—to come up with a study to investigate the link between PPA and stroke. The agency said that if the study, which involves two thousand people, shows there's a documented risk of stroke, the FDA will pull PPA products from the shelves and make them available only by prescription.

While the FDA continues its investigation, people who believe the labels on diet pills—"Safe, effective weight loss," "Lose weight fast"— continue to take them. And rare, but tragic, side effects continue to crop up. On May 27, 1992, Tracie Vandivere, a single mother from Amarillo, Texas, took three "Go Power" diet pills, which was two more than the recommended dose. Only a few hours later, Vandivere suffered a stroke. At the age of twenty-one, she was left mute, quadriplegic, and in need of round-the-clock care for the rest of her life.[16]

Despite terrible stories like this, diet pill manufacturers contrive to maintain that their products are safe and effective. They say that the fact that teenagers—who are under constant pressure from advertisements, parents, and peers to be thinner—are vulnerable to abusing diet pills is no reason to put them behind the counter. "People with eating disorders are abusing anything they can get their hands on," says Alison Mann, product manager for Thompson Medical's Dexatrim. "These people have psychological problems, and taking an over-the-counter diet aid away from the majority of people who can use it rationally is not fair to the rest of America."

Again, these are the very people the company is marketing the products to—people who are obsessed with their weight and are likely to try too much of anything to get thin. No matter what the price in terms of young women's lives, it seems that drug companies and the FDA don't think it's fair to take millions of dollars in sales away from companies that profit from—and encourage—Americans' irrational weight obsessions by pushing over-the-counter speed.

Chromium and Other Supplements

One of the hottest weight-loss supplements sold today is called chromium picolinate. It's sold in supplements, shakes, and nutrition bars, in health-food stores and through magazines, with labels and ads promising that it will increase lean muscle tissue, burn fat, and give you a higher metabolic rate. Americans seem to be believing the hype: 9 million took chromium supplements in 1995.[17]

What is this miracle mineral? Like many other essential nutrients, including carnitine, arginine, ornithine, and other amino acids that are touted as "fat-burners," a little chromium is necessary for proper metabolism, but more than a little goes to waste. Chromium plays a role in the way food is burned in the body, and helps insulin do its job of making sugar in the blood available to the cells for fuel. Receptors that live on the surface of cells are responsible for bringing sugar and protein inside the cell walls, and chromium helps increase the number of those receptors.[18] No one really knows exactly how much chromium people need—the National Academy of Sciences has proposed 50 to 200 micrograms a day, and some surveys have suggested that most Americans get less than 50 micrograms a day—but there are very few documented cases of chromium deficiency in the medical literature, and most of them are among elderly people who don't get enough to eat.

Chromium can be found in a smorgasbord of foods: broccoli, brewer's yeast, ham, beer, black pepper, mushrooms, shrimp, potatoes, peanut butter, fortified cereals, whole grains, drinking water, and anything cooked in a stainless-steel pan. Nevertheless, promoters of chromium picolinate suggest that no one gets enough of the mineral; if they did, their metabolism would increase, and they'd lose weight. The logic here is that if a little chromium helps burn fats and sugars, then a lot of chromium will burn them faster and faster.

Chromium tablets are being advertised in many fitness, body-building, and health magazines with some rather extraordinary claims. In one typical ad, featuring a super-fit woman in a bikini leaping in the sand, Chroma Slim promises it is a . . . "new advanced approach to weight loss, clinically proven to help you lose weight naturally." The ad maintains that Chroma Slim contains "clinically-proven thermogenic ingredients that help keep the weight off while promoting a trimmer, firmer, leaner body." Other products make even more inflated claims: "Melts the fat away," and "Plays a key role in reducing fat through better appetite control." Nutrition 21, which owns the patent to chromium picolinate and has sold the mineral to several manufacturers, has an ad featuring two bodybuilders with the headline, "Lose the Fat; Keep the muscle." The ad bases its claims on scientific research: "Studies show that 200–400 micrograms of chromium daily, as Chromium Picolinate, results in significant fat loss while muscle tissue is maintained or even increased."

The studies this last ad mentions were done by Gary Evans, a chemist at Bemidji State University in Bemidji, Minnesota, who formerly worked for the USDA. Prior to 1988, no one paid much attention to chromium. Its important role in nutrition was only noticed when patients who were being fed intravenously, with a solution that didn't contain chromium, began to have problems metabolizing sugar. Physicians then found that some diabetics were able to tolerate sugar better when they were given some chromium.

Evans promoted the idea that chromium supplements may be useful to people who aren't diabetic. In a 1991 study involving forty-one college athletes, he showed that those who received a 200-microgram dose of chromium—the amount in most supplements—had increases in muscle mass above and beyond those who didn't get the supplement. Those who took chromium also reduced the percentage of fat on their bodies.[19] Evans patented the idea of dietary supplements with chromium picolinate and other trace metals, and the USDA leased the exclusive rights to the patent to Nutrition 21, a San Diego–based company.

Nutrition 21 and Evans quickly began promoting the mineral as a fat-burner and muscle-builder. In 1990, Jeffrey Fisher, a physician and pharmaceutical company consultant, encouraged sales of the supplement with his diet book, *The Chromium Program*, in which he claimed that chromium might not only be helpful in controlling blood sugar and increasing lean muscle mass, but might even slow down the aging process. Fisher spread the news, based on a very loose estimate, that 90 percent of Americans are deficient in chromium. Women's and fitness magazines picked up on the story, quoting Evans and Fisher; *Cosmopolitan* wondered if at long last the "miracle mineral" had arrived.[20] Consumers, particularly bodybuilders and dieters, began buying quantities of chromium picolinate. Many are taking several times the dose recommended. In 1994, Nutrition 21's chairman Jim Bie reported that the retail sales of the supplement had reached $100 million.[21]

Meanwhile, several less dramatic studies on the trace mineral were ignored, mainly because they showed that the chromium claims are hugely exaggerated. Though researchers know that the body needs chromium, and that a deficiency can decrease the body's ability to use sugar properly, there is no strong evidence that supplements can help you burn fat more quickly or increase muscle. Once the body gets the chromium it needs, it seems it has no use for the excess, and discards it.

Three studies have shown that chromium has no beneficial effects. In one study of football players undergoing intensive weightlifting training, there was no difference in either body composition or strength between those who took the chromium supplements and those who didn't. The only difference between the two groups was that the men who took the chromium had five times as much chromium in their urine as the others. In a study at the U.S. Department of Agriculture Human Nutrition Research Center—where Evans did his original research—Hank Lukaski and his colleagues put thirty-five men through a rigorous weight-training program for eight weeks. "We were unable to find any significant effect of chromium in gain of muscle mass or loss of body fat," says Lukaski. It's likely, he adds, that chromium supplements can't hurt you—the toxic dose is about 750 milligrams per kilo of body weight, or several million times the recommended supplement dosage—but they probably can't help you, either. "The bottom line is this stuff is being sold all over the place, and we really don't know that it has any beneficial effect at all."

In 1995, researchers at Dartmouth College and George Washington University Medical Center did a study on chromium picolinate which indicates that too much of the mineral may actually be carcinogenic. The researchers tested the effects on cells taken from a hamster's ovary. The chromium picolinate caused damage to the chromosomes in the cells, which is often an indication that a substance could cause cancer.

At this point, it isn't certain that chromium supplements are dangerous. One test on hamster cells doesn't mean it's going to hurt humans. But just as uncertain is whether anyone needs to take chromium at all. The only thing you can say with any confidence about chromium is that taking 200 micrograms a day of a trace mineral isn't likely to make you lean and muscular. It's more likely to give you expensive urine.

In 1997, the Federal Trade Commission ruled that Nutrition 21, which holds the exclusive patent on chromium picolinate, can no longer advertise that the substance burns fat, causes weight loss, increases muscle mass, reduces serum cholesterol, regulates blood-sugar levels, or can treat or prevent diabetes. There's simply no evidence to support those claims.

Thigh Cream

In the fall of 1993, ads for a miracle fat-reducing thigh cream seemed to appear overnight in newspapers, on cable TV shows, and tacked up on signposts and grocery-store bulletin boards. "No more thunder thighs!" promised one newspaper ad. "Lose 2–6 inches a week, 100% guarantee, liposuction alternative," read another. A banner in the window at one discount cosmetics store near my office announced: "Finally! Thigh cream is here!" Inside, the saleswoman told me that at $39.95 a jar they could hardly keep the product on the shelves. Everyone wanted it.

Who wouldn't? It would be wonderful to rub some lotion on your thighs and watch your fat disappear. But thigh cream seems about as plausible as those expensive European creams advertised a few years ago that promised to smooth away cellulite. Not only didn't they work, it turned out there was no such thing as cellulite, which is just normal fat; it was a condition advertisers invented in order to cure. The idea of a fat-reducing thigh cream raised a lot of questions. Would the cream dissolve fat on contact or penetrate the skin? Where would the fat go, anyway? To the stomach, ankles, the bloodstream? Would it be dangerous? Would it last? If you took a bath in thigh cream, would you emerge thinner all over?

Given how incredible thigh cream seems, it probably never would have become a marketing sensation had not someone with a lot of authority in the weight-loss field vouched for the product. And he did: One of the most prominent obesity researchers in the country, George

Bray, director of the Pennington Biomedical Research Center at Louisiana State University and editor of the prestigious medical journal *Obesity Research*, gave his word that thigh cream worked. Like Alan Howard's Cambridge Diet, thigh cream is an example of how consumers can be persuaded that an implausible weight-loss product works if a prominent obesity researcher tells them so—without disclosing his financial interest in the product.

At the October 1993 conference of the North American Association for the Study of Obesity, held in Milwaukee, Bray and his colleague endocrinologist Frank Greenway presented a short report to the four hundred weight-loss experts on a study they had done. They explained that they had tested a cream containing an asthma drug, aminophylline, on twelve women's thighs. For six weeks, the women, all of whom considered their thighs pudgy and dimpled, slathered a teaspoon of aminophylline cream on one thigh, and a similar cream without the active ingredient on the other. When their thighs were measure at the end of the study, the women lost an average of 1 centimeter from the treated thigh—less than half an inch, a difference so small that even a woman who was extremely critical of her body might fail to detect it in the mirror.

The study was small, and the results weren't very impressive. But the researchers didn't hedge their findings with words of caution, the way scientists often do when they describe very preliminary studies, calling for more research and begging reporters not to jump to any conclusions. "The women liked the cream base and the results," the researchers told the audience. "We conclude that 2 percent aminophylline cream applied topically causes regional fat loss from the thighs of women." They even suggested that this new medical treatment might accomplish some of the same goals—getting rid of dimply thighs—as liposuction.[22]

Associated Press science editor Paul Raeburn, the only journalist at the conference, hurried off to write the story.[23] In it, he revealed some information that hadn't been disclosed at the conference: Greenway and Bray, who patented the topical use of aminophylline on fat in 1985, had already sold the rights to use the thigh cream idea to an entrepreneur in Los Angeles. Greenway told the reporter that the cream would be available as a cosmetic "relatively soon," and indicated that a marketing scheme had already been worked out to avoid the lengthy process of having to get the FDA to approve a new drug. "If you make cosmetic claims," he said, "you could market it as a cosmetic."[24]

In that first story, Greenway explained that the women's thighs probably shrank because the aminophylline had changed the fat cells to make it easier for them to release fat in the bloodstream. In subsequent weeks, Greenway, Bray, and other researchers fleshed out their theory. Since 1985, Bray had been working on how to decrease the amount of fat in women's thighs using the asthma drug. Several researchers had shown that in petri dishes, at least, aminophylline, like caffeine, causes fat cells to release their stores of fat. The fat cells in women's thighs are the most stubborn in the body, programmed to hang on to fat stores long after fat cells in the rest of the body burn theirs up, so that women have extra energy supplies on hand in case they need to produce breast milk. In interviews with several science writers, Bray explained that the hormones that regulate fat storage act on adenosine receptors, which inhibit fat cells from burning their stores. Thigh fat cells have many more adenosine receptors than other fat cells, and Bray believed that aminophylline would block those receptors, tricking the cells to release their fat.[25] But would a thigh cream that was only rubbed on the skin work the same way? To many researchers, it didn't seem likely.

Overnight, the thigh cream story spread to other newspapers and television. *USA Today* reported, "The dream of a cream that melts away fat may come true." National Public Radio did a morning show on the cream, and interviewed the endocrinologist Wayne Callaway of George Washington University about the new discovery. Callaway was skeptical that the thigh cream worked the way its inventors said it might work, especially since the study didn't even begin to prove how it worked. Because aminophylline is also used as a diuretic, releasing water from cells, Callaway suggested that it was more likely the thinner thighs may have been caused by water loss.

But before anyone really understood how the thigh cream worked, or whether it worked at all, it was being marketed to consumers. By January 1994, several thigh creams were being sold, some with the inventors' blessings and some without. Bray and Greenway had now sold the idea for thigh cream two more times. First, they sold it to Herbalife International, which marketed the product as Thermojetics

Body Contour Cream. Then, working with an entrepreneur lawyer, Dr. Bruce Frome, the researchers made their own version of the cream, called Smooth Contours, which was sold by the Nutri/System weight-loss chain (Bray is on the scientific advisory board for Nutri/System). They also signed an agreement with another company that marketed a cream called Cellution. Several copycat versions of the thigh cream appeared almost immediately, such as Skinny Dip. Some of the ads, which were not approved by the researchers, made remarkable promises: "I lost 1½″ off my thighs in 5 weeks!" claimed one Herbalife testimonial.[26] Most of the companies sold the cream for about $40 a jar or tube.

It didn't take many weeks of rubbing in slimy cream, however, before a number of consumers and science writers realized they'd been had. In February 1994, twenty-one employees of the *Boston Globe* tested out the thigh cream in much the same way as the women in Greenway and Bray's experiment did. For five weeks, they slathered the greenish cream—one likened it to "strained spinach baby food," and another to "frog snot"—on one thigh, leaving the other alone. The *Boston Globe* nurse weighed each woman and measured her thighs before and after the experiment. Of the seventeen women who completed the experiment, the thigh measurements of nine of them didn't change at all. Of the eight whose measurements did change, three had fatter thighs, partly because they gained weight. One woman lost more weight on her untreated thigh than the treated one. Only two of the women who lost weight lost more—a quarter to half an inch—on the treated leg. "Disappointment," wrote reporter Judy Foreman, "was acute."[27] Magazines including *Health* and *Vogue* took a closer look at the thigh cream, and were skeptical; the emperor had no clothes, it seemed, and he still had fat thighs.

The manufacturers of the thigh cream had never actually *promised* it would work, however. In order to escape FDA regulation, the aminophylline in the cream was watered down—to 0.5 percent, not the 2.0 percent used in the research—and so were the promises. Smooth Contours didn't say the product would burn fat, just that it would help "achieve smoother appearing thighs." In fact, the cosmetic version of the cream was diluted down so far that if it ever worked in research to reduce fat—which is a big if—it no longer worked in the same way by the time consumers got their hands into it. "If it has any effect on physiologic function, then legally it should be sold as a drug," says

Wayne Callaway. "If it doesn't have any effect, why should people buy it?"

People did buy it, and lots of it. One diet industry analyst, John LaRosa of Marketdata Enterprises, noted that the sales of thigh cream helped the flagging weight-loss chain Nutri/System revive itself during a tough time. "The thigh cream is literally flying off the shelves," LaRosa said. "By the time the FDA investigates amino-phylline and pulls it off the market, Nutri/System and others will have made millions."

What galls some professionals in the weight-control field is not just that another diet product has fooled the public into parting with its money, if not its fat, but that the whole fiasco was made legitimate by the participation of well-known obesity researchers. The *Tufts University Diet and Nutrition Letter* reported that Bray and Greenway had sold the legal right to use their thigh cream concept to Herbalife a full six months before they ever presented their research at a medical conference. "George Bray has been regarded as one of the foremost metabolic researchers in the country," says Susan Wooley, the internationally known eating disorders expert. "And suddenly he's selling thigh cream. It's a scandal."[28]

Bray counters that he had been studying and publishing work on aminophylline cream since 1987, and that he had nothing to do with the thigh cream sensation that jammed the country's 800 lines in 1994. "I'm not in business, I'm an academic," he says. "Nobody paid any attention to it before, and I had no expectation that anyone would pay attention to it again." Bray blames the media—not the thigh cream promoters, with whom he had financial agreements—for making a big deal out of the product. "If it weren't for the sweet press, nobody would've cared," he says, testily. Still, Bray claims that the product does work, at low concentrations, as a cosmetic that will improve the appearance of the skin, though he admits he hasn't proven how it works. "We know that small doses of aminophylline in a cream on your skin will smooth it—by whatever mechanism. It's not important," he says. "We don't know how most drugs work, and the mechanisms for most cosmetics aren't known, either." But cosmetics, by definition, aren't supposed to have mechanisms, or else they'd be drugs, subject to regulation. Bray says he's certain, at least, that at low doses aminophylline isn't toxic.

Bray claims he has only made about $3,000 on the thigh cream, and spent some $50,000 on patent costs. He doesn't view his involvement in the product as a conflict of interest, nor does he think there's anything wrong with selling a product that only "smooths the skin," even when it's been widely claimed that it reduces fat. "If you want no conflict of interest, the government pays for everything," Bray says. "Is that what you want? Let's close the cosmetics industry down and let women be au naturel."

By March 1994, the National Association for the Study of Obesity had received so much criticism about the way the thigh cream was introduced and marketed that it printed a half-hearted apology. The organization's journal, *Obesity Research*, assured its readers that the authors of the thigh cream abstract agreed it had been an "oversight" that the abstract did not include a disclosure statement; but this slip, it said, "probably would not have been noticed without the attendant publicity the abstract received."[29] In other words, there wouldn't have been a problem with scientists selling bogus thigh cream if they'd been able to slip it by the press—and the public.

Hypnosis

Weight-loss scams aren't limited to products sold through the mail, infomercials, health-food stores, or over the counter. All over the country, people with questionable credentials are willing to counsel you in person about nutrition and dieting or sell you tapes of their weight-loss visualization tips. It doesn't take much training to become a food therapist or a diet counselor. Some of these pseudonutritionists and fake psychologists hold huge hotel seminars across the country that claim to help people lose weight in a single evening.

In March 1994, I opened up the *San Francisco Examiner* and read the headline on a quarter-page ad: "Lose Weight with Hypnosis." For only $39.99, I could attend a seminar that would, *guaranteed*, make me lose weight. "You can lose the weight you've been wanting to—and keep it off permanently, without hunger, without dieting, without willpower." Once and for all, it said, I could lose unwanted cravings, eliminate the addiction to sweets, and break the impulsive/compulsive eating habit. The ad was rather specific in what it promised: "You can expect results ranging from 30–60 pounds in three months to 120 pounds in one year." A smiling photo of Ronald B. Gorayeb, certified hypnotherapist, dominated the ad.

That week, I went to a hotel in San Francisco to attend one of the seven Gorayeb seminars held in the Bay Area. After offering up my Visa card, I went into a conference room where about a hundred people were already seated, most of them women who were only 20 to 40 pounds over the ideal weight. A banner festooned on the wall showed a picture of an iceberg, depicting how only 10 percent of our mind is conscious, the rest subconscious. We were here to change the subconscious.

A neatly suited woman, Helen Frances, who looks like a younger version of California Senator Dianne Feinstein, stepped to the front of the room. According to literature passed out to the participants, Frances has experience as a human resources specialist, and as a director of two hypnosis centers in Denver and Salt Lake City. She had a bright presentation style and knew how to get a crowd of dieters on her side. "Tonight's not about weight loss," she told the group. "In this room we probably have some of the world's foremost authorities on weight loss." She quickly discredited every other diet program, trotting out well-known statistics about how 95 percent of those who diet gain the weight back. She asked for a show of hands of people in the room who had lost weight on diets only to gain more, and half the room waved. Then she asked everyone to repeat a pledge after her: "If I ever want to gain weight, I will go on a diet."

The subconscious method of losing weight, according to the literature that was passed out by assistants, doesn't involve dieting. Instead, the Gorayeb system involves exercise, drinking more water, chewing slowly, reducing fat, avoiding snacking, and making dietary changes. (Sounds like a diet to me.) The "behavior modification" changes listed in the material were like those suggested by many psychologists and commercial weight-loss centers who give grown women infantile advice about how to pick up their forks, chew their food, and drink their water. The Gorayeb technique placed an almost Horace Fletcher–like emphasis on chewing. "Chew each bite of food slowly, at least 20 to 30 times (if that means you have to count, then count)."

Frances reassured the group that the hypnosis session wouldn't be like those we imagine from TV and movies: no one was going to have to get up and bark like a dog. Nor would it be aversion therapy, where we would be told disgusting stories about food (as my psychologist did to me when I was thirteen years old). Instead, we were simply going to go into our subconscious file on weight loss and change the contents. "When you leave tonight you'll have everything you need to keep your weight down for the rest of your life," she said.

The lights dimmed, and we all got comfortable, shifting around on our hotel chairs. Frances began speaking in a soothing voice, telling us to relax our bodies from our heads to our toes. We were to imagine a beautiful, white cloud gently touching our faces. The cloud floated on down our bodies, caressing our thighs, knees, and toes. We were to repeat to ourselves the mantra, *"soothing and relaxing, soothing and relaxing."* Now presumably in a state of deep relaxation, Frances had us repeat several messages to ourselves, over and over. "I am in control of my eating habits. I am a thin, healthy person. I exercise three times a week. I chew each mouthful of food at least twenty to thirty chews per bite." Limp and relaxed, my jaw was beginning to twitch.

Frances led us through several different "visualization" scenes. In one, we were to imagine foods we desired, with a big, red international symbol for "no" circling it. "No desire," she intoned. "No desire." I conjured up visions of wild mushroom risotto, *tiramisu*, Cherry Garcia ice cream, and currant scones. The international symbol for "no" was having a hard time competing, and kept fading into the background. "No desire," I repeated to myself, drifting off. "No desire. No Cherry Garcia. Desire Cherry Garcia." I floated into the corner store and hovered over the ice-cream case, trying to decide whether I'd rather have chocolate almond fudge.

Frances redirected my attention with instructions for the next scene. We were to imagine ourselves going into a magical clothing store, where we could try on a special outfit that would make us look and feel the way we wanted. "Go four sizes more slender. Find the perfect outfit. Make it daring and lacy if you want," she told the women. "Anything goes. Men—be Tarzan!" I was having a hard time imagining myself four sizes smaller, in Nancy Reagan's body, so I concentrated instead on the magic outfit. I conjured up a lovely Donna Karan dress I'd seen in *Vogue*. The problem was, the dress was on a size 6 body. I worked hard at picturing the dress on my size 12 body, and instead imagined a whole line of size 12 models in the pages of *Vogue* wearing terrific dresses. It was a wonderful fantasy. "Shoe," I heard

Frances say. I focused on the feet, shod with witty little black Italian shoes. "Shoes," I repeated to myself. "Shoes, shoes, shoes."

Now she was saying, over and over, "Chew, chew, chew." I tried to tune out, to get back to eating ice cream in my Donna Karan dress. "Use the 800 number," Frances said in that soothing voice. "This is your number." I shook myself awake. She was repeating an 800 number to call. In our somnolent state, she was selling us as many products as she possibly could. "You can buy the nutrition and permanent weight-loss tape, special tonight, two for the price of one," came the soft, even voice. "The stop-smoking tape, the freedom-from-stress tape. Buy the whole collection for only $330. . . ."

The people around me were nodding their heads up and down. Buy, buy. It was as if they'd been told to bark like dogs after all.

The next day, I called the Gorayeb 800 number and insisted I get my money back. It was a real scam, I told the woman on the line, to hypnotize people in order to sell them weight-loss products. She told me that, instead, I could go back to any seminar I wanted for free, as guaranteed. Why would I want to go back? I asked. In the end, she promised to credit my account, which she did.

That month, the FTC accused Gorayeb seminars of making false and misleading claims, which violated the Federal Trade Commission Act. Specifically, the FTC said that claims that attendees would lose weight and maintain it after a single seminar, that thousands of others had lost weight that way, and that the seminar was more effective for weight loss than other methods, were misleading. Two weeks after the seminar I attended, on March 22, 1994, Gorayeb signed a cease-and-desist agreement, agreeing to stop making false claims about weight loss.[30]

A year later, in April 1995, I called Gorayeb's offices again and asked them if they were holding another weight-loss seminar in my area. "Absolutely," said the man on the line. "We do them all over the country. We'll be back in the Bay Area in May."

Weight-loss fraud will continue as long as women continue to want to lose weight at any cost, and as long as entrepreneurs are willing to exploit that desire by selling bogus products. Every month new mail-order products are being developed; a few recent ones include Erinasole, a shoe insert designed to help people lose weight by massaging the feet; Stay Trim, an "all-natural" tablet whose main unmentioned ingredient reportedly helped dieters lose 72 pounds in ten weeks (something usually only accomplished by amputation); and InstaTrim, a "new wonder pill," which makes it possible "to lose 6–10 pounds per week, while eating foods like fried chicken, double burgers, pancakes, etc."[31]

A few things might help prevent some of the most outrageous and unhealthy scams. The FDA needs to be able to investigate diet fraud more aggressively. Herbs that act like drugs should be regulated like drugs, carrying warning labels that tell exactly how much of the active ingredient the product contains and what side effects a user might expect. The FDA should place potentially dangerous herbs and over-the-counter drugs, such as ephedrine, in a position that is somewhere between an outright ban and total availability to consumers: behind the counter. PPA is useless and harmful and should be banned, despite the fact that well-paid pharmaceutical lobbyists disagree.

To prevent physicians from using their influence unfairly to persuade consumers to buy questionable products, medical journals and conference committees should require that researchers divulge any potential financial conflicts of interest they have before they present their studies, and make those interests clear to the public. Newspaper and magazine editors would do their readers a great service if they made sure their stories about new diet "breakthroughs" were informed with broad research and deep skepticism.

But the bottom line is that consumers need to stop being so gullible. As long as consumers continue to hold out hope that somehow magic herbs, pills, and potions will make them thin, they'll keep reaching for their charge cards. Many know the products won't work, even as they're dialing the 800 number. Their desire to lose weight—to be accepted, loved, and successful in this culture—is so strong that it's worth $79.95 just to buy into the fantasy, just to imagine themselves with thin thighs in thirty days.

Even if American customers become wary of diet scams, they'll be snatched up by dieters in other countries. Herbalife's worldwide revenues for 1994, says Frances Berg of *Healthy Weight Journal*, were estimated at $884 million, two-thirds coming from foreign markets.[32] In Moscow, according to *Working Woman* magazine, it's nearly impossible to ride the metro without seeing someone wearing an

Herbalife button that says: "Lose weight now. Ask me how."[33] Influenced by America's diet mania, these countries are also importing our weight-loss remedies, with all their false hopes, promises, and potential dangers.

Chapter 4

No Satisfaction:
Fat-Free and Fake Foods

It was mid-afternoon, my energy was lagging, and I wanted something sweet. Browsing at the corner store for just the right little something—a piece of creamy chocolate, a chewy ginger cookie, a handful of ripe raspberries—I noticed two women in the cookie aisle. "There they are," said one, reaching for a bright green box. "Get another," urged the other, conspiratorially.

They had SnackWell's Devil's Food Cookie Cakes in hand. These are the cookies that were, for a time, famous for being widely unavailable, for driving cookie-starved women to descend upon deliverymen and grocery-store managers demanding their chocolate and marshmallow-covered fat-free cookies, and devouring them.

Guiltily, as if I were buying pornography, I picked up a box. At home alone, I bit into a cookie. It was chocolately smooth and sweet, then suddenly—it was gone. It had dissolved in my mouth, leaving only a dreary aftertaste. Somehow, I hadn't gotten what I'd been after. I brought the box to the table and had another, and another. The first row of four cookies in the box was gone. Usually I stop after one or two cookies. But not now. I kept wanting satisfaction, thinking I might find it in the next row. Then there were only four left. They're fat-free, said the devil on my shoulder. Go ahead.

I had eaten the whole box. I felt miserable, like the woman in a

SnackWell's commercial who attends a Snack Eaters Anonymous meeting, confessing her sins. "Yesterday I faltered," she says, grief-stricken. "I couldn't resist these cookies! I've ruined everything!" She is redeemed and happy at the end of the ad, however, when she realizes the cookies she ate were fat-free and couldn't possibly harm her.

Unlike me, she didn't read the label. No fat, to be sure, but *600 calories per box*. I could have had a real meal with dessert instead. And still I didn't feel satisfied.

Whether or not we get any real pleasure from them, Americans are buying fat-free snacks with such zeal you'd think eating them would make us thin. Nabisco's SnackWell's did more than $400 million in sales in 1995, making it the number-one brand of cookie and cracker in the country, leaving old favorites like Oreos and Ritz behind in the crumbs. The SnackWell's phenomenon attests to our enormous taste for diet and fat-free products. Ninety percent of Americans regularly consume low-calorie, sugar-free, or reduced-fat foods and beverages, according to the Calorie Control Council, a manufacturer's group, compared with 76 percent three years ago. "Fat-free" is now the label consumers say they most want to see on boxes in the supermarket, replacing "healthy" from a few years ago. And they see the label everywhere—on cereals, granola bars, yogurts, pasta boxes, and probably, somewhere, on banana skins and broccoli. The fat-free craze has become so widespread that Americans have actually succeeded, in the past decade, in cutting their average fat intake from 36 percent to 34 percent of their total diets, according to the National Center for Health Statistics (since the 1960s, we've actually dropped the fat content of our diets from 40 percent). You would think, then, that Americans would be getting thinner, too.

But we aren't. Adult Americans have gained an average of 8 pounds apiece in the past decade. We may be exercising less than we used to, and many people have quit smoking and put on weight (becoming, on average, 5 to 7 pounds heavier and a whole lot healthier), but something else is going on, too. It's a paradox: We're eating less fat and getting fatter.[1]

The usual explanation for why Americans are putting on pounds is that we just eat too much of everything, fat-free or not. There's some truth to this view; many of us do overeat. Not all individuals who are fat overeat, however; many people who are genetically obese eat far less than their skinny friends. But as a group, we can't blame our collective weight gain over the past decade on a changing gene pool. We're not breeding that fast. It's hard to resist the explanation that we're eating more and exercising less. And in fact, though the percentage of fat in our diets has gone down during the past decade, the total number of calories we eat has gone up, from 1,969 calories per person per day to 2,200. We've become accustomed to jumbo portions and frequent snacks.

But *why* are we eating more? Many of us believe it's because we're gluttons, we have no willpower, and we don't know when to stop. We're wallowing in food here in the United States, and we just can't resist the pleasure. We like to eat, and fat-free foods just give us license to eat even more.

This belief that we overeat because we love food and can't resist temptation raises a few questions. If we love food so much, then why do so many of us often eat on the run, grabbing a snack or a fast-food burger and stuffing it down quickly, without really registering how it tastes? Why do we eat standing up, by the light of the refrigerator, grazing aimlessly through cartons of cold and soggy leftovers? Why are we content to settle for second-rate flavors, fake chocolates, no-fat cheeses, and chemical-tasting artificial sweeteners?

If it's pleasure that makes us overeat, then it's a guilty pleasure. Since the time of the Puritans, Americans have believed that eating too much is sinful; since the Victorian age, women in particular have been warned that a hearty, sensual appetite is unladylike and improper. Our desires to eat have been repressed, and so they surface in extreme and perverse ways. We've become obsessed with food, and fixated on how much we eat. We're afraid of food, and imagine that if we don't restrain ourselves, we'll go wild and end up being huge.

Americans tend to think of food in moral terms. One survey showed that eight out of ten Americans think that foods are inherently "good" or "bad," never mind the context in which you eat them; even just a small dish of chocolate mousse, we believe, is apt to be permanently polluting, glomming onto our artery walls for good. More importantly, we think that eating "bad" foods makes us bad ourselves—undisciplined, weak-willed, and piggish. But believing that foods are bad doesn't make us stop eating them; it just makes them that much more alluring. We intensely desire all the bad foods we can't have, and eventually break down—out of rebelliousness, hunger, or overwhelming feeling—and eat too much of them. Meanwhile, we take little pleasure in the "good" foods we might otherwise be happy to eat.

It's our guilt about eating, and our restraint, that end up backfiring and making us overeat. Several studies have shown that restrained eating—dieting, in other words—causes bingeing; when we starve ourselves, our bodies call out for help with hunger pangs and cravings, and our minds plot a rebellion.[2] Diet foods, in particular, make us want to overeat. They're both "good" and "bad" at once, and so they're irresistible. We also binge more on diet junk foods than we do other "bad" foods because they aren't as satisfying. When we eat diet foods, they're usually a cheap substitute for "bad" foods, and we aren't really fooled. We end up overcompensating for our desires, eating more of the diet food than we should, looking for satisfaction.

Our eating habits in America are extreme: We diet and then we binge; we obsess about fat grams and then give in to half a cheesecake; we buy fat-free cookies and then eat the whole box. Bulimia is an apt metaphor for the way we eat in this culture. The food and diet industries appeal to our binge-purge eating habits, seducing us with the guilty pleasures of food, then selling us quick remedies for our overindulgence. This is nothing new; the food industry has always promoted overconsuming food. In 1995, it spent $36 billion on advertisements. Its ads, coupled with diet industry ads and media images that promote slenderness, are a recipe for bulimia. In 1957, the eating disorders expert Hilde Bruch noticed this trend in her book *The Importance of Overweight*: "Parallel to the enormous pressure toward slimness runs the advertising of powerful interests who want to sell food. The popular women's magazines are examples of truly split personalities. The cover picture may show tempting and luscious food, and new and exciting recipes are one of the selling points of each magazine. Yet at the same time, a magazine will carry articles on the dangers of overweight, and offer prescriptions for keeping thin and beautiful." Ads in magazines and on television today are even more blatantly bulimic, one minute enticing us to eat, and the next to lose weight. Sometimes ads contain both binge and purge messages at once: "How much Chocolate Mocha Supreme will it take to get you into these jeans?" asks an ad for Nestlé's Sweet Success meal-replacement drink, featuring a very thin model.

No wonder we're overeating and gaining weight. It makes perfect sense that we would take these conflicting cultural messages to binge and diet to heart, and that, given the opportunity, we would binge on diet food.

Low-Fat Snack Foods

Fat has become the latest of many nutritional villains in the United States. At one time it was sugar, at others it was starch or cholesterol; now it's fat. Everywhere, people are counting fat grams, checking labels on cracker boxes, complaining loudly in restaurants if vegetables have a hint of olive oil on them, and grilling baffled Mexican waiters about whether the beans were cooked in lard. Given the recent emphasis on how terribly bad fat is for us—a "heart attack on a plate," the Center for Science in the Public Interest warns us about fettucine Alfredo; "Fat makes you fat!" screams Susan Powter—two out of ten Americans now believe that all fat should be eliminated from the diet entirely. The government recommendation for a healthy diet, meanwhile, is about 30 percent fat, though many moderate obesity researchers recommend that people who have a tendency to get fat should cut their fat intake back to about 20 percent.[3]

Food companies have taken advantage of our fear of fat by marketing fat-free versions of nearly everything we eat, including things like pretzels and fig bars that never had much fat in them to begin with. The word being spread is that it's the demon fat that makes you gain weight, but you can eat no-fat foods with total abandon. This message is seductive because, like a fat-free chocolate cookie, or French Vanilla–flavored Slim-Fast, it promises sin and repentance all at once.

No company has been more successful at selling these sinfully indulgent fat-free snacks than RJR Nabisco, maker of SnackWell's. The giant cookie, cracker, and tobacco conglomerate sits atop green rolling New Jersey hills that were once a golf course. Inside, posters of Oreos loom with a one-word message: INDULGENCE. Display cases show off the company's many products—it is responsible for nine out of ten of the top cookies and crackers sold in this country. Nestled in the middle of one display case is a box of Uneeda Biscuits, the product the National Biscuit Company launched in the 1890s with one of the first mass-marketed ad campaigns, selling Americans on the idea that "Uneeda Biscuit."

Over the years, Nabisco and other companies have been so successful in convincing Americans that we need to snack that we seem to eat constantly. Weight-conscious dieters tend to skip meals and fill up on snacks instead, resulting in an average of twenty "food contacts" per day, as they call them in the industry.[4] This in itself may be one of the reasons Americans tend to gain more weight than the French, who eat scrumptious butter-saturated meals but don't snack much (we get 22 percent of our daily calories from snacks; the French, 7 percent). To address this snacking problem, which it created, the food industry's marketing strategies have shifted. The new message isn't that we need to snack, but that we need to "snack well." In the end, it will just make us snack more.

At Nabisco, inside the laboratory research building, office cubicles circle airy stainless-steel kitchens where flour and sugar bins are labeled with names like "natural starch H-50," "potato granules," "defatted wheat germ," "MSG," and "high gluten flour." In one room, the SnackWell's product development team is gathered around a conference table. Casually dressed and lively, these six people have the relaxed and confident air of a team that has gone through an arduous battle and emerged victorious. In fact, what they have accomplished by making fat-free cookies that don't taste terrible is, in the history of food science, a dramatic feat.

"Diet food had really gotten a bad rap," says Richard Gill, senior manager of the group. Anyone who has ever tasted Tillie Lewis Tasti-Diet low-cal chocolate sauce (introduced in the 1950s), or early versions of fat-free cake, knows what he means. Technological improvements have improved diet foods in the past two decades, but most still don't please the palate. Even recently, fat-free snack manufacturers have had a problem: People would buy the products, but only once. One bite of coffee cake that tasted like a syrupy old sponge and they knew better the next time.

It's tough to make good-tasting snacks without fat, because fat carries flavor, texture, creaminess, moisture, and keeps things fresh. Fat has a certain "mouth feel," as they call it in the business, that's hard to replace. Fat is basically what we like about cookies, cakes, and muffins. So coming up with fat-free cookies that consumers would actually consume was quite an accomplishment.

It wasn't easy. After Nabisco's marketing department told the team it wanted indulgent, fat-free snacks, the scientists went through numerous versions trying to come up with something palatable.

Consumers had identified cheese, chocolate, and chocolate chip as the flavors they wanted—all of which rely on fat. Those were the flavors the team targeted. Rich McFeaters, the scientist responsible for the Devil's Food Cookie Cakes—he is the man behind the "Mr. Cookie" character in the ads—tried everything from cottage cheese to plum paste to make a fat-free product. "The early ones were horrid," recalls Marilyn Lamb, who is in charge of the "sensory" department, where employees spend eight-hour days tasting snack products, spitting them out, and rating them for their numerous qualities. SnackWell's early version of the fat-free graham stars, she says, were referred to as "dog treats" around the office.

Some of the cookies went through as many as two hundred formula changes. With the Devil's Food Cookie Cakes, McFeaters hit on using a variety of textures to impart more flavor and creamy texture—the marshmallow, cake, and smooth chocolate combination. The product was nearly shelved at first because tests indicated consumers didn't really like them. But once they heard the cookies were fat-free, they liked them just fine. In the stores, the cookies, which take over four hours to make on a rolling-trolley assembly line because the fat-free glaze has to be air-dried instead of chilled, were a hit. The initial forecast was for 2.5 million pounds a year, but consumers were clamoring for more. Caught short, Nabisco hurried to build more trolleys, but still, at 50 million pounds (which comes to nearly 4 million cookies *a day*), they haven't been able to make enough to keep up with demand. "People want to have their devil's food cake and eat it too," explains McFeaters. The team gleefully tells stories about women's groups that were formed to scout out the cookies, fights erupting in the stores over the boxes, and grocery-store managers who kept the snacks under lock and key.

But do people really like these cookies, or do they eat them because they're low-fat? Lamb says the only cookies in the line that score as well on taste as full-fat versions are the vanilla-cream sandwiches. "For others, there's a bit of a trade-off," she says. "But [consumers] say they feel satisfied eating a SnackWell's. They eat boxes of them because they like them so much."

Maybe. Or perhaps they're eating boxes of ersatz cookies because they *don't* feel satisfied, physically and psychologically, the way they would eating real cookies. Without fat, the cookies don't really satisfy a craving for something creamy; without substance, they don't fill you up or stick with you. Whatever the reason, people who believe that eating quantities of fat-free cookies is a smart nutrition strategy are deluding themselves.

One reason people fail to lose weight eating fat-free snacks is that in most of the products, the fat that's taken out is replaced with sugar to make up for the lost taste. Sugar, while not the nutritional enemy it was considered a couple decades ago, isn't widely renowned for its weight-reducing properties. "As much as we don't like to say it, these are not calorie-free products," says McFeaters. That's an understatement: fat-free products, such as fat-free Newtons, contain virtually the same number of calories as the regular version. SnackWell's Double Fudge Cookie Cakes have 50 calories apiece, the same as a regular Chip's Ahoy chocolate chip cookie.

The point of low-fat diets, say those who advocate losing weight on them, is to eat fewer calories. (Fat-free snacks make more sense for people who aren't trying to lose weight, but who have to avoid fat because of heart disease.) The logic with the low-fat weight-loss diet is that since a gram of fat has 9 calories compared to a gram of carbohydrates, which has 4, you can eschew the fat, eat more carbohydrates, and feel full on fewer calories. This may hold true if you're eating fruits, pastas, vegetables, and other foods that fill you up with fiber (and, not incidentally, vitamins). But highly processed, sugary foods don't have much bulk for their calories; Devil's Food SnackWell's have very little fiber (less than 1 gram each), and your stomach doesn't feel full. The sugar in the cookies is quickly absorbed into the bloodstream, where the body tries to burn it off as fast as possible, leaving other stores of energy in the body—fat—to sit unused.

All that concentrated sugar can be dangerous for a person who has insulin resistance, and is at risk for diabetes. When you eat a big load of sugar, your blood sugar levels rise. You use insulin to store the excess sugar away until your blood sugar levels drop. But with people who are resistant to insulin, the more insulin they produce, the more their bodies become resistant to the effects of insulin, so they have to produce even more to take care of the sugar levels in the blood. This situation can cause them to store away more fat than normal people, and can eventually lead to diabetes. Most people, of course, don't have insulin resistance—though purveyors of recent high-protein diets would like to have us believe that's true.

For most people, the sugary snacks simply add calories, while making you want to eat more. Fat-free snacks are also "empty" calories, in that they don't deliver any vitamins or minerals along with the sugar. The 600 calories in a box of SnackWell's isn't going to do the good for your body that a 600-calorie plate of vegetables (sautéed in olive oil), pasta, and a little sprinkled parmesan will do. People who are on low-calorie diets and eat a lot of these snacks end up getting very poor nutrition. It's even worse than sipping chocolate meal-replacement drinks, which at least have some added vitamins and minerals. But many people believe that diet food is not only going to make them lose weight, it's healthy. "I don't doubt that some people eat two boxes a day of SnackWell's and call it a 1,200-calorie-a-day diet," says John Foreyt a psychologist and obesity researcher at Baylor College of Medicine in Houston.

Foods that are low in fat but still taste like fat can be defeating, too, because they don't help you shift your tastes to prefer lower-fat foods. If you do eat a lot of fat in your diet (more than the 30 percent recommended by the government), it's sensible for a variety of health reasons—particularly to avoid heart disease—to try to learn gradually to feel satisfied with less fatty foods, the way people who switch from whole milk to low-fat milk eventually find the higher-fat stuff tastes too greasy. In one study at the Monell Chemical Senses Center in Philadelphia, Richard Mattes, a researcher in nutrition, put two groups of people on low-fat diets. In one, they were allowed to eat products that simulated fat. In the others, they ate foods that were naturally low in fat. After a couple of months, the group that didn't eat no-fat products didn't miss the fat; they began to prefer foods with lower-fat levels. The group that ate the fat-free cookies and cakes never weaned themselves from their preference for fats, however, and started eating high-fat versions of the low-fat products right after the experiment was over.

There are psychological reasons why people overeat fat-free products, too. If you think you're being "good," eating low-fat foods, then that gives you permission to be "bad" later on in the day. Barbara Rolls, a professor of nutrition at Pennsylvania State University, gave a group of women yogurt before lunch. Though each container had the same number of calories, some had labels that said "high fat" and others said "low fat." The women who ate the "low fat" yogurts ate significantly more food at lunch and throughout the rest of the day than the others. "Some people eat low-fat foods as an excuse to eat other high-fat foods," says Rolls. "It's the diet Coke and donut strategy."

At Nabisco, no one minds that people are eating boxes of their cookies. In fact, the promise of overindulgence is SnackWell's biggest selling point. SnackWell's ads, featuring women stalking men for cookies, tacitly encourage bingeing: "So good, can we ever make enough?" Those devouring women can certainly never eat enough. Yet the cookie team feels they're doing the public a service; they believe, as the package says, that the snacks "fit into your healthy lifestyle." Healthy, it seems to me, is something that improves your health when you eat it, like broccoli or kale.

Nabisco, along with a number of other food companies, has made the term "fat-free" seem synonymous with healthy nutrition, when in fact taking something *out* of a product doesn't necessarily make what's left in it any better for you. Life Savers has an ad comparing a donut with a donut-sized ring made of Life Savers; the caption points out there are "0 grams fat" in the Life Savers, as if eating a pile of candy is any better for you than a donut. Some ads imply that fat-free food can even take the place of exercise. Guiltless Gourmet—what name could be more appealing?—has an ad that features a woman swearing off of those boring exercise classes because she can now just eat fat-free snacks instead. Hägen-Dazs urges you to try their 0 percent fat sorbet and "Skip the gym."

At Nabisco, I asked the SnackWell's group what makes their cookies so darn "healthy." I read the list of ingredients, which included quite a lot of sugar. "Sounds like candy to me," I said.

There was a pause. Richard Gill, the senior manager, spoke up. "Candy is usually a hundred percent sugar," he said. "The use of wheat is not associated with candy." He says the company doesn't hide the fact that there's sugar in the cookies; they're just providing another choice for people who are concerned about reducing their fat intake. "We don't call them a health food. We don't talk about weight loss," he says. "We talk about wellness."

"Wellness" is a marketing buzzword that means something short of "healthy." The products are aimed at people who are not necessarily actively health-conscious but more passively "health-aware," as SnackWell's business manager Jean Thomas puts it. The idea seems to be that it's the absence of unhealthy things (like fat) that makes something fit into a "wellness lifestyle," and that the more you take out of a product, the better. This marketing strategy has been successful; last year, says Thomas, "wellness" cookies and crackers did over $1 billion worth of sales, up 70 percent from the year before.

The people at SnackWell's are working on getting the calories out of the cookies, too. Getting the fat out of a product was a great challenge, says McFeaters, but making a cookie with no fat or calories—essentially nothing in it at all—will be even more of a challenge. "Will there ever be a fat-free, calorie-free Oreo?" asks McFeaters. "No." Gill isn't so sure. "We've gotten out of the black box of diet food having to taste like cardboard," he says. "I think someday we'll have a fat-free, low-calorie, indulgent cookie product."

SnackWell's Devil's Food and Double Fudge Cookies are already so unlike a chocolate cookie that legally they can't be called "chocolate." Without fat and without calories, could they still be called "cookies"? Or even "food"?

Fake Sugars and Fats

Artificial sweeteners and fake fats definitely are not food; they're chemicals and substances we've concocted to try to fool ourselves into thinking we're eating what we really desire. The idea behind fake sugars and fats is that if you substitute them for the real thing, you'll lose weight. That might happen if people replaced all the sugary and high-fat drinks and foods they consumed one-for-one with artificially sweetened drinks or fake-fat foods. But they don't. Despite years of attempts to formulate new technologies to foil our appetites, we seem to compensate for fake foods by eating more of other things. The net result is that artificial sweeteners and fake fats haven't helped us lose weight; they've just left us with a bad aftertaste.

Artificial sweeteners are the oldest of the fake foods we use; saccharin was invented accidentally by a graduate student at Johns Hopkins in 1879, and is about three hundred times as sweet as sugar. At the turn of the century, a St. Louis factory opened up to make saccharin, and was successful; eventually, it became the giant Monsanto Chemical Corporation. For a number of years, artificial sweeteners were mainly used by diabetics, who bought the products in drugstores. But sales of artificial sweeteners and saccharin-sweetened foods expanded to dieters in the 1950s, particularly after 1951, when Tillie

Lewis launched her Tasti-Diet line of artificially sweetened peaches, puddings, jellies, and chocolate sauce. By 1957, Avis De Voto, a cookbook editor, wrote to Julia Child saying she was depressed by the manuscripts she was getting for diet cookbooks. There wasn't a single honest recipe in the bunch, she wrote. "Everything is bastardized and quite nasty. Desserts . . . are sweetened with saccharine and topped with imitation whipped cream! Fantastic! And I do believe a lot of people in this country eat just like that, stuffing themselves with faked materials in the fond belief that by substituting a chemical for God's good food they can keep themselves slim."[5]

From 1959 to 1961, sales of those chemicals—saccharin and cyclamates—tripled. Over the years, as dieting became more popular, the market for artificial sweeteners kept on growing, despite occasional health scares. Aspartame, the sweetener in Equal which is 180 times sweeter than sugar, was introduced in 1981, and by 1984 Americans were drinking its equivalent of 400,000 tons of sugar. During that time, actual sugar consumption fell about 1.15 million tons, to 8 million tons. Fake sugars haven't made much of a dent in the real sugar market; we've become so accustomed to artificial sweeteners that we use them in addition to sugar, and our real sugar consumption has climbed up again. Diet soft drinks have grown to take up half the soft-drink market (each of us drinks an average of 14 gallons of diet soft drinks per year), but soft drinks that contain sugar have never declined. Our appetites for sweets, real or fake, seem insatiable: last year, the average American ate 65 pounds of sugar, and 20 to 25 pounds of low-cal sweetener.[6]

Despite the fact that some health groups, such as the Center for Science in the Public Interest, remain suspicious of artificial sweeteners—studies feeding relatively large quantities to rats show that aspartame produces tumors and saccharin causes bladder cancer—most Americans accept the chemicals as safe. Today, according to John LaRosa of Marketdata Enterprises, we spend $1.4 billion a year on sugar substitutes, and $15.5 billion on artificially flavored soft drinks.

All the low-calorie soft drinks we're swigging seem to make no difference to our weight, though. In one study of almost 80,000 women aged fifty to sixty conducted by physicians associated with the American Cancer Society, those who used artificial sweeteners gained more weight over a year than those who ate sugar. The difference in weight wasn't very large—less than 1.5 pounds more—and may not show that the sweeteners cause people to gain weight (although some people speculate that the sweetness stimulates the appetite). Other studies have shown no difference in the amount of weight people lose on diets whether they're allowed to drink artificial sweeteners or not. What's clear, though, is that artificial sweeteners don't help people lose weight.

Animals don't lose weight on fake sugars, either. They seem to know how many calories they need to eat, whether or not their drinks are sweetened with artificial sweetener or sugar. In one study, monkeys were first given sugar solutions to drink, and they compensated for the calories by eating less monkey chow. When the animals were given a drink sweetened with aspartame, they ate less chow for a brief time, they quickly resumed eating the same amount they had before. Humans' eating habits aren't as finely tuned as monkeys'—what we think we've eaten and what we believe we should eat gets in the way of sensing how much food we've actually put away—but our bodies, too, know when we're being fooled. Our minds, however, keep on believing the ads for sweeteners and diet sodas, thinking that somehow these products will make us as thin as artificial sweetener spokeswoman Jamie Lee Curtis, or as that model in a bikini sipping diet Coke.[7]

By now, most obesity researchers have come to accept that artificial sweeteners make very little difference in how much people weigh. So they've shifted their attention to fake fats. The great hope, particularly since the fat substitute olestra was approved by the FDA in January 1996 for use in snack foods, is that people will fill up on fat substitutes and cut their intake of fat.

Fake fats have actually been a dream of chemists for years. Ever since the turn of the century, when a Chicago manufacturer, Frederick Hoelzel, ingested coal powder, chopped glass, and sea sand to find a non-fattening dessert, the search has been on. Hoelzel finally hit on a combination of surgical cotton and fruit juice, but his cookies didn't prove to be a hit. In 1955, American Viscose scientist O. A. Battista spun some rayon in a blender and found it looked and felt like fat. For a while, people were as enthusiastic about Avicel, as it was called, as they are today about olestra. "Tests show that the new product can be used, either as a fine flourlike powder or in the whipped gel state, in almost every kind of conventional mixed food," reported *Life* magazine. "It can replace a sizable portion of the calorie-laden ingredients in candies, pretzels, and snack items without at all affecting the flavor." But when testers tried a cellulose chocolate cake, they found those promises fell flat. "None of these revolutionary products was particularly tasty," said *Consumer Reports*. Nor did they keep people from wanting to eat more. "There is no clear evidence that the presence of a gelatinous mass . . . will really reduce the stomach's hunger contractions."[8]

Since the fake-fat technology was still half-baked, a few diet experts over the years advised readers to try indigestible fats to lose weight instead. In her book *Diet Without Despair* (1943), Marion White (also the author of *Sweets Without Sugar*) advised her readers to try making certain substitutions in their cooking. "It's an old trick to make mayonnaise with mineral oil instead of olive oil—for mineral oil adds no calories to the diet," she wrote. "So we use this same trick in other recipes. We use mineral oil, sparingly, wherever we can substitute it for heavy fats and shortenings."[9] Mineral oil is mainly sold as a laxative, causes gas, bloating, diarrhea, and other gastrointestinal distress, and is labeled with warnings to that effect. As unappealing as the thought of consuming mineral oil sounds to us today, olestra—while much more sophisticated and palatable—is based on the same idea, with many of the same effects.

Procter & Gamble, which spent more than $200 million getting olestra approved, has assured consumers that the fake fat is not only safe but will help them reduce the percentage of fat calories in their diet. It almost sounds too good to be true: brownie squares with only 50 calories instead of 185; a handful of potato chips with 67 calories instead of 155; chocolate ice cream with half the calories and all the super-premium fatty taste.

Olestra—the trade name is Olean—is unlike any other fake food ever invented. Instead of being a small additive to something we're used to eating, as artificial sweeteners are, it's a major new component of food and, potentially, of our diets. It's a whole new food group—or non-food group, actually—which is why the FDA approval process took several years. Olestra is not food, in the sense that food is something you eat that gives you energy. Olestra is just something that travels through your digestive system for the sake of the ride. It is fat, however: olestra is a synthetic chemical composed of sugar and vegetable oil, so it tastes, heats, and smells just like fat. "Olestra delivers virtually identical taste and textural properties in foods as fat," says

Wendy Jacques of Procter & Gamble (though some tasters at *Time* magazine reported that olestra potato chips have an aftertaste and feel "cloggy" going down the throat). But the chemical is so large that it can't be digested like ordinary fat. "The enzymes in the stomach can't wrap their arms around the olestra molecule, so it isn't absorbed," she explains. So as far as the body is concerned, olestra has no calories.

But will olestra actually help people lose weight? As with fat-free products and artificial sweeteners, people will probably compensate for olestra by eating more calories elsewhere in their diets. Procter & Gamble hasn't studied the question extensively; there's only been one study, lasting three weeks, on olestra and weight loss in lean men, and never a study involving target consumers, who are women who want to lose weight.[10] In the study on young lean men, Barbara Rolls of Pennsylvania State University found that when the men ate biscuits and margarine made with olestra for breakfast, they ate more carbohydrates later on in the day to make up for the calories they missed. Allowed to choose fats at lunch, they ate the same amount as they usually would, but no more. The total calories they ate were the same, but the fat content of their meals declined. "Fat substitutes help you reduce your fat intake, but if your goal is to reduce calories or try to watch your weight, they're not going to help very much," says Rolls. She said no one knows whether olestra will actually reduce the fat content in dieter's daily totals, since many dieters regulate their eating habits differently from lean men. As with fat-free snacks, olestra may get in the way of people trying to change their preferences from high-fat to low-fat foods, and encourage them to eat more fat elsewhere in their diet. "We have to be aware that some people will eat those foods as an excuse to eat other high-fat foods," Rolls says.[11]

Beyond the question of weight loss, olestra raises some messy health issues. As it passes through the digestive system, olestra doesn't leave the body unchanged. It vacuums up fat-soluble vitamins—A, D, E, and K—along the way. Procter & Gamble has convinced the FDA that it has solved this problem by fortifying olestra products with these vitamins; there are only so many nutrients olestra can absorb, so if it's satiated from the beginning, it won't absorb any more from the body on its way through. However, olestra also keeps the body from absorbing carotenoids, nutrients found in vegetables and fruits that many researchers believe help lower the risk of cancer and heart disease. Procter & Gamble isn't adding carotenoids to their products, though, because they say there isn't enough solid proof that they really prevent disease. Fifty researchers raised their concerns about how olestra may undo the health benefits of carotenoids to the FDA before the substance was approved, pointing to a stack of epidemiological studies that have found that diets rich in carotenoids are associated with lower risk of cancer. The FDA approved olestra anyway, with five out of twenty of the committee members expressing strong reservations about its safety.

The problem with olestra that will be most obvious to consumers is that its ride through the digestive tract is a rather bumpy one. Because olestra isn't asorbed in the intestines, the gastrointestinal tract protests its presence there loudly, with cramps, flatulence, loose stools, and sometimes severe diarrhea. In one study, volunteers who tested olestra found that their bowels became so loose they ended up with stained underpants. To counter this concern, Procter & Gamble made olestra more solid, but there are still complaints about the underpants problem. Two words frequently overheard at the FDA hearings on olestra sum up why it may be wise to avoid the fat substitute altogether: anal leakage.

Procter & Gamble says that anyone who experiences gastrointestinal distress after eating olestra will just stop eating the products, so it's really no problem. But perhaps they don't know dieters very well: Some women who thought that drinking laxative-laced dieter's tea would help them lose weight, for instance, didn't stop, in spite of severe diarrhea, until they died of potassium depeletion.

Olestra may be an example of one food—a non-food—that really is inherently "bad." But it does offer the promise of guilt-free bingeing. "Olestra won't do much in terms of the national diet or the national weight," says Harvey Levenstein, a social historian who writes about eating. "It will for a while at least do something about the national feeling of guilt."

Real Food

There is so much emphasis on faux fat foods and "wellness" snacks in this country that it sometimes seems hard to find real, healthful food—fruits, vegetables, grains, and good bread. Anyone who travels much in this country outside of big cities knows that it's often difficult to find a nutritionally satisfying meal. "You can practically starve to death on the road," says a vegetarian friend of mine who travels frequently.

On a recent trip in the rural Southwest, a friend and I were having a hard time one day finding anything we wanted to eat for dinner. We aren't especially picky eaters, but we don't usually eat fast food or anything deep-fried, and we like fresh fruits and vegetables. One restaurant in the small town we were visiting seemed promising because it advertised a salad bar; on closer inspection, the "salads" were all drenched in mayonnaise and seemed to contain nothing that had ever been picked from a plant. Deciding to cook instead, we stopped at a small grocery store where the only fresh produce we found were onions and some elderly bananas. The shelves were stocked with several low-fat, "healthy" cookies and breakfast bars, but we weren't in the mood for sugary snacks.

On the way out of town, we passed another store. "Lo-cal fruit," the hand-lettered sign said. I was outraged. Can you *believe*, I asked my friend, that we're so obsessed with low-calorie and fat-free foods in this country that way out here in the middle of nowhere they're advertising fruit, which has never had many calories to begin with, as *lo-cal* fruit?

He nodded at me, pulled the car around, and stopped in front of the store. "It's *local* fruit," he said, not trying very hard to suppress a smile. Sure enough, inside we found some beautiful zucchini and tomatoes, freshly picked from a nearby garden.

So it is possible, after all—whatever our obsessions—to find real, healthful food in this country. But fruits and vegetables, which offer a cornucopia of health benefits, fade in the nation's nutritional consciousness because no one's pouring money into ads for red peppers or broccoli. In 1992, the National Cancer Institute spent $400,000 on a campaign to get us to improve our health by eating more fruits and vegetables. That year, Kellogg's spent $32 million just to advertise Sugar Frosted Flakes. As a result, while Americans have gone wild eating fat-free products, they aren't eating any more fruits and vegetables, which contain disease-fighting properties that can't be bought in a bottle or box. The U.S. government's food pyramid recommends we eat at least five servings of fruits and vegetables a day; most Americans eat only three.[12] On any given day, one in ten adults doesn't eat any fruits or vegetables at all.[13] If we focused on the positive foods we could add to our diet, instead of the negative ones we should take out, we'd be in much better shape, physically and gastronomically.

But the food industry is much more interested in making snacks that have no fat—and less and less taste—that we can guiltlessly over-consume, buying boxes galore, but still feel we're indulging ourselves. The goal is to someday make a "food" that has no fat or calories at all so we can eat with absolute promiscuity.

In a small town just outside New York City, in her garden that stretches to the banks of the Hudson River, I visited Joan Gussow, a professor emeritus of nutrition education at Columbia University Teachers College. She studied a SnackWell's Devil's Food Cookie Cake I had given her. "Do I have to eat this?" she asked. "I'm not sure I'll have an appetite after this." She read the list of ingredients. "They've got no fat, no cholesterol, no saturated fat, less than one gram of fiber. . . . They don't have anything in them! It's amazing!"

She called to her husband Alan, an artist, who was harvesting egg-plant, chilies, and pumpkin-colored habanero peppers from their tidy, overflowing garden. "Do you want to taste this? I know you don't. Come taste it." She bit off a piece. "It's not awful," she said. "It's not anything. At least it's not artificial." Her husband tried a bite of hers. "Three of the first four ingredients are sugar," she informed him. "It's very sweet," he said, contemplating. "Where's the plastic? It has plastic overtones." He shook off the taste and showed his wife two per-fect, gleaming peppers with hints of red, explaining that one was a *corno de toro* and the other a *poblano*.

Joan Gussow, strong, youthful, and sun-weathered at 70 (Alan died in 1997), doesn't eat much that comes in boxes and cellophane. She grows most of her own vegetables in her garden, eats seasonally, and fills out her diet with fruits, some meat, cheese, butter and olive oil, and grains. "I just eat food, real whole food," she says. "I never count calories or nutrients."

She knows that most people can't grow their own food, but she insists that if Americans could just eat *real* food—the kind our ances-tors consumed, not the highly processed, fatty, sugary, artificial snacks and convenience foods we're used to—we would get perfectly adequate nutrition and probably be thinner, because our bodies seem to be naturally programmed to crave the kinds and amounts of foods we need. But when foods are not what they seem—when a fat-tasting food has no real fat—our bodies get confused. Ultimately, we stop trusting our bodies and start relying on other information, such as counting calories and fat grams, to determine what to eat, which throws everything out of whack. We end up eating mentally, instead of relying on our body's regulating signals that tell us we're hungry or satisfied.

One of the reasons some people overeat, Gussow said, pointing to the bright green SnackWell's box on her lap, is that processed foods are so deeply unfulfilling; when the body doesn't get what it wants, it keeps trying, eating until it feels satisfied. She recalled an essay back in 1954 by Philip Wylie, in which he described how one teaspoon of his mother-in-law's wild strawberry jam entirely satisfied his jam desire. "But, of the average tinned or glass-packed strawberry jam, you need half a cupful to get the idea of what you're eating," he wrote. People overeat, he said, out of an unconscious hope of trying to satisfy the cravings of their frustrated taste buds. "In the days when good-tasting food was the rule in the American home, obesity wasn't such a national curse."[14]

Americans are starving for real food, hungry for meals that are prepared soulfully, are eaten with others, and satisfy more than just a momentary desire to relieve boredom with a hit of sugar or salt. Why is it that the French and the Italians don't have the problem with obesity that Americans have? Some claim the answer's in the wine or the olive oil. They may also be less sedentary, and certainly have different genes. But those cultures also have a tradition of eating food with love, not promiscuity; they eat with ritual, not haste; they understand that food comes from the ground, not the grocery store. My Italian friends, for instance, wouldn't dream of touching a SnackWell's cookie. They would shake their heads at the poverty of our taste and technology; they would much rather not eat at all.

The next day, for lunch, I grilled the eggplant, *poblano* chilies, and green peppers the Gussows had given me with some olive oil, garlic, salt and pepper. Each mouthful was loaded with crisp, complicated, intense flavors that took me back to the expansive light in their garden by the river. After lunch, full and content, I still wanted a little something sweet. I went to the corner store and found a fresh, unpackaged brownie, made with real vanilla, butter, and Belgian chocolate.

One bite and I knew the rich, smooth, creamy brownie with bursts of slightly bitter chocolate chips was exactly what I'd desired. Three bites and I was satisfied. It was enough; I put the rest away for another time.

Chapter 5

Were You Good This Week?
Commercial Diet Groups

The first time I went to Weight Watchers, I was in junior high. Each week, I lined up in front of the scale with women who wore flimsy summer dresses and thongs in the dead of winter in order to weigh less. Actually, the line started at the bathroom, which everyone visited first to make sure they didn't weigh an ounce too much, some of them even spitting in the sink. At Weight Watchers, I entered a world where food is measured in exchanges, and feelings are charted on worksheets ("where and why I ate"). I learned a rigid system of eating and behavior; some foods were "legal," others were "illegal." If you strayed from the eating plan, the consequences were clear. You could end up like the really fat women in the class, sentenced to be "lifetime members" not because they'd succeeded at getting to their goal weight but because they'd failed, over and over again.

I joined—and dropped out—several times, and each time, I would start out being good. I liked coming to the meetings, at first, because I was serious about losing weight and wanted some support, and also because Weight Watchers was the only place where I felt thin. I would listen intently to the leader's *Good Housekeeping*-style nuggets of advice, participate in the discussions ("How to Avoid Sabotaging Yourself," "Staying Legal on Vacation"), clip coupons for Weight Watchers products, and, after a few weeks, proudly go up front to collect my 10-

pound pin. But soon after, I would hit the dreaded Plateau. I stopped losing weight and lost interest instead. I got tired of weighing, measuring, and writing down every little thing I put in my mouth, all the while dreaming of ice-cream sandwiches. At the meetings, I would move to the back, or show up just long enough to be weighed. Then I would quit, gain the weight back, and, when I was disgusted enough with myself, think about joining again.

It took a long time before I realized that the regain was an inevitable part of the whole deal, and that Weight Watchers, Jenny Craig, Nutri/System, and all the other commercial diet centers are making a fortune out of yo-yo dieting. Commercial diets, like most other diets, don't work in the long run for most people. Despite the scales, rules, rewards, and outside vigilance offered at diet centers, most members eventually end up dropping out and regaining the weight. They keep coming back, though: Each time they've joined, they've felt the first flush of success that comes with losing a few pounds, so they think the program works. Later, when they stop losing weight, they blame themselves—not the program—and resolve to try harder next time to follow the rules.

The commercial weight-loss companies know that this is how people use their services. Jenny Craig even had an advertisement once that compared dieting with having your hair done, something you just have to keep doing over and over again to keep it up. But yo-yo dieting isn't a very healthy form of weight control. It takes its toll on your pocketbook, your self-esteem, and your body. Several studies have shown that the physical stresses of repeatedly gaining and losing weight are linked with early deaths. Other studies have found that yo-yo dieting inevitably leads to bingeing and depression.[1]

Recently, though, I heard that diet programs had changed since I dropped out. There was a new emphasis on "healthy eating," "lifestyle changes," and sensible, long-term health habits. Friends were praising Weight Watchers for its sound nutrition advice and flexible eating plan. Indeed, a personalized Weight Watchers ad that came in my mail—"Make the decision that can change your life forever, Laura!"—promised that its new plan offered more care, more help, and better, more flexible choices. "Weight Watchers suits your lifestyle even more, Laura! You really owe it to yourself to give it another try . . . today!" Other friends swore by Jenny Craig because it was so convenient.

Just from the looks of their promotional literature, I could tell that diet programs had changed. They aren't just diets anymore. Diet has become a four-letter word in the commercial weight-loss business; now they're all "food plans" or "lifestyle programs." Their pitches emphasize permanent changes instead of quick fixes, backed up with classes on behavior modification, exercise tips, and individualized counseling. Weight Watchers has an ad describing "Why Weight Watchers *doesn't* want you to diet," featuring a woman who lost 88 pounds and kept it off for six years ("Results not typical"). It has added a simple "fat and fiber" food plan for their members who, like so many women, are more interested in counting fat grams than weighing cheese slices. The "New" Nutri/System offers more meal choices at a cheaper price, a "Personal Solutions" counseling approach that covers stress and coping techniques, and optional sessions with personal exercise trainers. The Diet Center monitors your body composition and works on improving your ratio of lean body mass to fat. Jenny Craig offers weekly lifestyle classes, exercise tips, and extensive behavior worksheets to go along with its prescribed meal plans. All of them sell maintenance plans, where clients switch from diet foods and are supposedly taught how to eat "normally" for the rest of their lives.

The repackaging certainly looked sophisticated. It had to: the commercial diet center industry has taken a dive in recent years, with revenues slacking off by about 15 percent per year. In 1994 alone, Weight Watchers lost $50 million, though attendance at meetings began to pick up again in 1995 after the company spent $30 million on an ad campaign featuring former TV anchorwoman Kathleen Sullivan. The commercial weight-loss center industry—of which Weight Watchers is by far the leader—made $2.1 billion in 1991, which dropped to about $1.6 billion by 1995. The bigger companies are squeezing out the small ones, and several franchises are closing. But commercial diet programs aren't about to die out: there are still 10,018 weight-loss centers in the country, or one for every 25,953 people.[2] To put that in perspective, Sondra Solovay, a writer for the San Francisco–based *Fat!So?*, recently counted fifty-five weight-loss centers listed in the Oakland, California, Yellow Pages, compared with one battered women's service.

One reason commercial diet companies are having problems is that they received a lot of bad publicity in the early nineties. In 1990, as we saw earlier, Senator Ron Wyden of Oregon held congressional hearings about weight-loss centers, exposing their unfair business practices, poorly trained employees, high failure rates, and the health problems experienced by some people who had enrolled, such as gallstones and bulimia.[3] Those hearings led to a Federal Trade Commission investigation of commercial diet companies' deceptive ads—especially those misleading "Sixty pounds in sixty days!" testimonials—which resulted in new guidelines for those ads. Companies can no longer claim that an extraordinary weight loss is typical, or promise that weight stays off permanently (now they put "Results not typical" in fine print at the bottom of the ad).

In 1991, in New York City, the Department of Consumer Affairs (DCA) sent undercover investigators to commercial weight-loss centers and found that they counseled underweight individuals to lose weight, refused to discuss the potential risks of weight loss, and made false and misleading health claims. The DCA issued a report showing that although commercial weight-loss sales representatives lead consumers to believe they'll have long-term success in losing weight, most gain the weight back. "A plan for long-term maintenance is nearly always stressed by the weight loss centers," the report described. "What is not discussed, however, is that studies have shown that the majority of overweight people who lose weight regain it back within a few years." During the 1990s, hundreds of people also sued Nutri/System, claiming that the diet caused them serious gallbladder problems (rapid weight loss can cause gallstones when cholesterol-saturated bile collects in the gallbladder). Most of the cases were either won by the diet company or settled out of court, but they didn't help the company's reputation—or its coffers.

More than anything, though, the commercial diet industry is flagging because consumers are tired of prepackaged diet food, weekly meetings, and food exchanges (two milk exchanges per day, three fat exchanges, five protein exchanges, etc.), and many have become convinced that diets don't work. It's the fresher approaches—the gurus who market diets in the guise of not dieting, the doctors who sell gimmicky high-protein diet books or promote prescription diet pills—that are attracting attention. Those who devise commercial diet programs are learning that they have to adapt to the current consumer climate, in which monitoring grams of fat and minutes on the exercise machines have replaced counting calories, and come up with aggressive new marketing strategies to survive.

Some are trying to squeeze into the health care industry as part of "wellness" teams, making deals with health clubs, hospitals, and health care professionals. Weight Watchers, for instance, had a deal with Blue Cross in Philadelphia in which the health care company reimbursed clients for part of their membership if they reached their goal. In 1995, Nutri/System started NutriRX, where clients can get prescription diet drugs along with their weekly weigh-ins. Unfazed when the fenfluramine-phentermine combination they were prescribing to anyone with about 20 pounds to lose was pulled off the market, doctors there immediately began prescribing phentermine and Prozac (phen-Pro) to clients—though it, too, is an untested drug combination.

The diet companies are targeting new markets outside their traditional client base of fairly affluent, young to middle-aged white women. They're reaching out, in particular, to African American and Latina women, and, to a lesser extent, men. An increasing portion of the $78 million diet companies spend on advertising is being directed toward these groups (company representatives won't say how much, only that they're doing more ads aimed at minority women). African American and Latina women are more likely to be overweight than white women, several studies have shown, and are less likely to attend commercial diet groups, so the diet companies see them as a lucrative potential market.

Black and Latina women tend to be much less obsessed about their weight than white women. In one University of Arizona study of teenage girls, for instance, 90 percent of the white girls were unhappy with their weight, but 70 percent of the African American girls were satisfied with their bodies the way they were.[4] The white girls defined "beauty" as being five foot seven and 100 to 110 pounds—the size of waif model Kate Moss. The black girls had much more realistic attitudes, describing proportions that were closer to what real women look like, with big hips and strong thighs. More importantly, they said that looking good has more to do with having the "right attitude" than the right body. If the diet companies have anything to do with it, women of color will change their largely positive attitudes about body size. Many Weight Watchers and Jenny Craig ads now feature black women, encouraging them to become as neurotic about their weight as upper-middle-class white women.

Since weight concerns are more closely correlated with class than race—professional black and Latina women tend to be thinner and have higher rates of eating disorders than poorer women—diet company advertisers are especially targeting upwardly aspiring minority women with the message that they're not going to make it in the professional world unless they lose weight. Like everyone else who goes to commercial diet programs, most of these women won't lose weight permanently, but the depressing feeling that they *should* will stay with them. One of Jenny Craig's TV commercials makes it seem that the well-educated, articulate, attractive, and barely overweight African American woman in the ad won't be able to find a job unless she loses weight to become the size of the predominantly white ideal.

Finally, in an effort to boost their credibility and expand their market, both Jenny Craig and Weight Watchers contributed $1 million to former Surgeon General C. Everett Koop's 1994 "Shape Up America" campaign, which loudly publicized the health risks of obesity, suggesting that more Americans need to diet (apparently 50 million of us aren't enough). In exchange, Jenny Craig was photographed smiling next to the eminent Koop in an eleven-page advertising supplement in *Time* magazine, and both companies began displaying the "Shape Up America" seal of approval on their ads. (Nancy Glick of "Shape Up America" admits that the Jenny Craig photo shoot was a mistake. "That was awful," she says, and explained that they no longer allow Koop to have his photo taken with sponsors.) The commercial weight-loss companies received other benefits from their generous contributions: the "Shape Up America" report gave the commercial diet industry a shot in the arm when it comes to their role in health care. It suggested that companies should pay for their employees' weight-loss programs, and that health insurance companies should give reduced premiums or rebates for those who enter these commercial programs.

With all this new hoopla about commercial weight-loss programs, I decided to check them out again. At Weight Watchers, the diet hadn't changed much, but the meeting was quicker and more business-like; the lecture seemed to be scripted by a team of psychologists instead of made up by the leader. Everyone received coupons for Weight Watchers products, and there was a pitch for the pre-made

Personal Cuisine products (Weight Watchers leaders get a commission from the products they sell). Still, there was an intimate group feeling at times, when longtime members stood up to show off their "before" photos.

At Nutri/System, the poor counselor had found her way into the wrong job: she told me I looked great the way I was, then went through the diet and foods available with a complete lack of enthusiasm. At the Diet Center, a white-coated counselor gave me a lecture about how it's body fat, not weight, that counts, then weighed me and gave me a diet. I spent the most time at Jenny Craig, where there is a strong emphasis on "one to one" support.

"Step up on the scale," said Suzie,* the young and hyper-cheerful Jenny Craig center director who was giving me my first consultation, which was free. As at the weight-loss programs I attended in junior high, the scale was king here. Suzie had just shown me her "before" photo, at 194 pounds, which she kept in the pocket of her white lab coat. I climbed up on the scale. I hadn't weighed myself in a long time, so I was a little nervous. The little marker crept past 140, 145, . . . then the big marker had to be shifted to 150. Fear welled up as the little marker kept sliding to the right, finally balancing at 165 pounds.

"One hundred sixty-five," Suzie announced brightly, as the guilty fat girl I grew up with suddenly took up residence in my body again. I forgot I was wearing thick-soled boots and a heavy winter jacket, cargo pockets stuffed with my wallet, keys, and a personal stereo. "Don't worry," Suzie consoled me. "You'll never see that weight again." Despite my years of swearing off dieting—my certain knowledge that it makes me obsess over food and ultimately eat more—all I wanted at that moment was to lose weight.

Suzie typed my height, weight, and wrist size (to determine my body frame) into a computer. "Your goal range is one hundred twenty to one hundred thirty-three pounds." The computer looked more sophisticated than the old Metropolitan Life height-weight chart, but it actually relies on the very same data. Most obesity experts these days say that chart, which almost all the weight programs use (because it makes more people look like they need to lose weight), is

*An asterisk indicates that names have been changed.

outdated and encourages the wrong people to diet. The government's 1995 *Dietary Guidelines for Americans* loosens the belt a little bit. The guidelines are based on research saying that for their height, women can weigh as much as men, so long as they carry their weight around their hips and thighs. (It's the apple-shaped people, not the pear-shaped ones like me, who face higher risks of cardiovascular disease, cancer, diabetes, and the like.) Many people dispute the notion of weight guidelines at all, saying that weight is very individual, and fat people who exercise can be as healthy as thin people. By the standards of the 1995 *Dietary Guidelines*, I could weigh up to 155 pounds and still be considered perfectly healthy.

"What goal would you like to pick?" asked Suzie. I had no idea; I thought my bones alone weighed more than 120. "Whatever you like," she said. "We're here for you." Given the choice, I picked the heaviest weight, 133 pounds. A graph of my projected weight loss appeared on the screen, and Suzie talked about it as if it were a done deal—she was selling me quick and easy weight loss. "Does March 12th ring a bell for you? Is that a special day, a wedding or anything?" she asked. "That's when you'll be halfway to your goal." She was assuming I'd automatically lose 2 pounds a week. She pressed another button. "On June 4, you'll be thin. Just in time for summer!"

Then Suzie showed me around the facilities, which had more of the atmosphere of a high-tech clinic than the homey Weight Watchers meeting rooms of my youth. That, along with the white lab coats, was supposed to inspire my confidence that these were trained professionals I was dealing with. Beyond the requisite bulletin board of "before" and "after" photos, there were examining rooms where counselors hold twenty-minute weekly sessions with clients to go over food diaries and sell new meals. The emphasis was meant to be on individual support, but it seemed to me most effective as an intimate sales technique. (At Jenny Craig, as at other weight-loss programs, counselors are paid $5–$10 an hour, and commissions from sales of foods and programs make up as much as 50 percent of their income.)

Next, Suzie pointed out the storage area with freezers full of prepackaged foods. You don't have the option of using real food from the supermarket on Jenny Craig, she explained; you have to buy their meals at first. If you follow the plan, Suzie told me, it adds up to about 1,000 to 1,200 calories a day. Later, on maintenance—if they make it that far—clients can add calories and begin including real food in the menu.

Jenny Craig's diet, like diets at other commercial weight-loss programs, is what researchers call a semi-starvation diet. For all the new packaging, these diets remain fundamentally unchanged from when I first went to Weight Watchers. Whether the calories are consumed in milkshakes, prepackaged microwave meals, or precisely measured exchanges of real food, they all add up to 1,000 to 1,200 calories a day. This is a level that is low enough to produce weight loss in most people, whatever their size, but high enough (over 800 calories) to avoid most of the negative health effects of low-calorie starvation diets, such as hair loss, fainting, weakness, headaches, nausea, aching muscles, cold intolerance, loss of lean tissue, muscle cramps, cardiac disorders, and sometimes death.

Most semi-starvation diets promise a weight loss of up to 2 pounds a week. All ignore piles of research which say that calorie levels should be individually tailored to people's different sizes, metabolic rates, and activity levels. The idea that a five-foot-nine-inch woman who exercises every day should eat the same number of calories, fat grams, or food exchanges as a five-foot-two-inch woman who never strays from her desk, car, or couch is absurd. Despite their emphasis on the latest scientific methods in weight loss, diet companies' pseudoscientific premise that everyone should weigh the same amount for their height and eat the same number of calories no matter their size or activity level is actually quite Victorian.

How many people who walk in the door reach their goal weight and keep it off? I asked Suzie. She smiled. "Oh," she said. "We don't keep statistics on that."

Since the emphasis at Jenny Craig is on one-on-one counseling, I asked Suzie whether any of the counselors were trained outside the company. Many, she said, had backgrounds in exercise, psychology, and nutrition; she herself was a college student with a minor in the field (and a major in business). Her grasp of nutrition was rather weak—she threw vague nutrition terms around with abandon and told me curious theories about why fat cells remain "open" for a year after one loses weight—but her business sense was much better. The point to her theory about fat cells taking a year to close down was that I should sign up for the more expensive, year-long maintenance plan.

"How many people who walk in the door reach their goal weight and keep it off?" I pressed her.

Suzie smiled. "You're going to do just great," she said. "Our success rate is much better than any other weight-loss program. It's ninety-six percent."

There are no statistics to back up Suzie's claim. In fact, there are no data behind any commercial weight-loss program's promises that for your money—and lots of it—you will lose weight and keep it off. The consensus among most obesity experts is quite the opposite: the overwhelming majority of people who go on semi-starvation diets will eventually regain their weight. In *Consumer Reports*' 1993 survey of 19,000 readers who had used a commercial diet program, most reported that they stayed on the programs for about half a year and lost 10 to 20 percent of their starting weight. The average dieter then gained back almost half of that weight six months after ending the program, and more than two-thirds after two years. In fact, *Consumer Reports* said its readers were less satisfied with diet programs than with any other commercial service they'd ever tested.

Weight Watchers can only point to its meeting leaders as representatives of its success. Despite numerous requests for data about their programs from government task forces and obesity researchers, diet companies have refused to let anyone know how many of the people who pass through their doors actually succeed in losing weight and keeping it off. "Weight Watchers has no statistics," said Barbara Moore, former general manager of program development for the company, who now works for Shape Up America. "We've never been legally required to collect such statistics, and it's very expensive to do. That cost would get passed along to the consumer."

But skeptics wonder that a billion-dollar company doesn't keep better track of its business. "Do you really think that Weight Watchers doesn't *know*?" the eating disorders expert and psychologist David Garner asked me, studying me from behind his little round glasses as if he'd just encountered a rare case of naïve dementia. "You think they don't collect data? If they had positive data, it would be the best advertising strategy possible. They could prove their long-term results. They could make critics like me shut up. So why do you think they say they don't have any data?" I shrugged. It would, um, be bad for business? Their statistics prove that their programs don't work? Garner nodded. It's likely that practically the only people who have kept weight off are the Weight Watchers leaders, the ones who have quite literally made a career of dieting.

Jenny Craig claims it has better success than other programs, based on dubious research. The company published one 1992 study, in the journal *Addictive Behaviors*, which found that 82 percent of their clients who reached their goals remained within 10 percent of that weight a year later.[5] But the study was based on surveys mailed to 517 clients a year after they completed the program. Of those, half responded, and you have to assume that the ones who threw their surveys in the trash were more likely to be the ones who weren't anxious to report that they'd gained weight. You also have to imagine that some of the other respondents were engaged in wishful thinking. The study (which was conducted by an employee of Jenny Craig, not independent researchers) relied on the self-reported weights of the clients; when Jenny Craig weighed some of those clients themselves, the success rate dropped to 64 percent. If they had continued to the study past a year, it's likely the success rate would drop much further. Most importantly, the study did not address how many people who began the program reached their goal.

From the view of ex-counselors, that's the significant number. One former counselor I talked with, who worked at Jenny Craig for over a year said, "Most of my clients quit well before reaching their goal weight. They dropped out from frustration, boredom with the food, and the work it takes to keep this up." Another ex-counselor estimated that in the year and a half he worked at the company, he saw nearly two hundred clients. "Three or five people reached their goal weight, and of those I don't know if any of them kept it off," he said. "The success rate is so low it's incredible."

Weight-loss companies are quick to attribute failures to a lack of willpower—how can you be successful if you drop out?—but more and more evidence suggests they may be blaming the victim. Physically, semi-starvation diets seem to increase the urge to overeat. The body isn't getting the energy it needs, and clamors for more food. The situation has very little to do with willpower, or how good you were at sticking to the maintenance program. "Rats that get put on Weight Watchers–type diets lose weight, too, and gain it all back again after they stop," says David Garner. Dieting may also depress the metabolic rate, he says, making it easier to gain weight the next time around.

Psychologically, telling people exactly what and when to eat often backfires. It makes them feel overcontrolled, and puts them out of touch with when they're actually hungry or full. "Diets require a person to ignore her body," says Janet Polivy, a psychologist at the University of Toronto who has studied how dieting causes bingeing. "In order to succeed at a restrictive diet, you have to ignore hunger, which means you also wind up ignoring satiety. Your eating cues and emotions get completely out of whack." Polivy says dieters who are out of touch with their hunger tend to overeat more frequently in response to emotional, rather than physical cues. They stray from the diet, feel they've "blown it," get upset, and overeat—often gaining weight.

Even Weight Watchers, which many people tout as the best of the diet centers because of its reliance on real, fresh food and flexible menu choices, doesn't help people learn to develop a sense of inner competence about eating. "What it comes down to is the issue of trust versus control," says the nutritionist Ellyn Satter, author of *How to Get Your Kid to Eat . . . But Not Too Much*, who treats what she calls "dieting casualties" in her practice. She believes that people need to learn to trust that they will get full, even on food they consider highly desirable, and know that they can reliably regulate their own food intake, rather than depending on outside rules to manage those choices. "Weight Watchers is pretty good at liberalizing food choices, teaching people how to eat attentively, and encouraging them to increase the variety of food in their diet," says Satter. "But it's still fundamentally a control stance they use." When people rely on outside rules, scales, and diet cops to regulate their eating, their relationship to food remains brittle. "It's easily disrupted. These controls are unrealistic, and they will break down. At that point, the person is likely to eat chaotically."

The psychological effects of being told what to eat can also be demeaning. It is humiliating to be treated like a child who doesn't know the first thing about feeding herself (actually, all children know how to feed themselves; it's dieting and deprivation that screw us up later on). From childhood, deciding what to eat is a very personal act of individual choice and power; for an adult to be told what and how to eat takes away that sense of power. Diets make women feel like children. No wonder that many grown women rebel against them.

Most commercial diet programs started out in the 1960s as support groups, where women could offer each other encouragement, company, and a sympathetic ear. In a society that was becoming increasingly intolerant toward obesity, these groups became refuges for fat women, where they could be among others like themselves, instead of being isolated. There, they were accepted—but only as long as they promised to change.

The group support offered in diet programs, though, has usually been mixed with a strong dose of group humiliation. The first weight-loss group, "TOPS" for "Take Off Pounds Sensibly," was organized with the idea that women need to keep an eye on each other—and often a competitive one at that—in order to lose weight. Esther Manz, a Milwaukee mother of five, dreamed up this idea in 1948 while she was in her doctor's waiting room, worried about what he'd say when she got on the scale and found out she was carrying 210 pounds on her five-foot-two frame. Flipping through the magazines, she came across an article on Alcoholics Anonymous. It got her thinking about a pre-natal care class she'd taken, where members in the group were able to keep their weight down by talking together and encouraging each other (losing weight during pregnancy was a widespread goal during the 1950s). Maybe the same thing would work in a weight-loss group.

Manz told her physician about the idea, and he agreed that group therapy might just do the trick. She rounded up three fat friends—they were all over 200 pounds—and started a group, meeting each week for a year over black coffee. They all went on low-calorie diets, and cheered each other on. After a year, all had lost weight: one lost 100 pounds; Manz was down to 163; the third, still quite fat, had lost 30 pounds. Manz, who was chair of the local PTA and quite an energetic organizer, found other mothers to join the group, and soon more chapters got started. She wrote a basic manual that explained the TOPS formula. "What it amounts to," she said, "is organized will power, sugar-coated with fun and relaxation and packaged in mutual under-standing and common sense."

At the meetings, members weighed in before class, then stood in three lines: the "Good Losers"; the "Turtles," who lost weight slowly; and the "Pigs." After singing the TOPS pledge—"The more we get together the slimmer we'll be"—each person's weight gain or loss was announced, accompanied by boos or applause. The person who lost the most weight the week before pinned cardboard pigs on the gainers. The leader would turn to the gainers and repeat the ritual disapproba-tion: "These I know 'cause they look so big; these are the winners of the shameful pig!" In some groups, a gainer had to sit before a Court of Weights and Measures, defending her weight gain, eventually pleading guilty (since there is no defense for gaining weight in this court), and paying a small fine.

But despite the humiliation, TOPS members tried to keep things light. They sang songs ("Show me the way to lose weight / I'm tired of dragging it around / I had a nice shape long, long ago / But now I'm much too round"), held striptease shows where losers shed layers of their old fat clothes, and played "Calorie Baseball," where a pitcher called out the name of a food to a batter, who had to say the correct calorie value in order to make a run. TOPS had a cornball approach to weight loss, which put more emphasis on camaraderie and acceptance than on shame.

Three years after Manz started TOPS, *Life* magazine reported ("A kind of Fat Ladies Non-Anonymous helps girls to fight for their figures") that 2,500 women had joined the clubs in six states. Fifteen years later, there were 2,481 chapters, each with its own name— Button Busters, Zipper Rippers, Food Addicts, Cast-A-Weighs, Shrinking Violets, Tops Not Tubs, and Do or Dieters. Manz herself, unlike later diet organizations, collected no dues, and made no salary; the organization was entirely nonprofit (today there are 11,700 chapters in the United States and Canada, and members pay $16 a year to join, with a weekly donation of less than a dollar).[6]

One of the reasons TOPS took off in the 1950s was that obesity was increasingly being viewed as an emotional problem, not just a physical one. More and more people believed that emotions were at the heart of overeating problems, so it only made sense that group therapy might help. This was a relatively new point of view. In February 1947, in the *Journal of the American Medical Association*, Charles Freed had argued that fatness was not caused by glandular disturbances, as was widely believed, but by emotional tensions, such as worry, fear, and insecurity, which led to overeating.[7] Later that year, the psychiatrist Hilde Bruch concurred; the popular theory that fatness was due to glandular ailments was, in her view, "mostly tommyrot."

Bruch painted a psychological portrait of the obese that contrasted sharply with the image of the jolly fat person. What made people overeat, she said, was insecurity and immaturity. Fat kids often come from families where the mother is domineering and overprotecting; she coddles and overfeeds the child, who grows up with a "fundamentally low self-esteem and with the conviction of his helplessness in a world which has been represented to him as a dangerous place." Further, she told *Time* magazine, fat was a protection for woman against men, sex, and the "responsibilities of womanhood."[8]

Bruch would be a strong defender of fat people in later years, and a voice of reason in a society that would become neurotically fat-obsessed. She argued that there is a great diversity of human size, and not everyone was meant to be thin. Not everyone got fat the same way, either. For some, overeating was a compensation for stress, but it was a fairly benign one. These fat people aren't emotionally disturbed, she said, just coping with stresses in their lives in a normal and understandable way by overeating. Far more harmful, she said, was to constantly struggle to lose more weight than is natural, to be a "thin fat person." Bruch also pointed out later that many of the negative personality characteristics associated with obesity, such as depression and lethargy, are actually caused by discrimination against fatness.

But Bruch's idea that fat people overeat because of their emotions became oversimplified and popularized by a society that already viewed fat people as morally suspect. The idea that they were emotionally damaged or deranged—which many people still believe—made their condition that much more humiliating. As Roberta Seid put it, "The psychiatric model added other, more pejorative, associations with overweight. The overweight also seemed immature and infantile, riddled with unresolved psychic conflicts."[9] Research now shows that on the whole, fat people have no more emotional problems than the rest of us, except, as Bruch pointed out, that they have to deal with the depressing consequences of discrimination. Interestingly, fat people commit suicide less often than the population as a whole. Some fat people do use food as comfort and to handle stress, but so do some thin people. Some fat people have binge-eating disorders—which are often caused by dieting—and need psychological help, but others eat the same amount as normal-sized folks.

Fat people, particularly fat women, began to be viewed as childish, impulsive, overemotional, incapable, and sexually starved. In 1952, *Newsweek* described how "The Fat Personality," as the article called it, worked: "Rich desserts, sauces, and bonbons offer a delightful panacea for boredom, unhappy home conditions, a lack of business or social prestige, or sexual maladjustment. The added poundage literally cushions the overeater against the onslaughts of a too-demanding world." By 1959, the *New York Times Magazine* was reporting that 90 percent of all obesity cases were caused by "psychogenic" problems.

If obesity was caused by emotional problems, experts now believed, then it could be cured by psychological therapy. Most fat people couldn't afford individual therapy, though—and it was still regarded by most Americans as something only people who were really crazy or who lived in Manhattan engaged in—so group therapy seemed more plausible. Obesity researchers and doctors, like Esther Manz's physician, were enthusiastic about the new weight-loss groups. Most people who joined the groups didn't think of themselves as being in "therapy," but the idea that something was emotionally wrong with them, and that they needed help with their problem, was clear.

In 1960, a Los Angeles housewife known only as Roxanne S. started Overeaters Anonymous (OA), a nonprofit group based on the 12-step principles of Alcoholics Anonymous. OA took the notion that obesity was caused by psychological problems to an extreme, viewing compulsive overeating as an addiction, and a chronic disease that could only be arrested by strictly adhering to a program of "abstinence" (a strange concept with food, since you have to eat to live). In her book, *Such a Pretty Face* (1980), Marcia Millman relates comments by OA members which showed their conviction that they were suffering from a serious psychological problem. "I've learned that overeating is a death wish, suicide," said one. "Most of us are victims of an emotional illness," said another. "Most of us have a tendency toward depression. Society puts the hang-ups on us and a lot of what we're blamed for isn't our fault, but it is in a way. . . . If we treat ourselves like crap so will others."[10]

Overeaters Anonymous has spread to 10,500 groups in 47 countries. Like other diet groups, it provides a social space for isolated fat people who need someone to listen to them and hear the very difficult emotional issues that arise for fat people in this society. (The National Association to Advance Fat Acceptance, NAAFA, provides the same social space in a much more positive, playful, and self-accepting atmosphere.) Unlike other diet programs, OA is cheap and makes no claims about weight loss. But it's hard to imagine how helpful a group can be that makes physical change a barometer of psychological and spiritual well-being. Like other diet programs, OA's "abstinence" plan, while flexible (it's often a low-calorie, low-carbohydrate diet, three measured meals with nothing eaten in between), imposes external controls on eating, preventing women from learning to regulate themselves. There isn't a single prescribed diet, but there is a rigidly prescribed approach.

OA members admit their powerlessness in front of food, in their words; they recognize that their problems have been caused by their compulsive overeating, and turn to a "higher power," God or a personal religious idea, for help. Yet compulsive eaters don't really have to be powerless. If they are overeating as a result of emotional distress, there are cures. Compulsive eating is not a permanent addiction. Nor are all fat people compulsive eaters. OA meetings, designed for support, can actually make fat people feel worse about themselves, encouraging them to assign all the problems in their lives to their obesity, which is something most know deep down cannot be cured. The meetings can be like Queen for a Day, where whoever has the most self-defeating, depressing story to tell gets the loudest applause. For some members, the need for "help," in the form of spending enormous amounts of time going to meetings and being involved with members, becomes a kind of addiction in itself.

In 1963, Jean Nidetch started Weight Watchers. She had gone to the New York City Department of Health's obesity clinic in 1961, where she received a diet written by Dr. Norman Jollife. She took the diet sheet home and, like Esther Manz, started holding meetings with local housewives like herself. "I lost all that weight on the obesity clinic's diet, but I added something," she said. "I added talk." It became an opportunity for these housewives to talk about the frustrations in their lives, with the common theme that their weight had somehow caused those problems. Unlike Manz, Nidetch was a savvy businesswoman: she charged for the meetings, and became an empire.

Nidetch, like others at the time, believed that obese people are emotionally disturbed. "The fat man who constantly stuffs himself is literally killing himself. He could drop dead from a heart attack or a stroke, but even worse, he could die emotionally," she wrote in 1970 in *The Story of Weight Watchers*. "I've met fat people who were emotionally dead. I've met people who looked as if life were all over. They've given up. They're ashamed and afraid." She believed that the motivation to lose weight could only come from people bottoming out emotionally. Nidetch herself decided to lose weight after a woman in a supermarket asked her when she was due. "Most fat people need to be hurt badly before they do something about themselves," she wrote. "Something's got to happen to demoralize you suddenly and completely before you see the light."[11]

Weight Watchers' growth was phenomenal, partly because so many people already felt quite demoralized by their weight, and partly because of Nidetch's gurulike zeal. "I want to reach every obese person in existence," she wrote. "To help them learn to live like human beings." In 1964, Weight Watchers made $160,000; in 1970, it brought in $8 million.[12] In 1978, the company was bought by the H. J. Heinz Company, which greatly expanded the products line. Today, Weight Watchers is a multinational corporation, with total company revenues of about $1.6 billion, of which 65 percent comes from product sales (the meetings have really become sales vehicles for the products). There are 29,000 Weight Watchers weekly meetings in twenty-four countries; 19,000 meetings are held the United States. Since it started, 25 million people have joined Weight Watchers—and many of us, several times.[13]

Noticing Weight Watchers' tremendous success, several other diet companies opened their doors in the late 1960s and early 1970s. Diet Workshop started in 1965, Why Weight in 1966, Weight Losers Institute in 1968, Diet Center in 1971, and Nutri/System in 1971. (Jenny Craig was a latecomer, in 1983.) One of the reasons for the growth of diet groups at this time was that many women, caught in the narrow world of homemaking described by Betty Friedan in 1963 in *The Feminine Mystique*, were anxious to get out of the house and talk to other women. Many wanted to share their strange feelings of malaise. Friedan identified the source of this "problem that has no name" as women's boredom and frustration at being confined in the narrow world of fifties'-style domesticity. Jean Nidetch, who always described herself as a Formerly Fat Housewife ("FFH"), was dealing with the same feelings of depression and listlessness. She identified the problem not as trying too hard to live up to a domestic ideal but as not trying hard enough. The real problem, for her, was being fat, not fitting the mold of the ideal wife and woman, and she marketed a solution.

Losing weight, of course, wasn't the answer to the dull plight of the *Father Knows Best* housewife. But in weight-loss support groups around the country, Weight Watchers and the other diet groups made it seem that way. In her book *The Obsession: Reflections on the*

Tyranny of Slenderness (1980), Kim Chernin points out that weight-loss groups and the feminist consciousness-raising groups that started during that era arose at the same time out of a common need. In both, women gathered to make confessions about their lives and find support from other women for changes they were making. But there was a fundamental difference. In feminist groups, the point was to increase women's power, and in the weight-loss groups, it was to decrease her size—and power. "In the feminist groups the emphasis is significantly upon liberation—upon release of power, the unfettering of long-suppressed ability, the freeing of one's potential, a woman shaking off restraints and delivering herself from limitations," writes Chernin. "But in the appetite control groups the emphasis is upon restraint and prohibition, the keeping of watch over appetites and urges, the confining of impulses, the control of the hungers of the self."[14]

There is a scene in the film *The Stepford Wives* that illustrates just what Chernin is talking about. A smart photographer trapped in suburbia, played by Katharine Ross, along with her women's lib buddy, decided to try to hold a consciousness-raising group for the neighborhood wives, who have mysteriously stopped all involvement in community groups in order to make their houses spanking clean. These wives are actually suburban robots, but the new women in the neighborhood haven't realized yet what's in store for them. When the ladies gather and the session starts, one non-robot wife, played by Tina Louise of Gilligan's Island fame, gets into the spirit of things by describing how disappointing it is that her husband only loves her for the way she looks, not for who she really is. The robots gape, uncomprehendingly, then gamely try their version. One complains that she has trouble cleaning and ironing her husband's shirts, and another whispers that she's found a new product that works wonders. They are sharing and confessing, but, as at Weight Watchers meetings, they stay well within the parameters of femininity programmed by a male-dominated society.

In weight-loss groups, women try to gain power—becoming more attractive and seeming, in our culture, more disciplined, controlled, and health-conscious—by losing weight. But it is the kind of power parceled out by a society that is profoundly distrustful of women: the power and privilege that come from attaining a body that fits the socially approved mold. It's the power derived from living up to society's expectations of women as objects, and of behaving in a manner—restraining one's desires and appetites—that fits the confining rules of proper female conduct. In other words, it's not much real power at all. Just as weight-loss groups teach women to follow external rules of eating, distrusting their internal hungers, they teach them to adapt to external notions of femininity, rather than express their internal sense of self. Women in such groups are encouraged to feel dissatisfied with themselves the way they are, which leads to depression when they find they cannot change. Ultimately, when these women fail to lose weight, they feel utterly disempowered.

The message that women will become more successful when they lose weight is even more disturbing in the "new" diet centers of the nineties than it was in the sixties. Now, it isn't just that a woman who becomes thin will win the traditional goals of romance and a happy marriage. Now, the fiction is that she, like the African American woman in the Jenny Craig ad, will be able to land a successful career if, and only if, she's thin. In the sixties, the differences between feminist consciousness-raising groups and weight-loss groups were clear. Now, things are murkier, as weight-loss groups have swallowed up some of the goals and language of feminism.

The most widely shared (and least threatening) feminist belief in the sixties was in equality of opportunity in the work world—"equal pay for equal work." The nineties Weight Watcher is definitely a working woman on the fast track (as well as a savvy consumer). She only has time to zip into thirty-minute meetings, and to pop her pre-made Personal Cuisine into the microwave. She has no more time for "talk," as Jean Nidetch put it. Whatever roots in "group therapy" these weight-loss centers may have had are gone, replaced by prepackaged lectures, videos, and meetings. "In 1963, eighty-two percent of households had a working dad, a homemaker mom and kids," said one of the company's executives in a speech tucked into a 1993 press packet introducing the "new" Weight Watchers. "The demands on her time, while never light, were finite—her home, family, and perhaps even some time for herself." Now everything is changed, including those leisurely Weight Watchers meetings.

"The new Weight Watchers meeting directly targets the consumer of today," the speech goes on. "You know, that lucky woman who has a huge number of leisure and entertainment choices, but no time to enjoy them." Weight Watchers now mainly targets women who have a cosmetic 20 to 30 pounds to lose—more than a quarter of the women in the *Consumer Reports* survey who'd been to commercial weight-loss centers wouldn't be considered overweight by even the most fat-phobic of obesity researchers—and so is no longer a social space where fat people can feel comfortable. One friend of mine, who weighs more than 200 pounds, says she and the other fat woman in her class always get ignored by the leader. "They figure we're hopeless."

Weight Watchers—and other diet centers—now promote weight loss as a way for mainly normal-sized women to sharpen themselves in order to get ahead in the working world. Losing weight, in their view, will give women the power, energy, and image they need for the competitive workplace. They aren't completely wrong: the work world is full of people who won't hire or promote people because they're fat. Being thin is seen as being lean and mean in a professional context.

In the seventies, the mainstream, "equal pay for equal work" version of feminism held that women should be just like men in the workplace, in dress-for-success suits and thin, masculinized, nonthreatening bodies. Women could be in the men's world as long as they kept their bodies under control. In the nineties, this idea has become stronger than ever. According to Susan Powter, Weight Watchers, and others in the diet industry, women can achieve power, control, and success in their lives only by becoming lean and aerobicized. Women who have a body that spills over the boundaries of the standard, safe, controlled image of success are apt to fail, and according to this individualist, power-feminist way of thinking, it will be their own fault.

It is a rare pleasure to see successful women go outside these boundaries. One who did—for a while—was Kathleen Sullivan. As a TV newswoman, Sullivan was always a little off. She defiantly refused to dye her hair to fit an image, keeping her streaks of gray. She resisted wearing corporate suits, choosing clothes with more personality, including short shirts and sweaters. Sullivan came off as a smart and sassy woman who was also sexy, not because she was thin in her short skirts, but because she was so defiantly female in a job where sexual neutrality is the rule. But then Sullivan disappeared, fired from CBS *This Morning*, replaced by the safe and blond Paula Zahn. At forty, Sullivan says, the gray-streaked hair that so many women found remarkable for a TV newswoman looked older than was acceptable. "It was remarkable, but I was unemployed," she told one reporter. "I couldn't get a job. When you don't fit that stereotype, you're damned."[15]

Four years later, Sullivan reappeared, sans gray streaks, subdued and contrite, as Weight Watchers' spokesperson. Hers is a cautionary tale for women who rebel, who think they can escape being measured by their appearance—and their weight. "Four years ago, I sat at an anchor desk, interviewed world leaders and looked pretty svelte," she says in Weight Watchers' ad copy. But then the worst thing happened. "Without the glare of the spotlight, I realized I had gained weight." Sullivan was photographed "before" for Weight Watchers in a dumpy sweater and baggy pants, with an embarrassed look on her face. Those of us on the Weight Watchers mailing list—forever, since they do a better job of following former members than do alumni magazines—watched Kathleen's smile brighten each week as she lost more and more weight. She especially pushed the Superstart! program for quick weight loss the first week, and the Personal Cuisine for those "stressful and hectic days" that busy career women like her endure.

In newspaper interviews, Sullivan defended her job as a Weight Watchers spokesperson, squarely facing accusations that she was promoting unreasonable appearance standards by claiming she was promoting women's health instead. "I don't think I send the message you should lose weight for cosmetic reasons," she said. "Obesity is a cause of three different types of cancer in women. Unfortunately, it's easy to say, 'Oh, I don't want to lose weight because I'm a smart woman.' If you're a smart woman, you care about your life and your quality of life."

But if you're a smart journalist, you don't take Weight Watchers at its word, and do a little research yourself. Then you find out that obesity doesn't cause three kinds of cancer. Instead, there is a very slight *statistical association* with certain cancers—endometrium, uterus, gallbladder, cervix, ovary, and breast—and the research is controversial. No one knows why this association exists; fat tissue could contain more estrogen, which can stimulate cell growth. It could be that fat people don't usually exercise very much, but it's the inactivity, not the fat, that's the problem. It could be the fat content of the diet. But whatever the cause, only women who are 140 percent or more above average weight—that means about 190 pounds for a five-foot-six woman—show this slightly increased risk.[16] A woman who is 20 to 30 pounds heavier than the media ideal, as Sullivan was, is not the one for whom the health risks of "obesity" are a cause for concern. The health risks of dieting should be more of an issue for her. Sullivan was perfectly healthy at her "before" weight. In her "after" ads, she is promoting Weight Watchers' vastly misleading advertising message that the diet is a "health care plan that works," and that you have to be very slim to be healthy. She's also sending the message that women have to be thin to be successful—and to be considered sharp.

After several months in the Weight Watchers ads, Sullivan emerged 30 pounds thinner, triumphant in a black jumpsuit and boots, sitting in a helicopter. The image of the light, fast, efficient, streamlined journalist was restored. Publicly shamed for her weight—and for showing her age—she had now redeemed herself by fitting the mold. It was disappointing to see a smart, spirited woman cave in completely to a culture that demands that women look thin and young to be acceptable. How much more encouraging it would have been if she'd fought the sexist standards she faced, as former anchorwoman Christine Craft did when she was fired for not being attractive enough, instead of becoming a spokesperson for her own defeat.

After Suzie showed me around Jenny Craig, I signed up, wrote a check, and had my first counseling session. I sat down in the clinic room with Amber,* a willowy weight-loss counselor (who, I learned, was trained in "visualization" techniques), and told her I wanted to reconsider my goal, which originally was 133 pounds. I'd be more comfortable aiming for 145 pounds. "One forty-five isn't grossly overweight, but it's not healthy," she said firmly. I explained that the only time I'd been below that weight was when I'd had a raging eating disorder; the thought of my pelvic bones protruding again frightened me to death. "Well," she said, "get down to one hundred thirty-three pounds, and then if you decide it's too low, you can always gain the weight back." The mention of my eating disorder didn't prompt concern at Jenny Craig, despite its policy to screen out such problems. A former counselor at Jenny Craig told me, "We get them all the time." Jenny Craig, he said, gave women with eating disorders a vehicle for their obsession; further, it encouraged competition among counselors and clients to see who could lose the most weight, making the obsession that much worse.

Amber started describing the diet restrictions: no salt, coffee, caffeinated tea, or alcohol. She gave me the prescribed menu, and said I couldn't deviate, even to add vegetables, because it was "portioncontrolled." The logic is that if you let yourself eat as many vegetables as you want when you're hungry, then when you go off the diet, you'll go wild on junk food. That didn't make much sense to me; it seems pretty obvious that it's never a bad idea to eat as many vegetables as you please. I scanned the menu, and found several things I dislike. "I'm not going to eat peanut butter bars or margarine," I told her. When I eat fat, it's usually olive oil to sauté vegetables—or a piece of good chocolate. She was unyielding: I had to eat everything. I made a face. "Your mother must've had a lot of fun with *you*," she said.

I asked Amber about going out to dinner. She leaned forward. "You need to make the decision to either continue going out or do something to lose weight," she said. "Is it worth it to lose weight?" It was looking less and less likely. At other diet programs there are at least tips on how to eat out without ordering high-fat foods; these days, many restaurants will gladly comply with a request for grilled or steamed vegetables. Amber's rigidity seemed to be a setup to buy more Jenny Craig food—and an incentive to blow the diet.

But that week, for $92.98, I tried the food. Each day, I started with an individual, foil-wrapped package of cereal, swallowed four vitamin supplements, drank six glasses of water, whipped up artificially flavored chocolate mousse snacks, and consumed prepackaged dinners that suspiciously resembled airplane food.

It was rough going—a chocolate drink and rice cake is not my idea of lunch. Nor do I think of pasta primavera as something to which you add hot water and stir. Breakfast one Sunday morning, before a six-mile hike, involved only a chocolate drink and an orange. I came out of the woods so famished I ran right into a three-egg feta omelette with a side of buttered raisin toast. I always eat a good breakfast in the morning, especially before exercising; now I knew why. That evening, when a can of pasta marinara was on the menu, a friend came over with a bottle of good wine and made wild mushroom risotto. I did not hesitate.

Despite these slip-ups, I came back for another visit. The counselor, a theater major named Jennifer* who appeared genetically thin (Weight Watchers at least uses real former fat people), instructed me this time to take off my sweatshirt and running shoes before I got on the scale. Nervous, I stepped up to judgment. The little marker went whizzing down: 151 pounds. "That's *great*," said Jennifer. "You've lost"—she counted on her fingers—"fourteen pounds! That's a new center record!" She stepped out of the office. "You guys," she yelled, "Laura's lost fourteen pounds in a week!"

I went home and weighed my coat, boots, and everything else I'd worn the week before. Eleven pounds.

Then I called Wayne Callaway, the obesity expert at George Washington University. "Is it possible," I asked, "for a five-foot-six woman who weights one hundred sixty-five pounds to lose fourteen pounds in a week?"

"Well, yes," he said. "Through extreme and catastrophic illness." My "weight loss" should have caused the counselors considerable alarm, he said. "The only thing you could possibly lose that fast is lean body mass."

In fact, Callaway says, people almost always lose lean body mass—those muscles you're trying to tone when you're working out—in the first few weeks of a 1,000- to 1,200-calorie-a-day diet program. (So much for Weight Watchers' first-week "Superstart!" program for that quick low-calorie "jump-start" to weight loss.) Unless a person is small and sedentary—a five-foot sixty-five-year-old woman, say—that isn't enough calories to lose weight without suffering the effects of semi-starvation. A larger, more active body will adapt to the food shortage by burning less and less fat; then, when you go back to eating normally, you'll store food more efficiently. In other words, you'll gain weight. "Our bodies have tremendously elegant mechanisms for surviving a famine," says Callaway.

The state-of-the-art advice on weight loss, according to Callaway, is to eat the way you would eat forever to maintain an appropriate weight; exercise more; and, if necessary, work with a therapist or support group to deal with emotional overeating behaviors. "You should never go through a diet phase." Not everyone, he says, is meant to be thin, either.

For people who need to learn the basics of healthy eating, Callaway says Weight Watchers might not be so bad. "Weight Watchers is a useful tool for someone who has not dieted a lot and doesn't have a lot of information." It offers people a basic idea of healthy nutrition in terms of the food's content—fresh vegetables and fruits, a good mix of protein, low fat but not drastically so—but not in terms of the calories, which should be higher. But you could just as easily consult the U.S. government's food pyramid, along with a few recipe books, to figure out how to eat better instead. If you're determined that a program like

Weight Watchers could be helpful for you, Callaway's advice is to add more food so you're not starving yourself, so you'll be more likely to keep eating that way permanently: "Cheat.'"

After the second week on Jenny Craig, I didn't feel so hungry, but I was listless and irritable. No longer so satisfied with my body, I kept pinching myself in the mirror, increasingly preoccupied with how fat I felt and how much weight I wanted to lose. I kept the program diary of my eating and exercise, checking off every glass of water I drank and writing down any deviation from the preplanned menu. My days became focused on food: Was it time yet for a snack? What would I get to eat? If I skipped the peanut butter on the celery, would I lose more weight? I became resentful of the control, and tired of feeling I couldn't have exactly what I wanted. One day, under stress, I found myself ripping the wrappers off of one, two, then three Jenny Craig snack bars, gobbling them at high speed. Stepping back from the pantry, I realized I had not binged with that feeling of panic in years.

I had to stop. I went to my last session, and the counselor weighed me. This time I was wearing jeans instead of leggings, and the scale showed I'd gained a pound. For a moment, I was depressed, angry that I couldn't be successful on a diet for even two weeks. "Don't worry," said Jennifer. "We lowered your metabolism last week, and now it's adjusting. You're still way ahead of schedule."

I wasn't really listening. My mind was already racing out the door, stopping at the grocer's nearby to pick up the things I would need—zucchini, onions, fresh oregano, asiago cheese, wine—to make some real pasta primavera later on, when I was hungry.

A few months later, when I attended a week-long cooking school in Tuscany, the problem with commercial diet programs really came home to me. In the large country kitchen, the chef, who had spent thirty years cooking at a fine restaurant near Florence, was artfully pouring olive oil on pieces of bread he was grilling. "We're afraid of oil in the United States," I told him in Italian. He nodded and shook his head, rubbing more bread with a clove of garlic. Then he told me the story of how the year before, La Signora Dieta—the diet lady—visited the school. She insisted that they make bruschetta without a drop of olive oil. Could I imagine? The chef opened his hands in a helpless gesture. *"Bruschetta senza olio non e bruschetta,"* he told me. It just isn't the same thing.

But, the chef said, he did the best he could, and made toast with tomatoes without olive oil. "But the thing that made me mad," he said, pausing to take a sip of wine, "was that as soon as her friends went into the other room, La Signora Dieta came back into the kitchen and secretly ate *six* bruschetta with olive oil." He made a gesture Italians use to indicate that someone is completely out of their head. Later, I asked the director of the school whether this story about La Signora Dieta was true. Oh, yes, she told me, laughing. She opened a photo book and showed me a photo of La Signora Dieta, tanned and smiling with her friends.

It was Jenny Craig.

Chapter 6

First, Do No Harm:
Diet Doctors

Recently, I came across a large ad in the morning paper featuring a slim woman in tight jeans who was jumping for joy. "If you've tried other weight loss plans without success . . ." the ad teased, "Try Dr. Ralph Alperin's weight loss plans. They mix medical care and great menu variety for safe, often *lifetime* weight loss. You don't *have* to be overweight—call today!" in big block letters, the ad proclaimed: "NOW AVAILABLE FENFLURAMINE/PHENTERMINE APPETITE SUPPRESSANTS, as shown on T.V. and Reader's Digest." There were phone numbers for each of Dr. Alperin's seven Bay Area offices.

Physicians in major cities across the country have been placing ads like this one, luring people into their offices with the promise of drugs and quick weight-loss treatments. I called to see what I could find out about Dr. Alperin's "safe, rapid weight loss under a doctor's careful eye." I told the receptionist at one clinic that I was just 15 or 20 pounds overweight, and she assured me that I could lose about 3 pounds a week on a program that included a 700-calorie-a-day liquid diet, prescription appetite suppressants, and vitamin injections. What time did I want to come in?

I was surprised: All of the medical literature on very-low-calorie diets suggests that they should only be undertaken by people who are very obese, not just a few pounds over the ideal, since extremely restrictive diets can be dangerous, burning lean muscle tissue, and sometimes leading to heart failure. The literature on prescription appetite suppressants agrees, on the whole, that no one should take the drugs unless they're at least 30 percent over a healthy weight, which is by no means just 15 to 20 pounds for almost any woman. As for vitamin injections, they don't even make it into the literature on weight loss.

I tried another of Alperin's offices to double-check. The receptionist there was busy; because of the ad, she told me, she was overwhelmed with phone calls. I got to the point.

"If I'm just fifteen pounds overweight, but I really want to lose the weight fast, could I still do the liquid diet?" I asked her.

"No problem, sure," she said.

"And how about the appetite suppressants?"

"That's part of the program, and the doctor will give you what he feels is medically safe for you."

"But you don't have to be a certain amount overweight to get the pills?"

"No, there's no limit."

It seems the line in the ad, "You don't *have* to be overweight," could be read two ways.

The most sensible advice you could give someone who wants to lose weight, it might seem, is "see your doctor." Or better yet, see a doctor who specializes in weight loss. Dieters who have tried everything else, or who are wary of faddish weight-loss schemes and diet centers where counselors are hired based on their experience as aerobics instructors, believe that their doctors, finally, know what's best for them. We trust in our physicians, and in their motto: First, do no harm.

Most of us think of physicians as being cautious and conservative in their practices, only prescribing potentially harmful treatments when necessary, if a person has such serious medical problems that the benefits of treatment outweigh the risks. In the case of obesity, we might think treatment would be appropriate for people who are fat enough that their weight aggravates other existing medical problems, such as high blood pressure, high cholesterol, or a family history of heart disease or diabetes. Most physicians, we trust, wouldn't prescribe treatments that involve serious risks just for cosmetic reasons.

But some doctors have a history of abusing that trust for profit, prescribing unnecessary and ineffective diet regimes to all comers. Diet doctors, who were notorious in the sixties and seventies for passing out amphetamines like handfuls of sugarless candy, and who flourished again in the eighties when Oprah Winfrey temporarily lost weight on a physician-supervised liquid diet, made another comeback with the enormously popular diet drugs fenfluramine and phentermine ("fen-phen") and Redux (dexfenfluramine) before they were taken off the market in September 1997.

From 1993 to 1997, diet doctors had a heyday selling fen-phen, with some physicians opening "pill mills," writing prescriptions to just about anyone who came in and didn't look blatantly anorexic. One doctor set up a tent at a flea market in Southern California, offering a week's worth of pills for $49.45. Other physicians marketed the pills on the Internet. Some doctors set up whole chains of diet-drug outlets. Fred Garcia, a Newport Beach, California, anesthesiologist, owned 24 medical diet centers; he and his partner saw 1,400 patients in a month, spending about 15 minutes with each patient at the first visit—and less at each subsequent visit. Like many other physicians, Garcia said he wouldn't prescribe the drugs to anyone who wasn't twenty percent over their "ideal weight," but he added a few exceptions: "There are some patients in the limelight—much of my practice is in Burbank or West Hollywood—who need to be at a lower level because it's necessary for their job."

At a time when commercial diet programs are faltering, Americans' weight continues to rise, and there's a glut of physicians in a managed-care environment, the diet-doctor business is becoming more and more attractive to some physicians. It's all too easy for a new physician in town to sign up with Nutri/System or some other diet chain. To legitimize the increase in diet-doctor services, physicians— and the pharmaceutical companies that offer them so many incentives to prescribe their drugs—have been spreading the idea that being even slightly heavier than "ideal" is a *medical* condition, not an appearance problem. There are now about 17,500 private physicians in the country who specialize in weight loss, as well as 3,300 hospitals and 540 health maintenance organizations that offer diet programs.[1]

It isn't just diet doctors who are cashing in on this trend, either. Countless family physicians, general practitioners, psychiatrists, and internists are treating their patients with diets and drugs during the course of their regular practice. One friend of mine who is 5'4" tall and about 120 pounds—slim, in other words—was offered, unprompted, a prescription for fen-phen by her gynecologist. While some physicians offer their patients sensible help in slowly changing their nutrition habits, exercising more, and learning to stop overeating, most prescribe drugs and very-low-calorie liquid diets (which are making a comeback after fenfluramine and phentermine were banned). Most diet doctors, though—despite their credentials, lab coats, and "medical" approach to weight loss—are no more successful in treating weight loss than diet counselors. They're just more expensive, and sometimes, as the fen-phen fiasco proved, more dangerous.

I decided to visit a couple of diet docs in person. No reasonable physician, I thought, could observe up close how strong and healthy I am and then prescribe me pills or put me on a liquid diet that is designed for the morbidly obese. I chose physicians who are members of the American Society of Bariatric Physicians (ASBP)—the Greek word, *barros*, means "heavy"—an organization of doctors who treat obesity. To most consumers, the ASBP sounds like a legitimate medical specialty, and the group says it's trying to change the pill-pushing image problem diet doctors have had in the past. "Bariatrics" is not recognized as a bona fide specialty by the American Medical Association, though, and no one needs to pass board exams or undergo a residency to be "certified" as a bariatrician, as one needs to do in order to become, say, a board-certified psychiatrist or pediatrician. The society issues physician guidelines for prescribing diet drugs, holds training sessions and conferences, and publishes standards of practice, which suggest that physicians should perform complete physicals on patients, weigh the benefits and risks of treatments, and keep up-to-date on the relevant medical literature. I randomly picked a couple of physicians to visit from the Bay Area section of the ASBP directory.

When I walked into the office of a prominent diet doctor in San Jose, California, I didn't walk in thin, but we're not talking obese here. At my last complete physical, at the well-respected Cooper Clinic in Dallas, the doctor congratulated me for exercising every day, eating a healthy diet, and having extremely good cholesterol numbers; on a treadmill test, I scored in the top fitness category for women my age. Though I am overweight by America's cosmetic standards, there's no medical reason for me to lose weight.

The San Jose doctor's nurse—like the counselor at Jenny Craig—weighed me with my heavy boots and jacket on, then led me to the examining room. "Who referred you?" she asked me. "If they refer five people, they get a free month." I blinked. For a second I thought I was in the sales office at a twenty-four-hour Nautilus gym. No: there's the examining table, the blood pressure cuff; it's a doctor's office. The nurse took my measurements, and, I noticed, added a generous 2½ inches to my relatively small waist; whatever my progress on the diet, it would seem like I'd lost some inches when she measured me again on my next visit.

The doctor came in and greeted me by staring at my hips. "You have a sit-down job, honey?" He reviewed my medical history, noticed I had allergies, asked me a few questions about them, and gave me—"at no extra charge"—a bottle of allergy pills. "These'll help you sleep," he said. Then it was on to weight loss.

"We have an injection program here," he said. "Is that what you had in mind?" This was a little odd: I'm used to having a physician evaluate my condition, discuss the options, and suggest a course of treatment. He apparently took my blank-eyed look as an assent. He explained that in addition to appetite suppressants and a 600-calorie-a-day diet, he gives his patients injections of vitamins and minerals three times a week. "My patients say, 'Doc, I feel wonderful.'" He promised me I'd lose 15 pounds in the first month. "A lot of docs charge twice what I charge," he said. "I give you a good deal."

He spent half an hour describing the evils of fats and heart disease, his yellow Hi-Liter flying through the pages of a booklet he'd given me. Halfway through, he stopped for a moment and looked at me. "You know, you don't look like you have much to lose. You don't look like you weigh that much."

"The scales don't lie," I said.

He nodded and continued apace, lecturing me about how I should drink no alcohol and eat no fat. He named a chapter in the Bible that exhorts us not to eat fat, and told me to go home and read the Good Book myself. Even though I'd told him I eat no meat and few sweets, he spent quite a bit of time lecturing me not to do those things, running his usual tape. He studied me. "You have nice teeth, so you must not be pigging out too much on sugar."

He did a routine exam, listening to me breathe and tapping on my chest. He pinched my calf, which is large and solid from bicycling. Again, common sense raised its head—"You exercise a lot?"—but not for long. He launched back into advice on how to stick to my diet—"It's mind over platter!"—and said he'd give me, free, a big bottle of appetite suppressants. Then he gave me a pitch for buying the protein powder soups the office had on sale, showed me charts of people who had lost 12 to 15 pounds in the first month, and dismissed me. "I want you to lose fifteen pounds for me, Laura," he said. "You have to be faithful to me. There's too much infidelity in the world."

At the front desk, when the nurse asked me whether I wanted to buy the B-vitamin injection program—at $150—or just the appetite suppressants, at $65, I wavered. I don't like injections, I told her. The doctor shot me a stern look from across the hall. "Injections," I said, compliantly.

As I left, rubbing the needle wound in my arm, I thought about all the women who squeeze three doctor's visits a week into their hectic lives, enduring needlepricks, just for vitamins. Then I drove across town, ate a nice sushi lunch, and went to the office of another diet doctor. The sign in the waiting room read, *Do You Know That You Can Lose Weight by Eating Chocolate Chip Cookies?*" On his scale—after lunch—I weighed 3$\frac{1}{2}$ pounds less than at Roth's office.

The nurse took my blood pressure, and the doctor came in. "Which diet do you want?" he asked, without really looking at me. "The liquid protein or the cookie diet?" I told him I wasn't sure, and he pushed the liquid protein. Because of the risks involved—gallstones, hair loss, anxiety, stress, rapid weight regain, depression—most physicians won't prescribe liquid protein for anyone who doesn't weigh about 40 pounds more than I do. The doctor, however, told me he'd prescribe the expensive liquid protein diet to anyone who was at least 25 pounds overweight. Only a modeling agent would say I'm 25 pounds over-weight. He asked to see my wrist, which is medium-size. Since I'm not big-boned, he thought I could handle getting down to about 130 pounds, which would make me 25 pounds "overweight" now. "You could get down that low," he said. "Sure."

The advantage of the liquid protein diet, he told me, is that it is "drastic," so I would lose at least 3 pounds a week. "It's the one Oprah Winfrey went on," he said, as if that were a recommendation.

I told him that since I'm an active person, I was concerned the 500-

calorie-a-day liquid protein diet wouldn't be enough to sustain me. That weekend, for instance, I said, I was going on a six-hour mountain bike ride on some pretty steep terrain. "That's great," he said. "That'll help you lose weight." When I demurred—no one can ride hard all day on the equivalent of two Power Bars without "bonking," as bicyclists call it, hitting a wall of exhaustion—he said I could add an extra diet shake that day, bringing the day's total to only 750 calories or so. That many calories might get me to the top of the mountain, all right, but not all the way back home.

Then the doctor launched into a pitch for a whole line of protein products I could buy, though I was under no obligation. "I'm not Jenny Craig," he said. "These are just here for your convenience." I finally insisted that I wanted the higher-calorie cookie diet (four fiber cookies and one frozen dinner a day still amounted to 400 calories a day less than a 1,200-calorie-a-day semi-starvation diet). The cookie diet costs less, since no lab work is needed, as it is required under ASBP regulations for the extremely low-calorie diets.

The physician gave me a quick physical. He didn't ask me for details about my eating and exercise habits, nor did he inquire whether I'd ever had an eating disorder. He gave me a package of prescription appetite suppressants, which he said had no real side effects. "These aren't like the ones in the past," he said. "They aren't addictive or anything." I told him that I'd read about the negative effects of crash dieting, and was concerned. "Well, it lowers your metabolism a bit, but if you exercise, you'll be fine." Finally, I asked him how successful his program was. He told me they didn't keep track, since most of his patients didn't stay with him after the two- to six-week maintenance period. "We can help you lose weight," he said. "But there's nothing we can do if you go back to your bad habits."

The visit cost $110; the nurse gave me a large bag of fiber cookies and told me to come back next week, for a $50 weigh-in, more cookies, and my next batch of pills. My take for the day, from both offices, was two sets of appetite suppressants (a large bottle of tablets of diethylproprion and seven tablets of phentermine); two bottles of multivitamins; a bottle of chromium, another of potassium; some over-the-counter allergy pills; a prescription for other allergy pills; and several cellophane bags of high-protein fiber cookies.

The next day, I tried a fiber cookie, which tasted like wood shavings and could be called a cookie only by someone starving. I took a diethylproprion tablet, and spent the morning antsy and nervous. I rapidly rang up Paul Ernsberger, a pharmacologist at Case Western Reserve Medical School, and asked him about the drug. "It's a stimulant, an amphetamine mimic," he told me. "It'll cause psychomotor stimulation, keep you awake, make you feel nervous, and raise your blood pressure. At high doses, it can promote heart arrhythmia. It's serious stuff." There have even been several cases in the literature of psychosis induced by taking diethylproprion. No wonder the first doctor had given me something to help me sleep. Ernsberger said he was astonished I'd been given a B-vitamin injection. "That's what they did in the early sixties," he said. "It was shown to do absolutely nothing about thirty years ago."

Interrupting him—this drug did nothing for my politeness or attention span—I asked several questions about his studies putting rats on very-low-calorie diets. The rats' metabolisms slow down when they're on the diet, he told me; when they're off the diet, they get fatter eating the same amount of food that maintained their weight before. They also produce more of the stress hormones that can lead to heart problems when they're dieting. Rockefeller University researchers recently demonstrated that humans have similar reactions to diets; their metabolism slows to help them regain weight back to the original "setpoint." "Put people on crash diets and they'll gain back more weight than they lost," Ernsberger said.[2]

The next day, I took a dose of phentermine, which was even speedier than the diethylproprion. I was so wired I had to drink a pint of beer with lunch in order to be able to sit still to work. I had a headache and was incredibly grouchy. In my agitated state, I became enraged thinking about all the people who trust their doctors to help them with a problem, pay them a lot of money, dutifully starve themselves, then blame themselves when the program doesn't work and they've gained the weight back. I imagined how frustrated many good physicians must be, too, to find so many of their colleagues motivated by greed.

As I threw away my bag of medical diet products, I considered the Hippocratic Oath: First, do no harm. I was sure, at the very least, that diet docs had done thousands of women like me no good.

Is Obesity a Killer Disease?

One of the reasons diet doctors like these are becoming popular again, and other physicians are treating obesity more often in their practices, is that obesity is increasingly being viewed as a killer disease. As we have seen, a hundred years ago, except in extreme cases, fatness was considered a simple physical trait, a natural variation in human size. Then, with all of the emphasis our culture put on discipline, restraint, and physical perfectibility, being fat became a moral problem. The more people tried to treat this problem—often unsuccessfully—the more it came under the auspices of the medical profession. Now, obesity is widely described as a disease, and, as Americans get fatter, an epidemic.[3]

Is obesity really a disease? Do people get sick and die because of the extra pounds they carry on their frames? Is it, as the *Oxford English Dictionary* defines disease, "a condition of the body . . . in which its functions are disturbed or deranged"? Are fat people always unhealthy?

Two prominent obesity researchers who recently formed the American Obesity Association (AOA), University of Wisconsin physician Richard Atkinson and University of California at Davis nutrition expert Judith Stern, say obesity *is* a disease, and many of their colleagues share their view. "Obesity is a disease that affects at least 70 million Americans: more than one-third of all adults and one in five children," the researchers state in their AOA brochure. "Some people are more susceptible to obesity than others. Each year obesity causes at least 300,000 excess deaths in the US and costs the country more than $100 billion. Obesity is the second leading cause of unnecessary deaths." The researchers describe obesity as responsible for increasing the risks of high blood pressure, diabetes, heart disease, stroke, gallbladder disease, and cancer of the breast, prostate, and colon. These very same statistics and lists show up frequently in the literature on obesity, as well as in books promoting diets, at FDA hearings on new diet drugs, in patient brochures in diet doctors' clinics, in medical weight-loss product sales packets sent to physicians, and in ads for commercial weight-loss centers. The campaign report for "Shape Up America," the C. Everett Koop Foundation's 1994 health crusade, for instance, uses these numbers, and calls obesity "one of the most pervasive health risks affecting Americans today."

These "facts" about obesity, however, are not as straightforward as they may seem. Most obesity researchers agree that like diseases, some people inherit a tendency to become fat (which is often encouraged by an environment where many people get little exercise and eat a high-fat diet). But beyond that, many researchers say obesity is not a disease, and does not, in itself, make people ill. There are, in fact, a number of questions about obesity and health that researchers are quite divided on: Does obesity lead to illness, and if so, how? How fat do you have to be to be at risk? Is being fat dangerous, or is it the sedentary lifestyle that often goes along with being fat? If you lose weight, will you be as healthy as a person who was never fat to begin with? There are no clear answers to these questions, and given the confusion, it pays to be skeptical when some obesity researchers call fatness a "disease" or fire off statistics about how many people it kills.

Take, for instance, the claim that a third of all adults are "affected by obesity." That number initially comes from a national survey: the National Health and Nutrition Examination Survey tracked the weights of between 6,000 and 13,000 adults from 1960 to 1991. "Overall," said researchers who reported on the data in the *Journal of the American Medical Association* in 1994, "approximately one-third of all adults in the United States were estimated to be overweight." What do they mean by "overweight"? In the report, researchers defined "overweight" as having a Body Mass Index of greater than 27.8 for men, or 27.3 for women. (BMI is weight in kilos divided by height in meters squared; you can calculate your BMI by multiplying your weight in pounds by 700, dividing by your height in inches, then dividing by your height again.) To translate that into real numbers, they're calling a five-foot-five woman overweight at about 165 pounds, and a five-foot-ten man overweight at 195 pounds.[4]

But does "overweight" mean the same as "obese"? For the most part, researchers say no. Most Americans who are overweight are only slightly so, with a BMI of 27 to 30. Some researchers call this "mildly obese," and others say it's just chubby. But whatever they call being about 20 to 40 pounds higher than ideal weight, there's very little evidence that it's bad for your health. In most studies, the health risks associated with being fat don't shoot up until someone is severely obese, or about 75 to 100 pounds over an ideal weight.

Body Weight (in pounds) According to Height (in inches) and Body Mass Index (BMI)
Body Mass Index

Height	19	20	21	22	23	24	25	26	27	28	29	30	31	32	33	34
								Body Weight								
58	91	95	100	105	110	114	119	124	129	133	138	143	148	152	157	162
59	94	99	104	109	114	119	124	129	134	139	144	149	154	159	164	169
60	97	102	107	112	117	122	127	132	138	143	148	153	158	163	168	173
61	101	106	111	117	122	127	132	138	143	148	154	159	164	169	175	180
62	103	109	114	120	125	130	136	141	147	152	158	163	168	174	179	185
63	107	113	119	124	130	135	141	147	152	158	164	169	175	181	186	192
64	111	117	123	129	135	141	146	152	158	164	170	176	182	187	193	199
65	114	120	126	132	138	144	150	156	162	168	174	180	186	192	198	204
66	118	124	131	137	143	149	156	162	168	174	180	187	193	199	205	212
67	121	127	134	140	147	153	159	166	172	178	185	191	198	204	210	217
68	125	132	139	145	152	158	165	172	178	185	191	198	205	211	218	224
69	128	135	142	149	155	162	169	176	182	189	196	203	209	216	223	230
70	133	140	147	154	161	168	175	182	189	196	203	210	217	224	231	237
71	136	143	150	157	164	171	179	186	193	200	207	214	221	229	236	243
72	140	148	155	162	170	177	185	192	199	207	214	221	229	236	244	251
73	143	151	158	166	174	181	189	196	204	211	219	226	234	241	249	257
74	148	156	164	171	179	187	195	203	210	218	226	234	242	249	257	265
75	151	159	167	175	183	191	199	207	215	223	231	239	247	255	263	271
76	156	164	172	181	189	197	205	214	222	230	238	246	255	263	271	279

Height	\multicolumn{16}{c}{Body Mass Index}
	35	36	37	38	39	40	41	42	43	44	45	46	47	48	49	50
	\multicolumn{16}{c}{Body Weight}
58	167	172	176	181	186	191	195	200	205	210	214	219	224	229	233	238
59	174	179	184	188	193	198	203	208	213	218	223	228	233	238	243	248
60	178	183	188	194	199	204	209	214	219	224	229	234	239	244	250	255
61	185	191	196	201	207	212	217	222	228	233	238	244	249	254	260	265
62	190	196	201	206	212	217	223	228	234	239	245	250	255	261	266	272
63	198	203	209	214	220	226	231	237	243	248	254	260	265	271	277	282
64	205	211	217	223	228	234	240	246	252	258	264	269	275	281	287	293
65	210	216	222	228	234	240	246	252	258	264	270	276	282	288	294	300
66	218	224	229	236	243	249	255	261	268	274	280	286	292	299	305	311
67	223	229	236	242	248	255	261	268	274	280	287	293	299	306	312	319
68	231	238	244	251	257	264	271	277	284	290	297	304	310	317	323	330
69	236	243	250	257	263	270	277	284	290	297	304	311	317	324	331	338
70	244	251	258	265	272	279	286	293	300	307	314	321	328	335	342	349
71	250	257	264	271	279	286	293	300	307	314	321	329	336	343	350	357
72	258	266	273	281	288	295	303	313	317	325	332	340	347	354	362	369
73	264	272	279	287	294	302	309	317	324	332	340	347	355	362	370	377
74	273	281	288	296	304	312	319	327	335	343	351	358	366	374	382	390
75	279	287	294	302	310	318	326	334	342	350	358	366	374	382	390	398
76	287	296	304	312	320	328	337	345	353	361	370	378	386	394	402	411

Source: Paul R. Thomas, ed. Weighing the Options: Criteria for Evaluating Weight Management Programs, The Nature and Problem of Obesity (Washington, DC: National Academy Press, 1994), Chapter 2, pp. 5–6.

Severe obesity means a BMI of 35 or heavier; that's 210 pounds at five-foot-five, and 244 pounds at five-foot-ten. Only 8 percent of the population has a BMI of 35 and over. So to say that one-third of the American population is obese and at some health risk for the condition is quite exaggerated.

It may be the idea that obesity is a "disease" that makes researchers and physicians use the terms "overweight" and "obese" interchangeably. The logic is that if being obese means being diseased, then being a little overweight means being a little diseased. A 1994 Institute of Medicine report on weight-loss treatment—written by a panel of obesity experts, many of whom are paid to sit on the scientific boards of weight-loss companies—reflects this idea that overweight people are in the first stages of serious obesity. The report explicitly says that being slightly overweight does not put people at any additional risk for disease, and that too many American women are preoccupied with their weight anyway; nevertheless, it sounds a warning: "This is not to say, however, that slightly overweight individuals who wish to reduce to improve their appearance and enhance self-esteem should be dissuaded from doing so. Some of them may be at the first stages of disease, and treatment might prevent further problems."[5] But why treat slightly overweight people who have no other signs of illness? By dieting, they run the risk of putting themselves in the first stages of a "disease" called weight obsession, which can lead to real health problems, such as eating disorders, and an endless cycle of dieting, bingeing, weight preoccupation, and despair.

The next claim worth examining is that obesity causes 300,000 excess deaths per year in the United States. This claim is based on an estimate, done by researchers Anne Wolf and Graham Colditz at Harvard Medical School, using data from the Nurses' Health Study (the same study from which the Harvard researcher JoAnn Manson claimed that being 10 or 20 pounds overweight led to an increased risk of early death). Based on the number of women who died from various diseases, and their body weight, the researchers extrapolated that obesity was the direct cause, nationwide, of 171,490 coronary heart disease deaths, 39,679 diabetes deaths, 53,087 cancer deaths, and 10,000 cerebrovascular deaths per year.[6]

But the problem with this kind of analysis, say other researchers, is that you can't make a direct cause-and-effect link between obesity and diseases. Just because people who are fat are more likely to die of cancer doesn't mean that their fatness *caused* the cancer. Other lifestyle factors that tend go along with obesity, which the researchers in the Nurses' Health Study did not take into account—such as a lack of exercise or a high-fat diet—may have contributed to the deaths, not the fatness itself. Studies on obese people who exercise, for instance— who live longer than lean people who don't exercise—may prove that *inactivity* is the cause of many of the problems we associate with obesity, not obesity itself. Steven Blair, an exercise physiologist at the Cooper Institute for Aerobics Research in Dallas has done studies that show that if you exercise, your weight (up to a BMI of 40) doesn't put you at any increased risk for early death at all. It may turn out that obesity is, for the most part, a red herring in the health debate.

"Nobody ever dies of obesity," says David Levitsky, a nutrition and obesity expert at Cornell University. Obesity, he says, is often a marker for other health problems caused by a sedentary lifestyle, but is itself not necessarily dangerous. "If you're a large person and you do not suffer from any other health problems, then there is no reason for you to lose weight."

If a person does suffer from other health problems, however, then serious obesity may indeed aggravate the situation. Almost all of the studies that look at the health risks associated with obesity— researchers call them "comorbidities," by which they mean high blood pressure, high cholesterol or blood sugars, diabetes, or other conditions that often go along with being fat—show that those risks do increase when people are very fat, meaning about 100 pounds or so overweight. In particular, researchers have shown that having abdominal obesity—an apple shape—can be dangerous.

Belly fat is rather active in the body, unlike fat in the hips and thighs, which sits there and causes no harm. Fat cells in the abdomen release fatty acids into the portal vein, which goes directly into the liver, where they interfere with the liver's job of breaking down insulin, thereby increasing the amount of insulin circulating in the body. This sets off a vicious cycle known as insulin resistance: with more insulin circulating, cells grow more resistant to what it does— regulate the metabolism of sugars, protein, and fat—and so produce even more liver-damaging fatty acids. Eventually, this can cause problems, including high blood sugars, high blood pressure, high triglycerides, lower HDL (good) cholesterol, and heart attacks. Regardless of BMI, many researchers say that having a waist-to-hip ratio (waist measurement divided by hip measurement) of less than 0.80 for women or 0.95 for men is likely to be healthy. So men with beer bellies are much more likely to have health problems related to their weight than women with big hips and thighs.

The bottom line isn't that obesity causes 300,000 deaths per year. It's more accurate to say that an unhealthy lifestyle contributes to those deaths, and that obesity sometimes goes along with an unhealthy lifestyle. Certainly there are people who never exercise, eat junk food, have high stress levels, and die of heart disease, who aren't a single pound overweight. Severe obesity does seem to make other health problems worse, but that's a far cry from the blanket statement that obesity is a killer disease. Extreme apple-shaped obesity is a special case (it's mainly men who have this condition), because researchers can show directly how belly fat leads to disease. But even belly fat isn't an argument for dieting; almost anyone, says Steve Blair, can fight off insulin resistance with regular exercise.

The claim that obesity is the number-two killer in America (after smoking) doesn't add up in other ways. If being fat is responsible for directly causing so many diseases that lead to early death, then it would follow that as Americans get fatter, more people would be dying from those diseases. But we're not; the Institute of Medicine report notes that while obesity is increasing in the United States, the rates of hypertension, high cholesterol, high blood cholesterol, and cardiac disease—all supposedly associated with obesity—are declining. (The authors mention this phenomenon only in passing, with no explanation, most likely because it undercuts their argument that obesity is a serious disease.) In other words, we're getting fatter, but we're suffering from fewer of the diseases traditionally associated with obesity. Clearly, the relationship between obesity and life-threatening health conditions is not as simple and direct as many people make it seem.

The statistic on obesity costing the country $100 billion a year is similarly suspect. That estimate was also derived, in part, from the Nurses' Health Study, and the same criticism—assuming that obesity directly causes disease—applies. The $100 billion figure also includes the estimated $33 billion Americans spend per year on dieting as a "cost," which is ridiculous; that money isn't a drain on national resources, but a spur to one particularly healthy sector of the economy—the diet industry.

The health risks of being *underweight* haven't been calculated into any of these equations, either. In a 1996 study, David Levitsky and his colleagues at Cornell University analyzed 60 previous studies involving weight and early deaths, involving 357,000 men and 249,000 women (many times more than the Nurses' Health Study), and found that the health risks of moderate obesity were exaggerated, whereas the risks of being underweight have been neglected. For women, there was little relationship between weight and early death at all. For men, after controlling for confounding factors such as smoking and disease, the data showed, if you drew a line on a graph, a U-shaped relationship between weight and early death. Those men who were very underweight were as likely to die early as people who were seriously obese. For everyone between the extremes, weight wasn't a substantial factor in their death. "The health risks of being moderately underweight are comparable to that of being quite overweight and look more serious than most people realize," Levitsky said.[7]

Another problem with calling obesity a "disease" is that it suggests that everyone who is fat must be suffering from the same disorder, with the same consequences for their health. In fact, people are fat for different reasons and should be treated accordingly. Some people who are fat, for instance, overeat; others don't. For some, being fat goes along with a constellation of other health problems; others are perfectly healthy. A measurement of body weight to height alone (BMI) is really too crude to make any conclusions about a person's health status. Still, most physicians accept that weight is an important indicator of health, and have us step up on the scale first thing.

Physicians warn us to lose weight, in part, because they hate fat just like the rest of us. Obesity, to them, is a disease in another sense of the word: "Absence of ease; uneasiness, discomfort; inconvenience, annoyance," as the *Oxford English Dictionary* puts it. Physicians, like many other people, feel uneasy in the presence of someone extremely large, and when they have troubles treating the patient, they feel inconvenienced and annoyed. A London physician in the 1920s expressed the opinion of many of his colleagues when he wrote that all obesity is caused by gluttony and leads to stupidity: "Every degree of alimentary obesity is contemptible, because it denotes self-indulgence, greed, and gourmandizing; and most are disgusting because they represent an unsightly distortion of the human form divine, and a serious impairment of intellectual faculties." In the 1950s, Hilde Bruch, the eating disorders pioneer, observed that these negative attitudes, while not so outspoken, persisted. "Many contemporary American physicians, even those who specialize in the treatment of obesity, consider their fat patients a somewhat lower type of humanity."[8] Several studies in the past decade have shown that many doctors still consider their fat patients weak-willed, ugly, and awkward. In one study of health care professionals, 84 percent thought obese patients were self-indulgent, 88 percent believed they ate to compensate for other problems, and 70 percent assumed they were emotionally disturbed.[9] These attitudes can be quite damaging, since many fat people prefer to forgo medical treatment altogether rather than be subjected to the humiliation that accompanies a doctor's visit.[10]

Doctors not only share our prejudice against fat, they have the added frustration of not being able to help their patients lose weight. Most physicians genuinely want to help, and all their training has made them believe that they should be able to help someone who seems only to need to eat less, exercise more, and get a little boost with some appetite suppressants. If only their fat patients would follow doctor's orders, they believe, they'd lose weight. "The physician," wrote Bruch, "has been indoctrinated with the conviction that obesity is a deplorable condition which should be corrected; and that it is easy to correct if only fat people would follow the excellent advice which is so generously offered to them."[11] Physicians are frustrated when their treatments fail. Rather than face the idea that the treatments may be ineffective, they blame their patients for being uncooperative, reinforcing their belief that fat people tend to be weak-willed.

But it's the diet treatments that fail. Fifteen years ago, the Yale University psychologist and obesity researcher Kelly Brownell observed that most people stand a better chance of recovering from most forms of cancer than losing weight and keeping it off. There is no standard way to treat obesity, as there are widely accepted ways to treat ulcers, diabetes, or appendicitis. Visit ten doctors and they'll give you ten different opinions about how much you should weigh and what you should do to get down there. One will recommend a liquid protein diet, another behavior modification, a third a 1,200-calorie-a-day diet, and a fourth diet pills. In the long run, almost nothing works. Despite the optimistic talk about successfully treating obesity, most honest researchers acknowledge that they are years away from really knowing what they're doing. "All current methods [for reducing weight], from thigh creams to stomach staples, are like gropes in the dark, and as such, are either totally ineffectual or are no more than counterforces to an incompletely understood regulatory disorder," says Jules Hirsch, a prominent Rockefeller University obesity expert. "There are no cures at this time."[12]

The idea that obesity is a disease, however, has given physicians license to keep trying unproven, unnecessary, and often dangerous treatments. In the imaginations of many physicians, obesity isn't as hard to cure as cancer, it *is* cancer. "To call obesity a disease," says the University of Cincinnati eating disorders expert Susan Wooley, "tends to suggest that we should keep all our treatments going even if the success rates are low and carry other risks." The disease concept makes it seem as if those risks are acceptable even for people who are hardly overweight. Before fenfluramine and dexfenfluramine were banned, for instance, I asked Steven Heymsfield, an obesity researcher at St. Luke's-Roosevelt Hospital in New York who is a paid consultant to Nutri/System and helped develop NutriRX, the company's medical weight-loss program, why the company considered people who were only 20 percent over ideal weight good candidates for treatment with diet drugs, despite evidence that the drugs could cause primary pulmonary hypertension and brain damage in laboratory animals and possibly in humans. (Nutri/System doctors, unswayed by the dangers of fen-phen, immediately began prescribing an untested combination of phentermine and Prozac to their patients.) Heymsfield took the long view, telling me that the process of developing diet drugs takes time and inevitably includes some occasional instances of harm, to the greater good. The situation reminded him, he said, of days in an early residency when he worked with children who had leukemia, who suffered terrible side effects from the treatment. "Obesity is not leukemia," I said. "No," he replied, "But you get my point."

The numbers of people who have become gravely ill as a result of taking those diet drugs shows how the balance of medical risks to benefits has become terribly skewed in obesity treatment. Being somewhat overweight is not a serious health problem, and obesity is not a terminal illness. And even if there are considerable health risks to severe obesity, there is no evidence that medical weight-loss treatments lessen those risks and improve patients' health in the long run. There are, however, good indications that those treatments can lead to depression, eating disorders, physically stressful yo-yo dieting, and with some treatments, serious side effects and even death. In no other field of medicine are patients routinely counseled to undergo a treatment that has a less than 10 percent success rate, except in oncology, where risky, last-ditch efforts are tolerated because in many cases the patients would otherwise die. "By ordinary standards of scientific discrimination, dieting might well qualify at best as experimental treatment, not valid therapy," says Andrew Lustig, a medical ethicist at Baylor University. In experimental treatment, there are different rules: patients are informed that there's a high probability the treatment won't help them. But with diets, he says, patients are often not informed that the chances of losing weight are low, and that they may be harmed in the process.[13] It's also profitable for physicians to keep on treating obesity as a disease. When people hear that obesity is a disease, it scares them into marching straight to their doctor's office. Inevitably, the more people believe that obesity is a disease, the more they will accept that dramatic medical treatments for the condition—very-low-calorie diets, surgery, and pills—are better for them than the healthier home remedies of exercising regularly and eating more vegetables.

Many physicians, especially those who specialize in weight loss, encourage, and sometimes advertise this idea that obesity is a medical condition that should only be handled by doctors. Their patients see them when they feel they've finally gotten serious about dieting (as if they were never serious when they plunked down hundreds of dollars at Jenny Craig). They believe that their physician will, at last, prescribe the safest diet, the strongest medicine, the most individualized weight-loss treatment, and the latest in "wellness," or "lifestyle maintenance," or whatever else is the current medical marketing phrase.

"The Truth in Bariatric Practice Marketing: What Works and Why!"

Most physicians don't make a business of dieting; they tell their patients to eat less and exercise, and leave it at that. It's the self-proclaimed obesity specialists—the bariatricians—who are really cashing in on the medicalization of obesity. They realize there are enormous profits to be made if all the weight watchers in the world decide they have a disease and go to their doctors for treatment instead. At least that's how it seemed to me when I attended an annual meeting of the American Society of Bariatric Physicians, which began with a two-day marketing seminar entitled "The Truth in Bariatric Practice Marketing: What Works and Why!"

Steve Cooper, a public relations consultant, makes his way through a hotel meeting room with a microphone as though he's a talk show host. He taps one man on the shoulder. "Why are you here, sir? Why did you come?"

"To make money," answers the man, and the audience laughs uneasily. Physicians aren't supposed to be so blatant about their desire to make money.

The participants at this seminar, many of them family physicians or general practitioners who have recently opened weight-loss practices, are here to learn how to sell their diet programs by such means as print advertising, discount coupons, sales brochures, free body-fat-composition tests at local gyms, and TV and radio spots. They're finding out, too, how to market their weight-loss practices as "wellness" programs in order to attract health maintenance organizations and large companies to their waiting rooms. "Wellness is the way to go," says Cooper. "You're going to see a wellness facility in every mall in America."

Many of these doctors offer weight-loss programs as a sideline to their regular practices of stitching up fingers and diagnosing strep throat. Their patients usually pay out-of-pocket, see them regularly (for about $50 a week after an initial $100–$300 visit), and purchase weight-loss products, such as protein powder shakes and fiber cookies, at a comfortable markup. One income prospectus for the Medifast liquid diet program promised doctors they'd bring in an extra $22,000 per year treating just twenty weight-loss patients with just one visit to the doctor each (the rest is handled by support staff).[14] Nearly half of all bariatric physicians eventually stop practicing regular medicine altogether, and some open several satellite diet clinics around town. "Bariatric physicians are definitely going to be the leaders in the weight-loss industry," says ASBP executive director James Mercker. "Even though we're practicing medicine, we *are* an industry."

And a growth industry at that. Membership in the American Society of Bariatric Physicians tripled from 1993 to 1997. One of the reasons more physicians are going into bariatrics is that at a time when it's more difficult to get into specialties, becoming a bariatrician isn't very hard to do. Any doctor can hang an official-looking ASBP certificate on the office wall for the price of attending a few meetings and a promise to follow the society's voluntary treatment guidelines. They don't need to have years of formal training in nutrition, much less endocrinology, as a really well-qualified physician who treats fat people would. They don't even need to have completed an internship or residency at all. For physicians who have difficulties passing their board exams, or who are disinclined to do more training after medical school, bariatrics is an attractive and lucrative alternative. There's no shortage of patients for them to treat. "More people are considering physicians as an alternative," says the diet industry analyst John LaRosa. "The advantage medical programs have over commercial programs is that they have more credibility. They're not just viewed as salesmen who are pushing diet food on them."

But in this marketing seminar, away from any patients, Steve Cooper is trying awfully hard to get these doctors to view themselves as salesmen. In a black suit and square wire glasses, Steve strolls with his roving mike among the tables of physicians, many of whom, I'm surprised to see, are fat themselves. I noticed at breakfast that for at least some of them, "wellness" includes eggs Benedict with bacon and fried hash brown potatoes on the side. "And why are *you* here?" Steve asks another physician.

"I want to learn how to market my business," the man says, more soberly than the first physician.

"Outstanding!" says Steve. "In medical school, they never talked about business. Business, money. Does that sound like medicine?" He nods his head vigorously. "Well, it is."

Cooper's wife, Sharon, a brightly made-up woman with a shiny black bob and a tight purple suit, takes the mike. She works the crowd, shaking hands and asking people their names. "Hi, Jim," she says. "Everybody give Jim a welcome." The physicians all clap, reluctantly. This is not like a usual medical meeting. "You know," she muses, back up at the podium. "There are three types of people. How many of you are pessimists?" A few docs raise their hands. "Optimists?" Several more lift their hands. "Then there's opportunists," says Sharon. "And the opportunist is the real winner."

There is no lack of opportunity in the medical weight-loss field, she assures the group. There are 50 million adults in the United States on commercial weight-loss programs, and all are potential patients. An average bariatric patient pays $1,000 to $2,000 over the course of treatment. "Gosh, that's a nice pool to market," she says. "Capturing customers is what it's all about."

Other physicians might not say so. Most doctors would rather mow lawns for a living than offer a free introductory exam to golf course members or advertise on the Rush Limbaugh Show, as the Coopers recommend. The traditional wisdom is that aggressive sales techniques exploit the trust inherent in a good doctor-patient relationship. "By and large, physicians don't need to market to be successful," says Thomas Murray, director of the Center for Biomedical Ethics at Case Western Reserve Medical School. "These diet doctors may sincerely think they're helping their patients, but it blurs the line between being a physician and peddling a product when you use the same marketing strategies you'd use to sell Veg-o-Matics."

But squeamishness about sales techniques, many bariatric physicians assured me, is old-fashioned. Douglas Cook, a tall, telegenic Louisiana physician who makes a presentation to the group about his successful marketing techniques, tells me, "In a consumer market, you're pretty much forced to participate. How can you invest all this money in an office, spending hundreds of thousands of dollars, and just put a little sign on the outside that says, 'Dr. Cook'?" He agrees ads must be done within certain boundaries of taste, however. "I wouldn't say, 'Bring a friend and get a Pap smear free.'"

Cook, who also treats patients for anorexia and bulimia, opens up his presentation with a joke about the late serial killer Jeffrey Dahmer's eating disorder. He soon gets down to the practicalities of building a successful practice. First is marketing the weight-loss program to overweight patients who come into your office for reasons unrelated to their weight—colds and allergies and such. You can put brochures in the waiting room, or gently suggest to them during the office visit that they might be interested in losing a few pounds. One physician in the audience questions whether that's being too pushy; another responds that the health risks of obesity are such that you're doing your patients a disservice if you *don't* offer them help losing weight.

Cook describes various strategies to attract outside patients, including joining community organizations, doing radio health shows, producing newsletters, and offering patients mugs, gym bags, and T-shirts bearing the office logo. Cook hired a public relations firm to create ads for his practice. "You want to evolve a response to an emotional need," he says. One ad is headlined: "Do you eat for emotional comfort?" Another is more traditional: "Patsy lost 54 pounds in 4¹/₂ months!" One is a bit frightening: "Bulimia Can Kill."

He advocates the personal touch with patients to keep them coming in, by initiating phone calls and sending concerned letters when they fail to show up for appointments. He makes videotapes of himself offering encouragement to patients for them to view during their weekly appointments. "They see me on tape every week even though I'm not there personally."

The diet doctors at this seminar are learning how to carefully manipulate their image. Their marketing techniques are becoming increasingly sophisticated, leaving their patients—who trust them, since they're doctors—more vulnerable than ever to their questionable treatments. One presenter was very sympathetic toward fat patients, describing obesity as a condition they couldn't help. He gave examples of the extreme prejudice and discrimination fat people face. But that prejudice, he said, was the best reason to convince patients they have to lose weight (this is the kind of logic that sells skin-lightening products to African Americans). By seeming to take an enlightened, sympathetic attitude toward fat people, and by using language that talks about the "whole patient" and "lifestyle changes," the diet doctors have appropriated the language of anti-dieters to sell their diets. Even their ads proclaim that "diets don't work," and that the real answer is long-term change with the help of doctors—who will inevitably prescribe a short-term weight-loss regime.

After several other presentations on easy financing schemes, building "club loyalty" among patients, and tips for handling troublesome reporters, Sharon Cooper wraps up the seminar by telling the group that, like it or not, the trend in advertising is toward scary ads. "It takes more, with the proliferation of advertising, to get people's attention," she says. "You have to scare 'em and grab 'em." Where, I ask her later, is this trend headed? "We'll see ads that say, 'Overweight can kill you,'" she says, then pauses, thinking hard. "Maybe with a tombstone."

Doesn't that kind of advertising give doctors an unfair advantage? I ask her. How can patients know they're not being exploited? There have been, I remind her, a whole lot of quacks in the diet doctor business. "Well," she says, blinking her heavily mascaraed lashes twice. "It's buyer beware."

Indeed. At lunch, I struck up a conversation with a Southern California physician who is a member of the ASBP and asked him what kind of a diet program he works with. "I 'work' at a 'weight-loss center' run by a lay person," he said, drawing quote marks in the air. "His main business is building boats, but he has some clinics on the side where he makes a lot of money selling diet pills. Without me, he couldn't be in business." This "physician"—the quote marks are mine—explained to me that he'd been out of a job, needed money, and answered an ad for a diet doctor. "I didn't know a thing about bariatrics, but I figured, why not?" He told me that he was hoping to get out of the operation soon, since he was just following orders from the boss, writing whatever prescriptions were required without actually seeing any patients. When I asked him to talk with me on tape, he clammed up. "I'm not sure of the legality of this," he said. "I don't want to go to jail, and I don't want to ruin the business."

The Diet Treatment Hall of Fame

Across the street, at the San Antonio Convention Center, the warehouse-sized exhibit hall was filled with vendors selling products to the group of bariatric physicians gathered for their annual meeting. There were body-fat-composition chambers, high-tech scales, protein powders, juices, psychological support booklets, weight-loss herbs, very-low-calorie diet shakes and bars, and mainly, a wide array of pharmaceutical drugs. A big rainbow-colored sign lists several prescription appetite suppressants, vitamins, and minerals. Everyone seemed to be selling chromium picolinate. When I asked the vendors how these various products work, I got the same answers from each one: "They help burn fat," or, "They curb your appetite."

Walking through the exhibit hall was like taking a stroll through the Diet Treatment Hall of Fame, with many old favorites on display. At one booth, a sign advertised thyroid. "It's commonly used," the exhibitor told me. "It speeds up your metabolism." A hundred years after its use as a diet aid was pronounced dangerous by physicians, here was thyroid being sold as a diet treatment. At another table, bottles of human chorionic gonadotropin (HCG) were on display, despite the fact that the AMA warned against its use three decades ago. At another booth, the tables were spread with bee-pollen capsules, coenzyme Q, chelation drip lopotropic combinations, and B-vitamin injections. The exhibitor refused to talk to a journalist, turning his face and aggressively shooing me away, as if my little notebook and I were a *60 Minutes* team with a TV camera and bright lights. Most of the other booths in the exhibit hall advertised pharmaceutical drugs. The American Society of Bariatric Physicians was actually formed by a drug company, Western Research Laboratories, some forty years ago.[15] Though the group split from the company in 1969, the strong pro-pharmaceutical spirit lingers.

Since nothing works to treat obesity in most people, physicians have, over the past century, tried almost anything. In the history of dieting, physicians have probably harmed dieters most, prescribing sometimes lethal liquid protein fasts, damaging and addictive amphetamines, strange potions of pig's thyroid and growth hormones, and dramatic surgeries that involve all manner of balloons, staples, and wires.

The methods doctors use to treat obesity do work in the short term, which is what keeps them going. But almost *anything*—lobster salad and champagne, pumpkin pie and amphetamines, or Optifast and appetite suppressants—works in the short term. Despite physicians' admonishments that their patients need to follow "maintenance plans" and "lifestyle changes," most haven't a clue how to help their patients keep their weight off long term. They say it's up to their patients to keep their dramatic weight losses off at a time when their bodies are fighting to get back to normal after a period of extreme starvation. When they almost inevitably gain the weight back, their doctors say they have no willpower.

Physician-Assisted Starvation

Several exhibits at the bariatricians' conference offered different varieties of very-low-calorie diets. Some had free diet cookies and bars on display to taste (the bariatrician standing next to me discreetly spat his sample into his handkerchief), and others featured powdered shakes and liquid diets. All promised safe, rapid weight loss. These cookie and shake programs that physicians use are called very-low-calorie diets, adding up to 400 to 800 calories a day (compared with 1,200 calories a day on a commercial weight-loss center diet). Diet doctors aren't the only ones prescribing these very-low-calorie diets; they are commonly prescribed in hospital-based weight-loss programs and by family physicians and internists.

Very-low-calorie diets starve people. Physicians have tried several means of starvation to get people to lose weight, from total fasting to modified fasts with protein supplements to more nutritionally balanced very-low-calorie diets. All of them eventually lead to the well-documented and unpleasant side effects of starvation—including fatigue, hair loss, cold intolerance, anemia, depression, loss of muscle tissue, dehydration, irritability, weakness, bad breath, gallstones, and cardiac arrhythmias—and all have been responsible for patient deaths. A Swedish study shows about 59 sudden unexplained deaths per 100,000 people on very-low-calorie diets, which is 40 times the rate of sudden death in the general population.[16]

Eating no food whatsoever will obviously cause people to lose weight quickly, though no one can keep it up for long without serious physical damage. "Fasting"—the term is a euphemism for starvation, as if the body can tell whether it is receiving no food on purpose or not—has been popular as a diet aid, off and on, since William the Conqueror. (In 1087, having difficulties riding on horseback because of his tremendous bulk, William the Conqueror took to his bed to lose weight with a "liquid diet" consisting mainly of alcoholic beverages.) Fasting had a recent heyday in the 1970s, when several diet doctors wrote books claiming that long-term fasting would not only help dieters lose weight, but would rid the body of impurities and give the organs a well-needed rest. Allan Cott, a Manhattan psychiatrist who wrote *Fasting as a Way of Life* (1977), for instance, advocated that fasting was the "healthiest way to lose weight," and believed that the body has at least a month's supply of food in reserve to feed on. But in reality, fasting for more than a day or two is hardly healthy. Instead of eliminating toxins from the body, it creates them, and puts a great strain on the heart, kidneys, and liver. The body not only burns up fat, but muscle and organs as well. No one can last for long on a fast, and at least five hospital patients who were put on fasts in the late 1960s died (others died during the course of treatment, or in the refeeding stage immediately afterward, but physicians claimed that the deaths were the result of obesity-related problems).

Obesity researchers, impressed by the quick weight losses

achieved by fasting, but dissuaded by the deaths, attempted to improve on the fast by adding enough protein to the diet to prevent muscles, including the heart, from being consumed by the body. In the early 1970s, a surgeon associated with Harvard University, George Blackburn, fed his fat patients 4 to 8 ounces of protein a day, about 300 calories' worth, enough to keep the body from cannibalizing itself. He developed what came to be known as the "protein-sparing modified fast."

The protein-sparing modified fast was popularized in the form of liquid protein diets. In 1976, a Philadelphia osteopath, Robert Linn, inspired by Blackburn's research, wrote a book called *The Last Chance Diet* that advocated a fast supplemented with liquid protein. Unlike Blackburn, who fed his patients plain meat or fish, Linn suggested people subsist on Prolinn, a formula he created (named for "protein" + "Linn"), which was only available through physicians. The New York state attorney swiftly ordered Linn's publisher to refund the purchase price of the book to buyers because it prescribed a diet that wasn't available except through the author. Linn responded by donating the Prolinn name to a nonprofit foundation and publishing the formula. Prolinn, it turned out, consisted of ground-up animal hides, tendons, and bones, useless slaughterhouse byproducts that were now going for a premium price. It was cooked into a gooey pinkish syrup and flavored with enough artificial cherry, orange, or pineapple to disguise the cowhide taste. Soon, liquid formula diets were available in drugstores throughout the United States.[17]

By the time some 4 million Americans had tried the ghastly liquid protein formula, the FDA began to get reports that people were dying of heart attacks after several weeks on the diet. For them, it truly had been a "last chance" diet. Physicians argued over whether it was the formula or the absence of potassium that had caused the fatalities (potassium gives the heart the electrical signals to keep pumping), and many thought the liquid protein itself was wrongly blamed. "It's the same kind of hysteria that surrounded Legionnaires' disease," Blackburn told *Newsweek* in 1978. The magazine quoted him saying that if the FDA took the liquid protein products off the market, reclassifying them as drugs that would require testing for FDA approval, it would be a "miscarriage of justice."[18]

Blackburn, however, distanced himself from the liquid protein formulas by 1979, after the Centers for Disease Control reported that fifty-eight people had indeed died on the diet. "It was fine as long as it was in the physicians' hands, because they could talk people into taking vitamins and minerals," he said, changing his tune somewhat. "But the exploiters just carried on with the connective tissue protein without the co-factors [vitamins and minerals].... A gullible public and exploiting industry added up to disaster."[19]

However, many of the people who died were under a doctor's care, and no one ever determined just exactly what caused the heart attacks. The protein itself was found to have little biological value, and didn't contain all the amino acids the body needs. The CDC identified a common pattern of heart failure among those who died. "This pattern is characterized by either sudden death or death due to intractable cardiac arrhythmias in individuals with no previous history of heart disease." At least fifteen of these deaths occurred in women aged twenty-five to fifty, who were healthy when they started the diet.[20] One study of seventeen of the fifty-eight deaths found that the deaths had nothing to do with the type of medical supervision received during the diet, the daily dosage of potassium supplementation, or the quality of the protein product used. The researchers concluded that based on the risk of cardiac arrest that occurred with starvation, "The use of very low calorie weight reduction regimens should be curtailed until further studies determine what modifications, if any, can insure their safety."[21]

Nevertheless, doctors continued to support the use of starvation diets. In the 1980s, because of the risks involved—and perhaps to corner the profits derived from the sales of the treatment—they insisted that such diets should be left in the hands of physicians. The diets were reformulated to include more vitamins, minerals, and carbohydrates. Medical versions of very-low-calorie diets became extremely popular after Oprah Winfrey dragged a wagonload of fat onto her talk show on November 15, 1988, and announced that she had lost 67 pounds in four months by consuming very-low-calorie Optifast. These diets are less dangerous than the liquid protein diets, because they are more nutritionally balanced, yet they still have problems of their own. Most obviously, they cause people to regain weight just as quickly as they lost it (à la Oprah). Even physicians who support the diets say they shouldn't be undertaken except by people who are at least 30 percent over a healthy weight. "Large losses of lean mass in dieters can have disastrous consequences, including disturbance of cardiac function and damage to the organs," wrote one group of obesity researchers, including Blackburn, in the *Journal of the American Medical Association* in 1990.[22] It isn't clear why, given the very low success rate of the diets, the researchers justify these risks for obese patients, either.

Some obesity researchers feel that very-low-calorie diets do no one any good—except the physician, whose financial health is vastly improved by prescribing the treatments to patients. In one journal article, John Garrow, an obesity specialist from St. Bartholomew's Hospital in London, said, "VLCD [the very-low-calorie diet] is not needed by the severely obese patient (because everyone would lose weight on a conventional diet), and still less by the mildly obese patient, but it is needed by diet manufacturers and physicians associated with commercial weight loss organizations." He noted that the cost of these diets, in time and money, is much greater for the patient, who has to pay for clinic visits and laboratory tests. Furthermore, these diets undermine patients' abilities to learn how to develop internal control over their eating habits. "The net effect is that obese people are put to additional expense to buy a product that they do not need, and their confidence in their ability to control their own diet is unnecessarily destroyed."[23]

Even though the serious health problems and deaths due to very-low-calorie diets were most publicized during the late seventies, they are still with us. Aside from the risk of death on these diets, patients who undertake a very-low-calorie diet will have a one in four chance of developing gallstones—about thirty times the risk they might expect if they didn't go on the diet. Patients who read the fine print before signing up for the diets would find, in the case of United Weight Control Corporation, which markets a medically supervised fasting program, that they're agreeing to a quoted risk: "Some reports have suggested a relationship between programmed diets and sudden death, probably due to irregularities of the heart. I understand that participation in this weight reduction program may entail a minute risk of fatal heart irregularities."

How "minute" that risk may be no one knows. Few deaths from very-low-calorie dieting are reported in the United States. "When a fat person dies, it's blamed on their obesity," explains the endocrinologist Wayne Callaway, who has testified in several court cases involving sudden deaths. "We don't know how many sudden deaths occur."

Dieting deaths aren't recorded in U.S. mortality statistics gathered by the Centers for Disease Control, and diet programs are not required to report such deaths. In most cases, diet deaths are simply listed as cases of cardiac arrest. In 1990, in the congressional hearings on the diet industry chaired by Congressman (now Senator) Ronald Wyden, Callaway testified that even known dieting deaths are quieted in court. "When the victim or his or her survivors have raised legal issues, in general, the cases have been settled out of court and the documents sealed," he said. "There is no registry for providing data on a national scale. As you can well appreciate, the companies themselves do not volunteer such information to outside researchers."[24]

Girth-Control Pills

Diet pills had a heyday in the fifties and sixties, when housewives around the country were downing amphetamines in the morning and barbiturates in the evening to put them asleep. For a while, people all over the country were optimistic that a cure for obesity had been discovered. As *Newsweek* put it in February 1949, "Many drugs have been used to correct obesity but only a few are safe and effective. One of the best is Dexedrine." In 1952, 3 billion 10-milligram amphetamine tablets were being produced annually in the United States. By 1970, 8 percent of all prescriptions were for these "mother's little helpers."[25] But diet pills fell out of favor when it became clear that the effects of amphetamines were sometimes disastrous: many women became addicted to the drugs, which rev up the nervous system, increase the heart rate and blood pressure, and cause anxiety, insomnia, nervousness. Long-term use led to heart damage, stroke, kidney failure, and psychosis in some cases. In 1979, the FDA reclassified appetite suppressants as dangerous drugs. For many years, most respectable doctors shunned the use of diet pills.

Diet pills became popular again among physicians in the early nineties—if only by default. "We've tried everything," explained Jules Hirsch, the obesity expert. "Nothing works, and people are desperate, so we're going back to drugs."

The pendulum started to swing back with a vengeance after a 1992 study showed that two old and fairly ineffective diet drugs—fenfluramine and phentermine—were more effective in combination than diet and exercise alone at taking weight off. The study, done at the University of Rochester by pharmacologist Michael Weintraub, was hailed by the media: "Drugs Found to Keep Lost Flab Off," read one headline in the *New York Times*. Nutri/System trumpeted the study in its ads for NutriRX, its medical weight-loss program, where diet center clients went down the hall for a quick visit with a doctor after they'd weighed in for the week. Wyeth-Ayerst, the company that makes fenfluramine, went into high gear, and was unable to keep up with the demand for the drug even with its workers on twenty-four-hour shifts. New prescriptions for fenfluramine (Pondimin) increased by 6,390 percent from 1993 to 1997, and unscrupulous physicians began opening "pill mills" to sell the newly nicknamed "fen-phen" to just about anyone, particularly in Southern California. After dexfenfluramine (Redux) was approved in April 1996, analysts predicted the market for diet pills would quickly reach $1 billion.[26] A few naysayers worried that the new era in diet drugs would end as the old one did: in disillusionment, or worse.[27]

Dieters, at first, seemed delighted with the drugs, saying that they finally felt in control of their eating and didn't even think about food. Aside from a few side effects—occasional dry mouth, a little nervousness, and vivid dreams—many said the drugs made them feel like they could stick to a weight-loss regime more easily. Cookies lost some of their interest, while stomach crunches took on a new appeal. Some patients went off the drugs quickly, however, when they found that they affected their moods or made them feel too antsy.

Fenfluramine works by toning down cravings for food by increasing the amount of serotonin in the brain. Serotonin is a chemical messenger that helps regulate not just appetite but impulsiveness, sexual feelings, and mood. The more serotonin, the calmer and more satisfied people feel. Fenfluramine is made up of a chemical package of dexfenfluramine (approved by itself in 1996 as Redux) and levofenfluramine. The levofenfluramine part can make patients feel drowsy, so phentermine, the amphetamine-like drug that speeds up the nervous system, was prescribed in tandem with fenfluramine to counteract the snooziness and further suppress the appetite.

Some researchers had reservations about the drug combination from the start—particularly since it was being over-prescribed. Cornell University psychologist David Levitsky pointed out that the long-term effects of the drugs were unknown, and that the drugs had not been tested together. More doubts about fenfluramine—and its cousin, dexfenfluramine (Redux)—emerged during the FDA hearings to approve Redux in 1996.

At the FDA hearings, scientists presented two main objections to the new drug. The first was that it caused a rare but serious condition called primary pulmonary hypertension (PPH) in about 18 out of a million users. In people who have PPH, the blood vessels that feed the lungs tighten up, and the heart must work so hard to pump the blood through the constricted vessels that it can fail. In France, where the drug had been used for years, some 20 women per year died of PPH after taking dexfenfluramine before the government tightened up prescription guidelines. Some researchers at the FDA hearings cautioned that some cases of pulmonary hypertension may have been overlooked. Ron Innerfield, an endocrinologist with the National Diabetes Center in Bethesda, Maryland, who was formerly a medical officer in the division of the FDA that regulates weight-loss drugs, said that the condition, which reveals itself through subtle complaints of weakness, shortness of breath, and debilitation, is very difficult to diagnose. "This is a tip-of-the-iceberg phenomenon," he told me. "For every patient you pick up with this, there must be one hundred more you're missing."

Another possible risk was even more insidious. Studies showed that with long-term use, fenfluramine and dexfenfluramine could cause subtle brain damage. Lewis Seiden, a pharmacologist at the University of Chicago, was one of several scientists who studied fenfluramine and dexfenfluramine in rats and monkeys and found that the drugs burn out the brain axons that release serotonin. The axons regrew, but in odd tangles. No one was certain what it meant to have tangled neural axons, but it didn't sound good. As Lynn McAfee, a fat activist, put it at the FDA hearings on the drug, "I don't like having tangles in my hair, much less in my brain."

George Ricaurte, a neurologist at Johns Hopkins University, showed that monkeys given high doses of the drug for just four days suffered substantial damage to the neural axons and that the damage lasted for as long as a year and a half. The drug's effect on the brain was similar to the kind that results from using the recreational street drug MDMA, better known as Ecstasy. "We have a need for a good appetite suppressant," Ricaurte said, "But when the animal data raise the possibility of neurotoxicity in humans, we have to be cautious."[28]

Other researchers argued that the animals in those studies were given very large doses of the drugs (recent studies have shown that the neurotoxic effects occurred in animals at doses equivalent to those humans take). Richard Atkinson, the obesity researcher at the University of Wisconsin (whose organization, the American Obesity Association, is largely funded by pharmaceutical companies), said that Ricaurte's findings probably had no bearing on humans. He, too, urged caution in prescribing the drugs, though. In his studies involving over two thousand patients on fenfluramine and phentermine, he saw significant mood changes, concentration problems, short-term memory loss, fatigue, and loss of libido—the kinds of changes that might, in fact, occur if neural axons that deliver serotonin were damaged. Atkinson also didn't believe the drugs should be used on people who only want to lose a few pounds. "It's a little scary to say everybody who's a little overweight ought to go take these things," he said.[29]

Outside the FDA hearings, other physicians voiced some concerns about the drugs. Jules Hirsch was wary of how frequently the drugs were being prescribed, warning that physicians should be careful to tailor obesity treatment to individuals, according not just to their weight but to their complete medical picture—other health risks, their history, their reasons for being obese. He pointed out that the drugs were hardly the magic bullets they'd been made out to be. In the short run, the fen-phen combination was as good as any diet: about a third of patients lost 5 to 10 percent of their body weight. In the long run, they're just as bad, because most of those patients regained the weight. The results of the Weintraub study, he pointed out, were really quite modest. Hirsch worried that physicians working for commercial weight-loss programs would have to follow company guidelines for prescriptions rather than judgments for individualized medical treatments. "I would consider this to be bad medical treatment," he said.[30] Other physicians suggested that the drugs might be helpful only to a small subgroup of dieters; one 1996 study suggested that for people with abdominal obesity (the "apples" among us), dexfenfluramine might help redistribute fat to a safer location on the hips and thighs.[31]

Given all the potential dangers of dexfenfluramine, the FDA advisory committee initially voted against approving the drug, six to five. Some obesity researchers were outraged. In an editorial in the

Chicago Tribune, Michael Fumento quoted American Obesity co-chair Judith Stern as saying that if the FDA panel recommended no on dexfenfluramine, "These doctors ought to be shot." Fumento (author of *The Myth of Heterosexual AIDS* and, more recently, *The Fat of the Land*) lamented, "In its caution the FDA panel refused to weigh the slight possibility of harm of the drug versus the very real harm caused by obesity.... What the heck is going on here? Is the FDA staffed at the highest levels by men who are into fat women?"

The pharmaceutical company presented evidence to the FDA that the risks of obesity outweighed the potential harm of the drugs. Much of that evidence was based on a study by JoAnn Manson of the Harvard University School of Public Health, a paid consultant to Interneuron Pharmaceuticals, the company that developed the drug. Manson, as previously mentioned, overstated the risks of obesity in interpreting her results. The FDA didn't question the numbers, though, and reversed itself, with the caveat that the manufacturer had to conduct another long-term study on the health risks of dexfenfluramine. Twenty-two research scientists sent a letter to the FDA protesting the approval, saying that the panel failed to take seriously the evidence that the drug could cause brain damage in humans. The FDA went ahead and approved the drug anyway in April 1996, making it the first new diet drug in this country in over 20 years.

Over the next year, serious problems with the drugs emerged. By May 1996, Mary Linnen, a 30-year-old Massachusetts woman, died after taking the pills, and her parents sued the drug companies for failing to warn potential users of the risks. Linnen had tried to lose 25 to 30 pounds for a wedding, but developed cardiovascular problems and died several months later. The FDA reported that 12 people total had already died after taking the drugs.

In August, a study in the *New England Journal of Medicine* reported that the number of people who developed primary pulmonary hypertension from fenfluramine and dexfenfluramine was higher than previously believed—about 46 per million instead of 18. In an editorial favorable to Redux in that issue, authors JoAnn Manson and Gerald Faich argued that Redux would still prevent 20 obesity-related deaths for every one person who died of PPH. The editors of the journal were soon embarrassed to learn that both Manson and Faich had undisclosed conflicts of interest; Manson, the lead author, was a paid consultant to Interneuron Pharmaceuticals for several months in 1995, and Faich was a paid consultant to Servier and American Home Products, companies that marketed the drug in collaboration with Interneuron.

In December 1996, the National Task Force on the Prevention and Treatment of Obesity concluded in the *Journal of the American Medical Association* that there was "little justification" for the short-term use of weight loss drugs. "Until more data are available, pharmacotherapy cannot be recommended for routine use in obese individuals, although it may be helpful in carefully selected patents." In January, Cornell University's David Levitsky published a meta-analysis of studies done on fenfluramine and dexfenfluramine in *Healthy Weight Journal* in which he found that the drugs caused a weight loss that was only five pounds greater, on average, than placebo pills, resulting in a daily difference of only 62 calories—about the same as taking the stairs instead of riding the elevator.

In July 1997, the Mayo Clinic reported that physicians had discovered an extremely rare valvular heart disease in 24 diet-drug users. The women, all previously healthy, had a condition where their heart valves were coated with a waxy build-up that prevented them from closing properly, causing blood to regurgitate; many had to have surgery to prevent heart failure. The FDA, which had received reports of nine additional similar cases, issued an advisory to 700,000 physicians, warning them that the safety of fenfluramine and phentermine used in combination was not established, and that serious concerns had arisen. The agency also asked five clinics to perform echocardiograms on patients who'd taken fenfluramine or Redux.

In August, a *Journal of the American Medical Association* report concluded that the doses of diet drugs believed to cause brain damage in animals were roughly equivalent to those taken by humans. Lead author Una McCann, a psychiatrist at the National Institute of Mental Health, said that relatively small amounts of the drugs "amputate the neurons" that deliver serotonin into the brain. The next day, August 28, an editorial in the *New England Journal of Medicine* called for a moratorium on the use of Redux and fenfluramine. The editorial criticized the FDA approval process for Redux, arguing that there wasn't sufficient evidence that the benefits of the drugs outweigh their risks for any but the seriously obese. Cardiologist Gregory Curfman, deputy editor of the NEJM called the side effects of the drugs "pretty scary," and told the *Wall Street Journal*, "It has never been shown that these drugs can make people live longer, [but] even short-term use has been associated with serious complications." The NEJM also reported on the case of a 29-year-old woman who died of pulmonary hypertension after taking the drug combination for only 23 days.

In September, Florida regulators put a 90-day ban on fen-phen prescriptions after the 53-year-old wife of the mayor of North Miami Beach died of a heart attack while on diet drugs. That month the FDA received results from the echocardiograms it had asked clinics to do to monitor heart valve damage. Nearly one-third of diet drug users—92 out of 291 tested—showed signs of heart-valve irregularities. In the face of these frightening results, the FDA requested a voluntary recall of fenfluramine and dexfenfluramine, and Wyeth-Ayerst complied. The drugs were, in fact, recalled worldwide.

By late September, American physicians were already prescribing phentermine and Prozac—"phen-Pro"—and one physician, Michael Anchors, was quick to publish *Safer Than Phen-Fen* about the new combination, which hadn't been studied in tandem, either. By November, undaunted, the FDA approved Meridia (sibutramine), another, though probably less dangerous serotonin booster—against the advice of its own advisory committee.

Instead of attacking appetite, the drug called orlistat is meant to work *after* you've eaten—by interfering with the body's metabolism of fat. Likely to be approved by the FDA soon, gossip columnist Liz Smith has already called orlistat a "dream drug," and *Self* magazine hailed it as "the miracle drug we've all been waiting for." The promise of orlistat is that it would allow us all to be on a low-fat diet without having to eat any less fat. It's the drug that does to the body what olestra does to food—both make it impossible for fat to be absorbed into the body.

Under normal circumstances, fat in food is broken down by an enzyme that allows it to pass through the intestinal walls and into the bloodstream, where it's either used as energy or sent along to convenient storage areas (like the thighs). Orlistat interferes with that enzyme—called pancreatic lipase—so that about one-third of the fat you take in passes through the body undigested.[32]

It's an elegant idea, if you don't think it all the way through. But there may be some uncomfortable side effects to blocking fat. "If you have more fat in the large intestine, you'll have more fat in the stool," says F. Xavier Pi-Sunyer, an obesity expert at St. Luke's–Roosevelt

Hospital in New York City. The effect, he said, would be bulky, greasy, foul-smelling stools. Anyone who has had weight-loss surgery to shorten their intestines, so that fat is not absorbed into the body, can attest to how nasty this particular side effect can be. There may also be health risks: Robert Eckel, a professor of medicine at the University of Colorado, speculates that the increase in fat could heighten the risk of colon cancer. (One theory has it that fat in contact with colon cells may explain the well-known association of high-fat diets with this cancer.) Another potential problem is that when fat isn't absorbed in the body, fat-soluble vitamins are lost, too.

Finally, it's likely that many patients on the drug would simply eat more fat. When people eat fake fat, which is now used in many foods, like ice cream and cookies, they don't lose weight; they eat more to make up for the loss. The same thing would likely happen with fat-blockers, says Wayne Callaway. "The fallacy here is that people are fat simply because they eat too much, and all you have to do is reduce food intake or digestion of a certain nutrient."

The human body is much more complex than that, and not likely to be fooled by such a crude trick as blocking fat. Over the millennia, the human body has learned to fight to hold on to its store of food; our survival has depended on it. "There are always compensatory mechanisms," says Callaway.

Until scientists understand more about the underlying causes of obesity, dieting with drugs is likely to be hit-and-miss—and sometimes dangerous. Despite all the optimistic reports about new diet pills, we're a long way from having a pill that would make us thin.

Weight-Loss Surgery

While I was at the American Society of Bariatric Physicians' Conference, I met a surgeon from Florida, Michael Butler, who performs weight-loss operations. I asked him about these surgeries, which are only recommended for people who are extremely obese. Butler motioned me toward a sixtyish blond woman who was wearing a cowboy hat and a glittery Western-yoked shirt. "I'd like you to meet someone," he said.

The woman was slightly fat, with loose sallow skin and a slow and uneven gait. She didn't look too healthy. Seven and a half years ago, Butler said, he had performed her surgery. "I lost one hundred twenty-three pounds," the woman told me, "and those one hundred twenty-three pounds are still off." She appeared to be delighted with her results. "This is the best thing that ever happened to me," she said.

Butler smiled quietly, proud of his work. He performs more than one hundred of these surgeries a year—at a cost to the patient of about $20,000 each—for people who are at least 100 pounds over average weight. "You really do something that changes a person's life," he said. "You have individuals who have been out of society, can't work, and now you can put these people back in society, and they feel positive about themselves."

Of all physician weight-loss treatments, surgery is the most drastic. On the whole, patients are pleased with the results—at least in the first few years. One study of patients conducted three years after their surgeries showed that almost all of them would rather be deaf, blind, or have a limb amputated then go back to being as fat as they were before.[33] But often, after those first few years, when the "honeymoon period" is over and many patients have begun to gain weight again, a number of them wonder whether the surgery was worth it, particularly in light of the very unpleasant side effects almost all experience, as well as the serious long-term medical complications many endure. Yet weight-loss surgeries are becoming more popular as obesity is increasingly viewed by the medical establishment as a dire health problem that needs aggressive treatment with drugs and other interventions.

The 1995 report issued by the Institute of Medicine, for instance, recommended that more attention should be paid to surgery as a viable option for weight loss when all else has failed. "There is compelling evidence that comorbidities are reduced in severely obese patients who have lost weight as a result of gastric surgery," the panel members wrote. "Therefore, it is puzzling that this treatment is not more widely used for severely obese individuals at very high risk for obesity-related morbidity and mortality."[34]

Weight-loss surgeons, like bariatricians, are starting to push their services more aggressively. There are about five hundred weight-loss surgeons in the country; they perform some 25,000 procedures per year, at $20,000 apiece, for a total of $500 million a year.[35] Although the medical literature suggests performing the procedure on people who are "morbidly obese"—the 0.5 percent of the population that is more than 100 percent over desirable weight—it is being marketed more widely. Some bariatric surgeons say the procedures are appropriate for anyone who is 100 pounds overweight, even though a 230-pound woman, for instance, may not have any health risks at all associated with her weight. Bariatric surgeons use television and newspaper ads, 800 numbers, telemarketers, and sophisticated marketing techniques to target potential patients. In San Diego and other cities, weight-loss surgeons advertise in local papers for the large hotel seminars they hold for prospective clients.

"They used very slick sales techniques," says Suzanne Szames, a San Diego woman who attended a seminar not long after she watched a good friend of hers slowly die from malnutrition and kidney failure several years after she had had intestinal bypass weight-loss surgery. The physicians, she said, began the presentation to the audience of 150 with a show of empathy and friendliness. "They said they knew diets don't work, they knew what we'd all been through, they understood us, and they were there to help," Szames recalls. Then they used scare tactics, telling the audience that fat people were apt to succumb to something called Sudden Death syndrome. They described obesity as a cancer, says Szames. "They said fat was a malignancy, and like any other malignancy, it required surgery." The rewards of the surgery were great, the surgeons said; not only would patients lose their excess weight, but their diabetes and asthma would be cured.

The surgeons didn't mention the side effects of weight-loss surgeries until audience members asked them directly, says Szames. When they were mentioned, they were usually made light of, or glossed over. One woman in the audience, she recalls, stood up and asked if patients had a problem with flatulence. "Oh, yes, there's flatulence," one of the surgeons told her. Then he laughed. "You have to always carry air freshener." Szames said the physicians downplayed the very real risks involved with the surgeries, and emphasized the fairy-tale promise of a morbidly obese person gaining a new lease on life by losing huge amounts of weight.

Two main types of weight-loss surgery are performed these days. Both sound a little like a bad home-plumbing job. With gastroplasty, or stomach stapling, most of the patient's stomach is stapled off so that only a small pouch is still usable. The stomach becomes about 5 percent of its original size, and its capacity to hold food decreases a hundred-fold.[36] Often gastroplasty is done with a band around the opening leading from the stomach pouch to the intestines, called vertical banded gastroplasty (the most common type of surgery), which keeps the stomach from distending again. With gastric bypass (the Rouxen-Y gastric bypass is the second most common surgery), the stomach is stapled, then the intestines are whacked off below the stomach and rerouted to the bottom of the stapled pouch, blocking off the rest of the stomach, the duodenum, and part of the small intestines, where food and vitamins are usually absorbed. Food goes straight from the esophagus to the tiny stomach pouch and directly into the lower part of the small intestines.

Both of these procedures can usually be reversed, although that requires another surgery that is potentially more dangerous than the initial one. With both, there is a slight risk of stomach juices leaking into the abdomen, resulting in severe infection and occasionally death. Both cause severe diarrhea, awful flatulence, foul odors, pain from the staples, skin eruptions, and occasional infections. Patients vomit if they eat more than a few tablespoons of food. Those who have had their stomachs stapled often turn to bland, easily digested foods; they often can't tolerate meat, vegetables, and fruits, and turn instead to ice creams, puddings, pastries, processed white breads, potato chips, and other nonnutritious fare. The gastric bypass surgery patients can't eat sweets because of "dumping syndrome," in which sugar passes into the small intestines too rapidly, causing dizziness, diarrhea, weakness, and sweating. Because the part of their small intestines that absorbs nutrients has been blocked off, many patients develop deficiencies in iron, calcium (leading to osteoporosis), and other vitamins; it's difficult to take enough supplements to make up for what isn't absorbed in the intestines.

Several other long-term complications arise with weight-loss surgery. Sometimes, food gets clogged in the outlet at the bottom of the stomach pouch, requiring that patients get their stomachs pumped (this happened to 22 percent of patients in one study). Others need several revisions to their surgeries, and develop painful masses of scar tissue. These scars can end up blocking segments of the digestive tract, so stomach secretions and bile continue to enter, with nowhere to go; this condition requires immediate surgery. About half the patients develop gallstones. Some develop cardiac arrhythmias. There is a higher suicide rate among weight-loss surgery patients than there is among the morbidly obese.[37]

Medical texts say there is an illness rate of 10 percent with the surgeries, and a death rate of 1 percent with most surgeries. But people who oppose weight-loss surgery—including the National Association to Advance Fat Acceptance (NAAFA)—say the side effects are more severe, and that the death rate from complications several years after surgery is higher. "Somewhere along the line, at five or ten years, the outcome of these surgeries is malnutrition and malabsorption," says Marty Lipton, a San Diego NAAFA member who had a friend die after weight-loss surgery. "Eventually, people's bodies cannot keep up with it." Usually, she says, insurance companies will cover the surgeries, but not the revisions that may be needed later on when these long-term side effects develop. NAAFA is a 4,500-member organization based in Sacramento, California, that works to educate people about obesity. About 10 percent of NAAFA's members have had weight-loss surgery, according to its founder, William Fabrey, and most gained the weight back and suffered health problems; several members have died after the surgery.

In one longer-term study, in 1993, Norwegian researchers looked at 174 cases of vertical banded gastroplasties (the surgery that reduces the stomach size without bypassing the intestines), following patients who had the operations for five years. They found higher rates of complications and deaths than are reported in shorter-term studies. During the first month, twenty-five patients reported complications, including severe wound infections, perforation of the stomach, peritonitis (inflammation of the abdominal cavity due to bacteria leaking from the stomach), and blood clots in the veins and the lung. One patient died of widespread infection and multi-organ failure.

Those numbers are in keeping with most statistics on the risks of weight-loss surgery. But after five years, there were sixty cases of severe complications. Twenty-six patients had to be re-operated on, half of them because they had continual vomiting. Fifteen had developed hernias where the incisions were, and four patients died (one death was unrelated). Fewer than half had kept their weight at or below 30 percent of the desirable weight; many had regained weight because the stomach pouch eventually expands. After the study was completed, the researchers changed their minds about gastric surgery; their "early optimistic view" became a more "realistic one," and they suggested that weight-loss surgery isn't the final solution to obesity.[38]

In 1989, an AMA panel of surgeons and gastroenterologists—not obesity experts, like the Institute of Medicine panel—was divided on the question of whether weight-loss surgeries should be considered safe and effective. Half thought that neither of the main techniques used—stomach stapling or stapling plus intestinal bypass—had established its safety or effectiveness.

Many people who have had the surgery have come to regret their decision. Karen Smith, an Albuquerque woman in her forties who heads NAAFA's Weight Loss Surgery Survivors group, underwent a jejunoileal bypass—a surgery, now rarely performed, in which most of the small intestine is bypassed, leaving it floating, unattached at one end, inside the body—when she was twenty-six years old and weighed about 375 pounds. She lost 90 pounds after the surgery, down to 285 pounds. After five years, her body adjusted to its shortened intestines, and she regained all the weight. The side effects, however, have stayed with her. She has fifteen to twenty bowel movements a day, many of which she can't control. She always has to carry an extra change of clothing with her in case she has an accident. Because the food she eats is improperly digested, her stools have a foul odor. One government office where she worked set up a special cleaning task force to try to identify the source of the tremendously bad smell on her floor. "It was me," she says. "It was terribly embarrassing."

Because of her bowel problem, Smith can no longer exercise, and, formerly socially active, she often avoids people. "They said if I had surgery, I would lose weight and do all the things I could never do because I was fat," she says. "Instead, I didn't lose weight, and I can't do any of the things that kept me healthy before." Smith lost most of her hair from nutritional deficiency, she had kidney stones, and a bacterial overgrowth at the shunt end of the useless portion of her intestines caused an arthritis-like syndrome in her body. She tried to lose weight by dieting, but gained weight even on Weight Watchers. "It isn't fair; I have only eighteen inches of intestines, and I can't lose weight," she says. She has since given up dieting and slowly lost weight to 300 pounds, where it has stabilized for some years. "I lost more weight by giving up dieting than by weight-loss surgery," she says.

In the past few years, Smith, a former minister, has devoted much of her time to counseling people who are considering weight-loss surgery. "I knew the surgery would kill me someday," she says. "I had to face that, and do what I could to tell people." She tries to provide people with information about the risks. "I was angry that I wasn't given all the details of my surgery," she says. "Everyone should have enough information to make an informed decision. Doctors over-emphasize the dangers of obesity, and minimize the risks and side effects of surgery."

Smith gives people who call her—some four hundred prospective patients a year—statistics on weight-loss surgery that she has gleaned from medical journals. Ten percent of patients, she tells them, don't lose any weight at all. People who are morbidly obese—100 to 200 pounds overweight—have a 39 percent chance of getting down to 130 percent of their ideal body weight. Super-obese patients, those more than 200 pounds overweight, have only an 8 percent chance of getting down to that "success" point. After about five years, 70 percent of patients regain all the weight. One in ten loses the weight and keeps it off. "Everyone goes into it with the hope that they'll be one of the lucky ten percent," says Smith.

Despite her efforts, Smith says she rarely talks people out of having the surgery. She knows how difficult it is to be extremely obese in this culture, and she understands their intense desire to lose weight when nothing else has helped them. Instead of changing their minds, many callers get angry with her. "They tell me," she says, " 'You're taking away my dream.' "

A Healthier Prescription

Not all physicians who treat fat people encourage them to diet, take pills, or have surgery. Like the physicians and weight-loss sur-geons at the bariatrics conference, Allen King, an endocrinologist in Salinas, California, has tried everything to help his patients lose weight. For twenty-one years, he treated thousands of obese and dia-betic patients, three-fourths of them women, with very little success.

At first he put patients on standard calorie-counting diets. They generally lost weight quickly and gained it right back. Then he pre-scribed very-low-calorie protein powder shakes for more than five hundred patients. "Our success rate would be fifty pounds lost in six months," says King, "and sixty pounds regained in three years."

Next came the gastric balloon. King worked with a gastroenterolo-gist who inserted the inflatable device, designed to make people feel

Chapter 7

Thinking Disorders: Obesity Researchers

When physicians need to figure out what advice to give their fat patients, or when magazine journalists need an expert to tell them the latest tips for losing 10 pounds after the holiday season, they turn to the same source: obesity researchers. These academic physicians and psychologists specialize in studying weight loss, and are largely responsible for shaping our beliefs about how dangerous it is to be fat and whether people should diet, count fat grams, exercise three times a week, take prescription weight-loss drugs—or accept themselves the size they are.

Like other scientists, obesity researchers are supposed to work by a process of consensus. They conduct studies with laboratory animals or human volunteers to test their theories or treatments for fatness. After they do a study on, say, how much weight people lose after twelve weeks on a combination of a very-low-calorie diet and behavior modification, they submit their findings to a medical journal. The journal sends the paper out to colleagues in the field to review to decide whether the results were interesting and significant enough to be published. If the study is controversial, a lively debate over the results usually ensues in the pages of the journals and at medical conferences.

Every so often, leading specialists or government-sponsored ta

full, into the stomachs of twelve patients who were markedly overweight. Some of them lost weight, but mainly because their abdominal pain was so intense they did not want to eat. Others experienced more extreme side effects: five developed stomach ulcers, two had obstructed intestinal tracts, and one required emergency surgery to remove the balloon.

After that, King and an oral surgeon wired two obese patients' jaws shut. "The patients started drinking high-calorie milkshakes," says King. "They *gained* weight." King then recommended even more radical surgery. First came the intestinal bypass; over half the patients developed kidney stones, arthritis, liver disease, and other serious illnesses. Then came stomach stapling: most of the patients would lose a third of their weight the first year, but it wouldn't stay off. "After five years, the weight would return to where they began," says King.

King finally came to the conclusion that there was nothing he could do to help his patients lose weight. Not only were the treatments unsuccessful—and risky—but they harmed his rapport with his patients. Ashamed of not sticking to their diets, they would miss appointments and fake their food diaries. They would binge and then fast like crazy before having to step on the doctor's scale. They would diet to comply with doctor's orders, and then, away from his watchful eye, go right back to their old ways. "I'm so tired of being ineffective as a physician," says King.

He's not the only one. In the face of a trend to medicalize obesity, a few physicians are going in the opposite direction. As more physicians are finding out just how hard it is to help obese patients, some have begun to wonder whether diets are merely exercises in futility and a setup for defeat. Instead, they are trying new approaches to obesity which, unlike dieting, don't make the problem worse. Some recommend no treatment, others much more moderate lifestyle changes. Wayne Callaway says obesity treatment needs to focus less on losing pounds and more on figuring out how the patient can gradually learn to live a more active, healthy lifestyle. For some, that might mean getting out and walking once a day. For others, it might mean therapy to root out the underlying causes of overeating. For a few, it might mean medication. "It's a much more complicated approach than putting people on 1,000-calorie-a-day diets," Callaway says. "I don't see any reason to do that anymore."

He says that physicians need better training to understand the limits of obesity treatment, as well as the complex reasons behind why people get fat. Obesity isn't just a simple energy-in-energy-out equation, as many physicians still believe. It may be a genetic condition, a hormonal problem, a psychological problem, or a lowered-energy requirement from long-term dieting. Callaway suggests that physicians who treat obesity need special postgraduate training in residency programs or at medical conferences in order to assess the genetic, emotional, motivation, and behavioral components of each case.

Allen King in Salinas has also adopted a new approach to helping his obese patients improve the quality of their lives. He and a nutritionist who works with him, Dana Armstrong, explain to patients that they're not going to restrict their diets. Basically, they don't tell their patients what to eat, leaving that to them. They explain what happens to the patients' health when they eat too much fat and sugar, and ask them to notice the changes they feel in their bodies when they eat those foods. But they tell them to decide for themselves what to eat.

This approach, called "demand feeding," is similar to the techniques advocated by Overcoming Overeating, Geneen Roth, and other feminist anti-dieters. It asks that patients sort out their true hunger—the hollow, rumbling kind—from emotional hunger, which may arise from stress or habit. When patients give themselves permission to eat, and don't feel deprived by a diet, says King, they're less likely to overeat. The approach also gives the patient, rather than the physician, responsibility for taking care of her eating habits. "Patients become self-directed, and they make their own decisions about their bodies. After time, they usually make good decisions."

Maren Martin, a diabetic in her forties, came to see King after a long history of yo-yo dieting and wildly fluctuating blood sugar levels. "I would always diet well and lose weight," she says. "But then I'd gain it back in a storm." With Armstrong and King's help, she gradually stopped dieting and started allowing herself to eat anything she wanted, making decisions based on when she was hungry. After two years, she no longer binges as she used to. "The foods that sparkled before because I couldn't have them just don't seem so special now," she says. Martin's weight and blood sugar levels have stabilized, though she is not thin.

After seven years of using this approach, King says he has finally succeeded in helping many of his patients to stabilize their diabetes,

sometimes to lose a few pounds, and, most imp[...] their problems themselves. Unlike diets or surg[...] approach is no quick fix. It takes one to five years[...] dieting, learn to eat what they want—and want wh[...] for their health.

"As a physician, you have to realize that you ca[...] obesity," says King. "All you can do is give her the[...] and confidence to do it herself."

forces conduct reviews of all the major research on a topic in the field—weight-loss surgery, for example, or yo-yo dieting—to determine some overall conclusions and guidelines. Journalists write about these studies and reviews for magazines and newspapers, sometimes analyzing them in context of other research in the field, and sometimes just presenting them as the latest fashion to come down the scientific runway. Eventually, this process, which is designed to be thorough and objective, is supposed to lead to a consensus that represents the closest thing to truth that science has to offer—at least until researchers publish new, conflicting studies that start the whole process in motion again.

But obesity researchers rarely agree with each other. As a result, the advice that physicians and the media offer people based on what these experts say is often confusing. For the most part, the researchers are split into two camps: pro-diet medical researchers and anti-diet eating disorders researchers. A few moderate psychologists and physicians who believe that slow changes in exercise and eating habits will help some people lose weight without starving themselves occupy the center. The medical researchers, most of whom are men, tend to favor strong interventions, such as very-low-calorie diets, drugs, and surgery. Even though many of them recognize that these treatments are often risky and short-lived, they believe it's better to do *something* than to allow people to remain fat. The anti-diet researchers, on the other hand—more of whom are female—often believe that the very treatments physicians recommend are doing their patients more harm than good. They've seen people whose repeated attempts at dieting have led to poor self-esteem and chaotic eating habits. Because researchers who study fat people hold such opposing points of view, there are many conflicting studies out on obesity treatments, and further, those studies get interpreted in very different ways.

Obesity researchers often fail to come to a consensus on even the most basic issues in the obesity field because strong cultural biases and business interests get in the way. Academic researchers don't stand apart from our weight-obsessed consumer culture, which spends billions on obesity treatments. They're right in the thick of it. Like anyone else, obesity researchers' attitudes are shaped by our society's deep-seated preference for slenderness, and even by their own worries about their weight (a few are well known for yo-yoing up and down, appearing at a conference slender one year and fat the next). More importantly, medical obesity researchers' studies are often bankrolled by drug and diet companies.

Like dieters, obesity researchers' thinking can be warped by their culture. Just as dieters feel they have to be thin to have meaningful lives, obesity researchers feel they have to continue to promote diets to have enriching careers. The social pressures they're under to make people thin are very strong. As anorexics and bulimics distort their body size, obesity researchers distort their own data to show that diet failures are really successes. In their study conclusions, obesity researchers show evident signs of distorted self-image. Anorexics look in a mirror and see a fat person looking back. Obesity researchers look at research that shows that diets don't work and come to the conclusion that people should keep on dieting. It isn't fair, perhaps, to suggest that obesity researchers, who work in a culture where their status, reputation, and livelihood depends on how well they promote dieting and diet drugs, are intellectually dishonest. Instead, we should probably say that many obesity researchers suffer from serious "thinking disorders."

Obesity researchers' thinking is distorted most by the fact that almost everyone who funds their work is in the diet business. Scientists' careers depend on publishing studies, and they often have to scramble to get the money to do them. In 1995, the National Institutes of Health spent about $87 million on obesity research (out of a total budget of $11.3 billion), which funded only a small portion of the studies done that year; the lion's share was funded by companies that are in the business of promoting diet treatments. "The so-called clinical research in this field has been largely paid for by the formula and drug companies," says Wayne Callaway, himself a moderate who opposes most diet treatments in favor of long-term lifestyle changes. Researchers who oppose dieting don't stand much of a chance of getting funding from companies who know the research will undermine their products.

Diet and pharmaceutical companies influence every step along the way of the scientific process. They pay for the ads that keep obesity journals publishing. They underwrite medical conferences, flying physicians around the country expense-free and paying them large lecture fees to attend. Some obesity researchers have clear conflict of interest, promoting or investing in products or programs based on their research. Others are paid to be consultants to diet companies, and sit on the scientific advisory boards of Weight Watchers, Jenny Craig, or other commercial programs—while they also sit on the boards of the medical journals that determine which studies get printed. What it comes down to is that most obesity researchers would stand to lose a lot of money if they stopped telling Americans they had to lose a lot of weight. "It's not always out-and-out bias," says Callaway, "but we end up with fuzzy thinking."

The fact that an obesity researcher accepts funding from a diet company doesn't necessarily taint that particular researcher, but there is a stain on the whole field. "It isn't diabolical," says eating disorders expert David Garner. "Some people are very committed to the belief that weight loss is a national health problem. It's just that if their livelihood is based in large part on the diet industry, they can't be impartial." A few of the conflicts of interest in the obesity research field seem quite obvious. Richard Wurtman, the MIT researcher whose company, Interneuron Pharmaceuticals, owns the patent to the obesity drug dexfenfluramine, for instance, was frequently quoted in the media as an expert on the drug prior to its approval, foretelling its rosy possibilities, without any mention of his financial involvement. Louisiana State University obesity researcher George Bray presented his study on thigh cream without divulging that he'd already licensed the formula for the stuff to three companies. Obesity researchers JoAnn Manson and Gerald Faich wrote an editorial in the *New England Journal of Medicine* downplaying the risks of Redux without disclosing that both had been paid consultants to the company that makes the drug.

Some obesity researchers, paid to be consultants to pharmaceutical companies, exaggerate the health risks of obesity in order to testify to the FDA that new diet drugs should be approved. Obesity researchers have been known to promote dieting or drugs in order to sell books—and to increase the numbers of patients flocking to their practices. Conflicts of interest make some researchers seem quite muddled about what they actually believe: When I asked one researcher, who has criticized dieting for being ineffective and psychologically damaging, about the policies of a commercial weight-loss program that pays him to sit on its scientific advisory board, he replied—not for attribution—"What can I say? I'm a consultant for them."

Other ways in which financial interests influence obesity researchers are more tangled and complicated. Looking at the connections between liquid diet companies and the researchers who are experts on liquid diets, as one example, sheds some light on the situation. One eminent obesity researcher, Theodore VanItallie, who is the founder of the Obesity Research Center at St. Lukes–Roosevelt Hospital in Manhattan, was also a co-founder, in 1986, of the Englewood, New Jersey–based United Weight Control Corporation, a liquid diet program used in hospitals and outpatient clinics. The company had big plans. In 1989, a business journal reported that venture capital companies had invested $3 million in United Weight: "The company wants to turn itself from a regional, $5 million entity to a national $100 million powerhouse by 1994." United Weight provided a liquid diet program to five hospital centers, including St. Luke's–Roosevelt Hospital.

VanItallie's participation in the company had something to do with its initial success. "A lot of companies didn't have good medical backgrounds," said Ashok Vaswani, director of Long Island's Winthrop University Hospital's weight-loss program, who told a business reporter why they'd chosen to use United Weight products. "Dr. VanItallie's association with the company put it in good standing." The company didn't achieve its goals; by 1990, when several liquid diet companies were having problems, John LaRosa of Marketdata Enterprises estimated its value at $1.5 million to $3 million.[1] (The company is no longer operating. VanItallie now directs the VanItallie Center for Nutrition and Weight Management at St. Luke's–Roosevelt, where some patients are still prescribed liquid diets.)

Meanwhile, VanItallie defended liquid diets to the media without revealing his own interests. An October 1988 *Newsday* piece on liquid diets quoted him as saying, "[Liquid] diets are nutritionally easy to control, you get all the vitamins and minerals you need." In that article, he conceded that few people who lose weight on liquid diets keep it off, but he had a ready explanation, placing blame on the dieters, not the treatment. "We tell people that if they're not willing to make a long term commitment to change their way of eating, to learn to keep that weight off, this is not for them."

In 1993, VanItallie, now a professor emeritus of medicine at Columbia University College of Physicians and Surgeons, was a member of the National Task Force on the Prevention and Treatment of Obesity, which determined physician guidelines for very-low-calorie diets. The panel also included University of Pennsylvania psychologist

Thomas Wadden and Harvard Medical School obesity researcher George Blackburn, both of whom have done several studies funded by Sandoz Nutrition Corporation. Sandoz makes Optifast liquid diets, sponsors medical conferences, has paid for at least sixty published studies on liquid diets and countless others that didn't make it into the journals (often because they showed no success), and is one of the three hundred largest companies in the United States. Blackburn was also a paid consultant to Sandoz, and Wadden, at one point, worked for Sandoz.[2] The panel concluded, in an article published in the prestigious *Journal of the American Medical Association*, that very-low-calorie diets are "generally safe when used under proper medical supervision in moderately and severely obese patients." The review didn't contain a whiff of suggestion that the authors each had personal financial ties to the liquid diet company, stating: "This position paper has been prepared . . . to provide a balanced overview of the scientific, published information on the safety and efficacy of [very-low-calorie diets] and to provide rational recommendations for their use."

In light of the research the experts reviewed, their conclusions were rather odd. They noted that the long-term treatment results of very-low-calorie diets were poor; the patients' metabolism dropped, they lost some body protein along with their fat during rapid weight loss, they gained the weight back, and experienced numerous adverse side effects.[3] But their conclusion was that fat people should try them anyway. It doesn't take a scientist to see that the argument for using very-low-calorie diets was not rational; it seemed it was being defended for some other reason.

Despite the biases and conflicts of interest in the field, once in a while obesity researchers take a long view of the terrain and agree on what they see. They may come to a consensus, as they have in the past, that such treatments as jaw wiring, amphetamines, or stomach balloons are harmful, and shouldn't be used. National medical groups write guidelines that oppose the treatments, and physicians who continue to use them may be shunned by their peers, no longer invited to speak at conferences in Hawaii or contribute articles to journals. The last time a strong consensus on obesity treatment was reached was in 1992, when a national task force agreed that diets don't work. That time, however, partly because of the epidemic of thinking disorders that has afflicted obesity researchers, the consensus didn't last.

A Consensus: Diets Don't Work

In the spring of 1992, a group of well-known researchers in the fields of obesity, nutrition, exercise, and metabolism gathered together in Washington, D.C., for a conference. Puzzled over the paradox that more and more Americans were gaining weight despite the fact that more were dieting, the National Institutes of Health (NIH) invited these experts to a summit meeting on the state of weight control in the United States. The purpose was to present evidence about who in America was dieting, and how safe and effective current diet methods were. An independent panel, chaired by Dr. Suzanne Fletcher, editor of the journal *Annals of Internal Medicine*, would evaluate the presentations in order to suggest new directions for obesity research.

For two days, this panel of distinguished medical professors, physicians, and public health experts—none of them, significantly, directly involved in the weight-loss field themselves—listened to presentations by the nation's leading obesity specialists. The list of speakers was a Who's Who of prominent obesity researchers: Reubin Andres, Richard Atkinson, George Blackburn, Steven Blair, George Bray, John Foreyt, Jules Hirsch, F. Xavier Pi-Sunyer, Judith Rodin, Thomas Wadden, David Williamson, and others. Some of these researchers are in favor of strong diet treatments and drugs, and some believe lifestyle changes are more effective. The NIH panel members heard the researchers present studies and papers on the benefits and risks of weight loss, and on the success and failure of various weight-loss treatments. At the end of the second day, and on the morning of the third, the panel members sat together in a closed session, deliberating.

On the afternoon of April 1, the committee members emerged from the room to announce their findings. Even though none of the internationally renowned eating disorders researchers who strongly opposed dieting had been invited to the conference, and even though many of the experts who presented studies were advocates of very-low-calorie diets, diet pills, behavior modification, and other short-term weight-loss methods, the conclusion the panel reached after hearing all the evidence on weight-loss programs was startling but inescapable: Diets don't work.

Despite all the time and energy spent on such programs and products, the panel found, very few people succeeded in losing weight and keeping it off. Some dieters had, in fact, developed serious health problems in the process of losing weight. The NIH panel ran through the list of the main treatments for weight loss—dietary change, behavior modification, drug treatment, and combination therapies—and pronounced each ineffective. Some of the regimes, they said, had disturbing side effects. Very-low-calorie diets caused patients to experience fatigue, hair loss, dizziness, and other short-term symptoms; more seriously, they greatly increased the risk for gallstones and gallbladder disease. Drugs seemed to be safe in the short term, but had potential for abuse and hadn't been adequately studied over time. The sole treatment to which the panel awarded a clean bill of health was exercise, which causes only a 4- to 7-pound weight loss in most people, but increases lean body mass and levels of good (HDL) cholesterol in the blood.

The NIH evaluators challenged the widely held belief that losing weight will improve your health. They agreed that being very fat can adversely affect one's health and longevity, since high cholesterol, high blood pressure, and diabetes are associated with (though not necessarily caused by) obesity, and can increase the risk for coronary heart disease, gallbladder disease, gout, and some types of cancer. But that doesn't mean, the panel pointed out, that if fat people lose weight, they necessarily lower their risk for these health problems. There is no evidence that fat people who become thinner—"thin fat people," as the famous eating disorders specialist Hilde Bruch called them—are going to be in the same shape, health-wise, as naturally thin people. It may be that people who have a genetic tendency to get fat may also have a tendency to get certain diseases, regardless of whether they lose weight. When fat people who have diabetes or high blood pressure lose weight, their symptoms do improve, the panel said; but that's only temporary, since the weight almost always returns.

Long-term studies on mortality showed that there was little evidence to believe that losing weight will prolong your life, either. Instead, the opposite may be true: "Several epidemiological studies raise the possibility that weight loss is associated with increased mortality," the panel members said. Most lengthy studies show that people who lose weight over the years seem to die earlier than those whose weight remains stable. Those studies are confusing, the members pointed out, since it's hard to tell whether people lost weight because they were dieting or because they had an underlying illness, which would contribute to an early death. The fact that people who stop smoking also tend to gain weight muddles the conclusions on weight and longevity even more. But the possibility that dieting itself can shorten one's life can't be ruled out, the panel said. Weight cycling—or yo-yo dieting—appears to have other ill effects, too, lowering the dieters' metabolism, which make it easier for them to gain weight the next time around.

The NIH panel described how dieting can cause psychological problems. They pointed to evidence which shows that people who diet may be at increased risk for binge eating and eating disorders. Anyone who is considering trying to lose weight, they said, needs to consider seriously a variety of possible negative effects: "These effects include the risk of poor nutrition, possible development of eating disorders, effects of weight cycling, and the sometimes serious psychological consequences of repeated failed attempts to lose weight."

These risks of dieting are especially important to bear in mind in a society where many of the people who are trying to lose weight—especially young women—are perfectly healthy and don't need to lose a pound, the members added. For them, the risks of dieting far outweigh the benefits, which are uncertain in any case. Many of the people in the United States who are dieting just want to improve their appearance, modeling themselves after an unrealistically thin cultural ideal. "For most people, achieving body weights and shapes presented in the media is not a reasonable, appropriate, or achievable goal."

The panel said that even for those who are far from the ideal, the range of "healthy weights" is probably much wider than most people realize. There *is* no clear definition of "overweight," but the committee noted that recent government guidelines had broadened the definition of healthy weight from the old Metropolitan Life height-weight charts to make allowances of the fact that people come in a wide variety of body builds, and tend to put on a few pounds safely as they age. Other factors come into play when determining whether someone is too fat, the panel said, such as where the fat is located on the body—in a pear, or, more worrisome, an apple shape.

Finally, the panel members looked at some of the assumptions underlying obesity research, and suggested that obesity needs to be approached from a completely new point of view. To date, most researchers have tended to lump all fat people together under the heading of "obesity," and then conducted experiments to see how they fared on starvation diets, pills, or other regimens. They pointed out that not all obese people are alike, and that obesity has many causes. "Evidence suggests that overweight is multifactorial in origin, reflecting inherited, environmental, cultural, socioeconomic, and psychological conditions." They noted that obesity has a "substantial genetic basis" in human beings, and is not a matter of mere willpower. They suggested that researchers should focus on the individual root causes of obesity rather than on the symptom itself; fatness means different things in different people, and they cannot all be studied or treated the same way.

The committee scolded obesity researchers for the short-sightedness of many of their studies. Most studies last only long enough for people to lose weight, and researchers report on that snapshot of success, without showing the whole picture—that after a few years, almost everyone gains the weight back again. "The paucity of well-designed, long-term clinical trials evaluating various methods for voluntary weight loss is disturbing."

The panel stopped short of suggesting that everyone should throw away their scales and burn their diet books, but the members sounded a clear cautionary note. They pointed out that despite years and years of research, we really know very little about how weight is regulated, why people get fat, and whether or not any intervention can change people's genetic body size. They concluded that because of the failures of most weight-loss treatments and the many possible health risks involved with these methods, there was a clear need for more studies—and not just on how to get people to lose weight. "Research on the biologic and social influences on weight and weight control and the health consequences of weight and weight loss should assume a high priority on the nation's health agenda," the panel concluded.[4]

Almost overnight, this new consensus that diets don't work changed people's views about weight loss. It was as if the weight-obsessed world had woken up sane, and people realized that human beings naturally come in different shapes and sizes, and shouldn't struggle with potentially harmful treatments to fit an ideal. For those who had long struggled to diet, the NIH report confirmed their suspicions that it wasn't a simple lack of willpower that had sabotaged their success. The report sparked the first nationwide debate over whether low-calorie dieting was now outmoded.

On April 8, 1992, the health writer Jane Brody reported on the NIH conference in a *New York Times* article, and suggested that people need to stop expecting weight-loss miracles, set reasonable goals, and focus more on exercise. On April 12, the *Times* writer, Molly O'Neill, went a little further in a front-page story about the new "anti-diet movement," as she named it. She freely quoted eating disorders experts who had long opposed dieting but had received little ink for their efforts. They described how a new paradigm was emerging, in which weight is considered less changeable and less unhealthy than had previously been believed. "The establishment clings to the belief that weight causes disease and death just as people once insisted that the world was flat," said Susan Wooley, who wrote some of the earliest academic journal articles opposing dieting.

The new anti-diet movement, O'Neill said, was emerging as consumers who were distrustful of diets met up with feminists who were fed up with women having to starve themselves to meet an unreasonable social ideal of beauty. Several anti-dieting groups had been organized, such as the National Association to Advance Fat Acceptance, which focuses on civil rights for fat people, and Overcoming Overeating, which teaches women to stop dieting, accept their size, and eat according to their body's hunger and satiety signals instead of a food plan. Traditional obesity experts, such as Theodore VanItallie, poohpoohed the new movement, calling the idea of allowing women to eat whatever they want "ridiculous." But women who had abandoned dieting described an enormous sense of liberation when they stopped wasting their time worrying about their weight and what they ate.

The *Times* article quoted a thirty-five-year-old paralegal in Manhattan who had stopped dieting at an Overcoming Overeating seminar in 1984. "Something clicked," she said. "When I understood how my life was almost ruined by diets, I started to understand something very basic about society. Nothing has been the same since." O'Neill made it clear that despite what male obesity researchers had to say, the women who were trashing their scales at anti-diet demonstrations around the country should be taken just as seriously as the women who had dropped their bras in a freedom trash can in Atlantic City in 1968.[5]

Other events that spring helped reinforce the consensus that diets don't work. In May, Representative Ron Wyden held further congressional hearings on deception and fraud in the diet industry. Wyden blasted all the segments of the diet industry—which did as much business in America that year as the American lumber and plywood industries—for cheating consumers with empty promises that they'd get thin. "Millions of Americans abused by this industry may as well burn their money on the curb for all the good they get," he said. Wyden called for more government regulation of weight-loss claims, asked that commercial centers be required to compile data about their programs, that the FDA be able to monitor ineffective over-the-counter diet products, and that a government obesity and nutrition program be developed, following the NIH conference suggestions about new directions in research.[6]

Later in May, several fat activists, anti-diet groups, and eating disorders researchers met in Virginia for the first anti-dieting conference, held by the new Association for the Health Enrichment of Large People (AHELP). That November, the *New York Times* published a three-part series, "Fat in America," which exploded many of the myths of obesity in this country. Numerous women's magazines followed with stories about the ineffectiveness of diets (mixed, in typically schizophrenic women's magazine fashion, with photos of that year's waif models and articles on how to get thinner thighs and perfect abs by summer). By the following May 1993, *Vogue* had declared "The Death of Dieting." In June 1993, *Consumer Reports* surveyed 95,000 American dieters, and found that most thought diet programs were a big rip-off. After sifting through the literature on dieting, the authors concluded that most people are better off focusing on health eating and exercise than trying to lose weight. "Dieting," they said, "may actually carry a greater health risk for some people than staying overweight."[7]

Backlash

Despite all of the activity and evidence against dieting that emerged during 1992 and 1993, the obesity research community remained largely unmoved. Some respected researchers began to take a few steps away from dieting, but others clung to the old methods even more tenaciously. They continued to study and advocate diets, but they did so with some new twists. First, they began coopting the language of the anti-diet movement, using such terms as "lifestyle changes" and "eating plan" to describe their diets instead of that now-forbidden four-letter word. Second, while they continued to present research that proved that diets don't work, they either misinterpreted their own data, claiming success when the numbers showed clear failure, or began to engage in what Susan Wooley calls the "P.S. phenomenon." The "P.S." she is referring to are the lines that began appearing at the end of research articles which suggested—illogically—that despite the obvious problems with dieting, it is better not to discourage fat people from trying anyway. It could almost be seen as a confidential line to drug or diet companies: "P.S.: Fund me again."

By 1995, it seemed that the April 1, 1992, NIH conference statement had been an April Fool's joke. A strong backlash against the anti-diet movement had developed in the obesity research community. The only problem with most diets and drug regimes, many researchers asserted, was that the treatments ended; any medical condition returns when a patient is taken off of treatment, so the solution is to have patients diet or take drugs for the rest of their lives. Several papers were published which not only defended the notion that being fat is unhealthy, but raised the stakes by suggesting, with very sketchy substantiation, that obesity had become one of the nation's biggest health problems—a "disease." Researchers who opposed dieting, who had been in the limelight briefly around the time of the NIH conference, found themselves once again underfunded, often ignored, and trying to fight what eating disorders specialist Joe McVoy, the founder of AHELP, only half-jokingly refers to as the "diet-pharmaceutical industrial complex." It wasn't long before consumers began to believe these obesity researchers, and to forget that many scientists had agreed diets don't work and can be harmful.

The backlash to the anti-diet movement was driven by an epidemic of thinking disorders among obesity researchers. Their opinions on dieting began to swing back and forth, and sometimes the conclusions to their studies would completely undermine their study results. "I spend most of my time trying to treat obesity researchers," says David Garner, who is an outspoken opponent of most diet treatments. "I try to get them to read the literature as they've written it, not with the distortion they've superimposed on the literature."

In 1993, in an overview of obesity treatment written for practicing physicians, for instance, Thomas Wadden acknowledged that there was a great deal of evidence that weight-loss efforts are ineffective, and that people who yo-yo dieted had a higher risk of health complications than people who were fat but maintained a stable weight, but still argued that there wasn't enough evidence to tell people *not* to diet. "The option of no treatment deserves serious consideration, particularly in the case of older individuals with lower body obesity who are free of health complications," he said. "It is an option, however, that cannot be universally endorsed until there are definitive research data."

Wadden is standing conventional medical wisdom on its head here. In medicine, the usual conservative and ethical thing to do, unless a person is gravely ill, is to prescribe no treatment unless that treatment is proven. A treatment that has been shown to be harmful is never advocated without some evidence that its benefits outweigh the risks of treatment. Wadden shifts the burden of proof away from those who are advocating a potentially harmful treatment to those who say it's best to do nothing until you have a good idea you're doing something beneficial. Based on a flimsy argument that people continue to gain weight as they get older if they don't diet (weight gain in an aging population is not unexpected or necessarily unhealthy), Wadden recommends that dieting, even when people regain the weight, is still better than not dieting. He did not weigh the proven risks of dieting with the unidentified risks of gaining a few pounds over the years, but made it seem that the "prudent" thing to do in the face of confusion is to undergo a demonstrably harmful treatment.[8]

A similar "P.S." was added to papers by psychologists Kelly Brownell and Judith Rodin in 1994. Brownell and Rodin are two of the most moderate obesity researchers who have been influential in identifying the risks of dieting. Brownell, a Yale University psychologist who is on the scientific advisory board of Jenny Craig, and is a shareholder and director of American Health Publishing Company, a corporation that markets many weight-loss books (including his own *"LEARN"* diet behavior modification manual, which, according to a company spokesperson, sold about 50,000 copies in 1994 at $22.95 each), was the first researcher to suggest that yo-yo dieting lowers the metabolism and makes it progressively more difficult to lose weight. Judith Rodin, a psychologist who is now president of the University of Pennsylvania, is the author of *Body Traps* (1992), a book on overcoming body image problems, and has done several studies showing how weight preoccupation and body image dissatisfaction are so common among women as to have become normal. In her book, she argues eloquently that women need to understand the genetic limitations of their bodies, and not be caught in the trap of striving for an unnatural, socially imposed ideal.[9]

Still, in their journal articles, these researchers are cautious about telling people to give up dieting. Many of their arguments to anti-dieters make a lot of sense: even though the human body isn't as malleable as we believe, some people *can* lose weight, and it's important to identify who those people might be, and how they do it. It's also necessary, they say, to identify who among the obese really is at risk for health problems, while accepting that not everyone can be thin. They suggest that lowering fat intake, increasing consumption of fruits and vegetables, and increasing physical activity might be a healthier approach than more aggressive low-calorie diets.[10] Even most anti-dieters would agree with these points; there's nothing wrong with teaching people healthy habits, which may cause some to lose weight. But that's not dieting, which involves restrained eating. Yet Brownell and Rodin still stick to the idea that although dieting can be "pathological" in normal-weight people, it shouldn't be discouraged in people who are heavier, and they take a slap at those who have been whipping up an "anti-dieting fervor."

In a 1994 review article in the *Archives of Internal Medicine*, Brownell and Rodin thoroughly damned yo-yo dieting. They described all the evidence that weight cycling, which is very common, puts people at an increased risk of an early death from all causes, and especially from coronary heart disease. They recounted studies which show that yo-yo dieting leads people to feel less satisfied with their lives, and puts them at greater risk for binge eating and eating disorders. Some people who lose and regain weight frequently, they said, become more prone to gaining weight in the abdomen, which is more dangerous rather than the hips and thighs. Weight cyclers even tend to learn to prefer fat and sugar. The only negative finding on yo-yo dieting that they were unable to confirm was the idea that the body adapts to cycles of weight loss and regain by lowering its metabolism; they said it seems that happens only in some susceptible individuals. Brownell and Rodin urged that, given the high numbers of people dieting, weight cycling should be a research priority. Then came the P.S.: "It is probably premature to urge all patients to stop dieting. The prudent stance is still to recommend that overweight individuals lose weight." Brownell and Rodin flipped their conclusion away from their own research, and prescribed the problem they'd described.[11]

Susan Wooley says Brownell and Rodin's articles ceded many of the most important points in a critique of dieting. But they tried to salvage dieting in the end. "They implied that the cautious, conservative thing to do is not to jump to the conclusion that diets are dangerous and ineffective," Wooley says. "I would certainly argue the other way, that it's more cautious not to offer treatment that might be dangerous."

That same month, the psychologist David Allison and F. Xavier Pi-Sunyer, who works at the Obesity Research Center of St. Luke's–Roosevelt Hospital in New York (and who sits also on the scientific advisory board of Weight Watchers), wrote another thought-disordered article on obesity in *The Sciences*. The article began by describing a pair of twins, Georgette and Gina, who were identical in every way except that Georgette had suffered brain damage in an accident. Georgette, as a result, never considered herself obese and didn't diet; Gina dieted all her life. Both weighed exactly the same: 475 pounds. The authors used the example to describe how fate determines our weight; between 50 and 70 percent of the variability in people's body weight, they said, is due to genetics. Genetic research may provide clues to overweight. They described, once again, how most people regain the weight on diets and how weight cycling leads to increased mortality.

One might imagine that their conclusion would be that until we know more about the genetic causes of obesity, and find a safe treatment for fatness, we should stop telling people to diet. No; instead, they add a P.S.: "Most of the obesity research community has deemed such data [on the risks of weight loss] compelling—but not enough to state that weight-loss attempts by obese people are dangerous." And a P.P.S.: "Nowadays it is not uncommon to hear 'Diets don't work.' In fact, diets do work. It is prescriptions to diet that fail, because the patients usually do not follow them."[12]

The most offensive argument these two researchers made for dieting—and one that crops up everywhere in the literature—was based on the fact that obese people suffer enormous social discrimination. "Obese people are less sought as mates and less likely to be rented apartments, to be offered jobs or to be given financial support

for college, all of which can, predictably, be deeply demoralizing."
That's true, but imagine recasting the article to talk about skin color:
First, the researchers give evidence to show that green skin is genetically determined. Then they say that the fact that people suffer from
discrimination because they're green means they should try to change
their color, rather than change society. They describe how being green
is a health risk, because green people have a higher chance of getting
polka-dot disease than people who are pink. They admit the treatment
for changing the color of your skin is potentially harmful and not very
effective. But if that treatment fails, they says it's the green person's
own fault for not sticking with it. In the end, the message is that green
people deserve to be discriminated against because they're not pink.

Some researchers use their social discrimination argument to recommend that black women, who are heavier in general than white
women but less obsessed about their weight, should start worrying
about their bodies. Many obesity researchers decry the "problem" of
how black women are much more satisfied with their large bodies than
white women in this society. In one study, researchers found that
black adolescent girls were seven times more likely than white girls to
say they were not fat. The black girls had much better body images
than the white girls, and a lower incidence of eating disorders, but
they were fatter. The researchers suggested that black women should
become as concerned about their weight as white women because of
the health risks of obesity. "These findings should be used in the development of culturally sensitive Public Health intervention programs to
help reduce the high rates of obesity within the black community and
encourage black youth to achieve a healthy and reasonable body size,"
say the authors of one article in *Obesity Research*.

Noting that the white girls' attitudes led them to eating disorders,
the researchers tried to have it both ways, adding that their findings
"should also be considered for eating disorder interventions for predominantly white female populations in which there is considerable
cultural pressure to be thin." Lost to the authors was the obvious
implication of their research, which was that encouraging black girls
to diet and be dissatisfied with their bodies would inevitably lead to the
same eating disorders the white girls experienced.[13]

One of the most influential backlash articles was a widely reported
review of weight-cycling studies that appeared in the *Journal of the
American Medical Association* in October 1994. A group of obesity

researchers, several of whom sit on the scientific advisory boards of commercial diet centers, reviewed forty-three reports on weight cycling published since 1966. Some of the studies showed that yo-yo dieting has clear detrimental effects, and others did not. In the face of contradictory research about the ill effects of weight cycling, the panel recommended that dieters stay the course. "Obese individuals should not allow concerns about hazards of weight cycling to deter them from efforts to lose weight," they wrote. Though they said it's "obviously distressing" to lose and regain weight, they said there wasn't enough evidence to say firmly that it can cause psychological harm. In a situation where some evidence clearly points to harm, they recommended ignoring the risk.

When the study was boiled down and reported to the media, the emphasis was even more pro-diet. "Weight cycling does not appear to have adverse health effects," the researchers wrote in the abstract, when in fact they had concluded that the evidence was mixed.[14] When Susan Yanovski, a physician who is director of the Obesity and Eating Disorders Program at the NIH, told reporters about the review, she made it seem as if a new consensus had been reached that weight cycling wasn't the concern everyone had previously believed. "It kind of flies in the face of current medical opinion," she said. Newspapers simplified the story: "Yo-yo Dieting Not a Health Risk."

Many moderate obesity researchers were distressed by the way the review was reported. Kelly Brownell told the *New York Times* that it was premature to dismiss the possibility that yo-yo dieting may slow down people's metabolism. "This report is being interpreted as 'weight cycling isn't important,' " he told the *Times*, emphasizing that more research needs to be done. "If you give up on research too soon, you might be missing something important." John Foreyt, who was on the review committee, was similarly peeved. "Do I believe there are serious problems with yo-yo dieting?" he asked me. "Sure, and a lot of people do. But does the literature support it? The conclusion was for more research." He said he thought the review left too strong an impression that there was nothing psychologically damaging about yo-yo dieting. "Clearly, the psychological effects of yo-yo dieting are horrible."

But that wasn't the impression the public got when they read the headlines. Most believed there was nothing wrong with yo-yoing up and down. For others, the review simply proved that obesity researchers are yo-yo thinkers.

On February 8, 1995, the Harvard epidemiologist Walter Willett undermined the NIH consensus even further when he published a study in the *Journal of the American Medical Association* which warned that women who were even a few pounds overweight were at increased risk for coronary heart disease. In a study of 115,000 nurses between the ages of thirty and fifty-five, Willett found that a five-foot-five woman whose weight was 170 had three and a half times more risk for coronary heart disease than a woman who weighed 120 pounds. Even those in the "normal" weight range of 110 to 150 pounds had an increased risk of heart disease if they'd gained weight since they were eighteen years old. Willett used the study results to argue that the 1990 *Dietary Guidelines for Americans*, which expanded the definition of "healthy weight," were "falsely reassuring" to women who fit within the guidelines but have an increased risk of heart disease because of their weight. The study made headlines everywhere, and newspapers printed a revised height-weight chart that reflected the lean weights Willett recommends. According to his study, women should have a Body Mass Index of 19 to 21 to be healthy; that means a five-foot-five woman should weigh less than 114 pounds, or about the same as a fashion model.

But in his study, Willett ignored many other factors that determine whether a person's weight is healthy—weight distribution, age, other risk factors for disease—and used weight alone as a simple and blunt instrument to measure whether a person is apt to get cardiovascular disease. Cardiovascular disease is a relatively rare cause of death in the women he studied, most of whom were under forty-five, and therefore not a very good predictor of mortality. Women at that age are more likely to die of breast cancer, and Willett's own data showed that a little bit of excess weight actually protected the women from that disease. Willett ignored the previous consensus on healthy weight, which was based on numerous studies, and made sweeping recommendations to change the weight guidelines for Americans based on a slight statistical association between weight and a relatively rare condition in the women he studied.[15]

After seeing so many news stories in the wake of the study that told me that I, as a five-foot-six-inch woman, should weigh 124 pounds, I called Willett and told him I took his study rather personally. By his lights, I was a good 30 pounds overweight. A woman like me could read his study and assume that her chances of keeling over from a heart attack were pretty good.

I told Willett my height and weight, which, according to the U.S. dietary guidelines, is healthy. I gave him a more complete picture of my risk profile. I am a pear, not an apple, so whatever fat I have is not likely to hurt me. My blood pressure is normal, and so are my blood sugars. My cholesterol level is a low 135, and the ratio of total cholesterol to HDL cholesterol (the good stuff) is 2.4, which is exceptional. The physician at my last checkup told me my cholesterol numbers were so good that even if I had coronary heart disease, I'd be reversing it. I told Willett I eat a healthy diet; I'm a wannabe Italian who eats lots of vegetables, grains, and no meat except fish; I have a steady hand with the olive oil, and I eat very little saturated fat (Willett is himself a great fan of this kind of Mediterranean diet). I exercise daily, and, like Willett, I try to ride my bike around town instead of driving. "Whatever I die of," I told him, "it doesn't look like it's going to be heart disease."

He agreed with me, and said he thought I had very healthy habits. "You're unusual, though," he said. "Unusual people don't get counted in studies."

I told him I wasn't sure I was so rare; a lot of women I know exercise and eat healthfully and still carry around more weight than he suggests. Besides, how would he know if I was unusual? In his study, he didn't determine what his subjects ate or whether they exercised, nor did he measure whether they carried their weight in their bellies or their hips and thighs. My case, rather than being irrelevant because I'm unusual, points to the fact that health is based on much more than weight.

Willett conceded that activity can change his formula. "If people are regularly engaged in vigorous activity, the rules may not apply to them," he said.

I told Willett that people will interpret his weight chart as an order to diet. "It's abundantly clear that dieting alone is doomed to failure," he said. So what is he suggesting people should do? "It's very hard to get those pounds off once they're there," he said, and recommended daily exercise, which can stabilize people's weight.

The bottom line for Willett, like other researchers, is exercise and healthy eating, as the NIH panel recommended. No one can argue with these recommendations. But their insistence on proving that everyone is at an increased risk of dying early if they aren't super-thin, frightening people into going on starvation diets to reach an improbable weight, and ignoring reams of studies that demonstrate there are much more sophisticated ways of looking at health risks, is a sign of a thinking disorder.

Rather then developing new ways to approach the issues of weight and health, many obesity researchers are repeating studies that have shown time and again that trying to get people to lose weight by starving them is an exercise in futility. They are clinging to an old view, insisting that people diet, partly because these researchers are susceptible to cultural biases against fatness and fat people, and partly because they are swayed by the financially driven biases of the diet and pharmaceutical companies. And they're not getting any closer to figuring out the different reasons people get fat and whether anything can—or should—be done to help them.

"Someone needs to say that the emperor has no clothes," says Wayne Callaway. "What we're dealing with here is cultural bias, not science. Obesity researchers have been ignoring everything we know about biology, which is that people adapt, and since for most of human history we've adapted to starvation, it's natural that some people are heavier now. Instead, we've been doing this weird ironic experiment in taking affluent people and making them starve." It isn't that researchers should give up looking at obesity altogether, he says, but just start asking more sophisticated questions. Callaway favors the kind of research that separates the different reasons people get fat, and illuminates why some people respond to some treatments, and not others. "The more we can look at the actual mechanisms of obesity, and get away from cultural stereotypes and the pseudoscience of thinking everybody should be the same weight, the better," he says. "But it's going to take a lot of work to get there."

The field remains deeply divided. Some researchers have accepted the NIH consensus, instead of fighting it, and are trying to find new strategies of making people healthier without dieting. But many others are intensifying the fight to lose weight, with a renewed interest in drugs and surgery. "Obesity is a chronic problem for which current treatments are not effective," says obesity researcher and thigh cream purveyor George Bray. "People need to look at it as a chronic condition, much as we look at high blood pressure. If you're going to treat high blood pressure, you're going to do it for the long term with drugs."

Perhaps it is no coincidence that as formula diet companies are losing money, the biggest new source of funding for weight-loss research is the pharmaceutical industry. Few companies are willing to support research on how to effectively make lifestyle changes, such as exercise and healthy eating, that don't require expensive treatment, even though the only real consensus researchers have ever reached on stabilizing weight is that people need to eat more fruit, fiber, and vegetables, and get outside and take a walk.

There *is* some new research in the area of obesity and genetics that may eventually help sort out why some people are fat, however, and genuinely help a selected few. When Jeffrey Friedman and his colleagues at the Howard Hughes Medical Institute at Rockefeller University discovered that certain mice had a fat gene in 1994, they found that the reason they got fat was that this "ob" gene couldn't produce a substance called leptin. Named after the Greek word *leptos*, meaning "slender," leptin helps regulate the body's "setpoint," telling the mouse brain how much fat is stored in the fat cells, so the brain starts sending messages to the appetite that it's had enough. When the scientists injected the fat mice with leptin, they became skinny minnies. Normal mice, too, slimmed down to utter sleekness when they had a little leptin.

It seemed, at least for a few weeks, that the answer to obesity had been found. Inject fat people—or even people who want to lose 10 pounds—with leptin, and they'll trim down right away. News articles called leptin a "flabulous discovery," a "magic bullet for obesity," "weight-loss nirvana," and hinted that it really could become the "thin pill" that Americans have longed for, allowing us to shed pounds with no exercise and no dieting. The potential for marketing a new drug was obvious; Amgen, the Thousand Oaks, California, corporation, paid Rockefeller University $20 million for rights to make a diet pill based on its discoveries, with an agreement to pay many times that amount if this eventually panned out.

It didn't take long, though, for scientists to realize that leptin was not the cure-all everyone had hoped. It turned out that, unlike the particular strain of fat mice, most fat people already make copious amounts of the substance—up to thirty times as much of it, one scientist has estimated, as thin people. The hormone is produced in fat cells, and since fat people have more fat cells than anyone else, they make more leptin, too. It's possible that there are some very obese people—and we're not talking garden-variety chubbiness here—who may have a gene that causes a deficiency in leptin, as the mice have the ob gene, but no one knows yet who those people are. Identifying them eventually and giving them the hormone could in fact make them leaner. But giving leptin willy-nilly to any fat person would likely be dangerous, although it would also likely make them thinner.

So much for an easy answer. The discovery of leptin has opened the door to other research possibilities, though. Scientists at Millennium Pharmaceuticals in Cambridge, Massachusetts, for instance, have found receptors in the brain and other parts of the body for leptin. Obesity, they believe, may not be due to an absence of leptin in the fat cells, but to a problem the brain has in tuning in to its messages. Some people, the Millennium microbiologist Louis Tartaglia suspects, may be resistant to leptin, unable to pick up the signals it sends. But no one knows whether it's the leptin receptor in the brain—a kind of satellite dish for fat signals—that may be having problems, or the relay stations along the way that deliver the message to the receptor. In other words, it will be quite some time before the kinks are worked out of the system.

And even if a drug to improve the way the brain receives the leptin signal is developed, that doesn't mean it will help all fat people. "I think it's only going to be a small percentage of obese people who will actually have mutations in this exact gene," says Tartaglia. Not all fat people are likely to have leptin resistance. The likelihood is that there are many other types of fat genes—as many as sixty, some researchers guess—and the cure for one type of genetic obesity won't work for others.

The hope is that the new research on obesity genes may lead to drugs that are more specifically geared to the individual taking them for their type of obesity, and have more pinpointed effects on the body. Most likely, they would only work for people who have serious genetic defects that make them fat, which are probably people who are severely obese. Instead of prescribing drugs that not only regulate appetite but affect numerous other systems in the body—as amphetamines do—these new drugs will only target the genes that regulate body weight. "We aren't just working with random drugs that made rats lose weight in the lab," says Tartaglia. "Other weight-loss drugs are things people stumbled on by accident. Here we're starting with the actual genes whose job it is to focus on body weight. I think in the end we'll come up with safer drugs."

These new discoveries about genes, hormones, and proteins that affect our weight and eating behavior may not lead to one cure for fatness, but eventually they may lead to many. The danger with such potential diet drugs, like all drugs, is that before they are thoroughly researched, they will probably be prescribed indiscriminately, to anyone with a few pounds to lose.

As long as obesity research is primarily funded by companies that make money by promoting short-term weight-loss methods, and as long as both researchers and their patients are strongly influenced by a culture that demands that people get down to unnatural and even unhealthy weights, the thinking disorders among researchers will likely persist.

Chapter 8

A New Paradigm: Anti-Diet Researchers

Despite the fact that there is intense interest now among obesity researchers, physicians, and public health officials in treating obesity as a disease—aggressively—a new view about weight is emerging. This view, which is shared by many eating disorders researchers, nutritionists, exercise physiologists, psychologists, and fat activists, holds that weight is not an accurate measurement of human health—or character.

The new paradigm about weight acknowledges that dieting is negative and most often doesn't work, and that a more positive approach to health is in order. This view encourages people to stop dieting, to develop lifelong healthy eating and exercise habits instead, and to accept whatever weight they end up with. Some people may shed a few pounds by eating better and exercising more, and others won't; whatever the result, there's nothing more anyone can realistically do about their size. The research that supports this point of view is compelling; whether science will overcome cultural prejudice in the long run, however, remains to be seen.

In 1992, when the National Institutes of Health task force announced that diets don't work and the news media discovered that an anti-diet movement was afoot, three groups of people were hardly surprised. One was the fat people, who knew from long experience that bouts of starvation did them no good; in particular, activist members of the National Association to Advance Fat Acceptance (NAAFA) had worked for years to try to persuade the public that their size was a reflection of their genes, not their willpower. A second was those feminists who had, since the early 1970s, met in groups to talk about how their failed efforts to lose weight left them feeling powerless, unworthy, and angry; some eventually wrote books describing how to stop struggling to be thin and come to peace with food. The third group was the eating disorders specialists, who had seen their waiting rooms fill with the casualties of dieting—bulimics, anorexics, and binge eaters—for years. "This is not a news flash," said David Garner, the internationally known eating disorders specialist, not long after the major newspapers ran anti-diet stories that year. "We've known this for twenty years."

Garner, like a handful of other eating disorders researchers, first became critical of dieting in the 1970s, when he encountered the only group of people he'd ever met who were actually successful at keeping weight off. "They're called bulimics," says the psychologist. "They're the only people who have discovered a cure for obesity, and bingeing and vomiting has made their lives a nightmare." Garner, Susan Wooley, Janet Polivy and Peter Herman, and a few other researchers early on challenged the traditional wisdom that fat people should diet.

Unlike obesity researchers, eating disorders researchers have been in a unique position to view the long-term effects of dieting. Most medical researchers, after they've put their subjects on liquid diets, drugs, behavior modification, or some combination regime for several weeks, don't stick around to find out what happens to the people later on when they regain their weight. Nor do they typically describe the psychological effects of dieting in their scientific papers. But clinical psychologists who treat eating disorders see what happens to people after they've tried, time and again, to lose weight. They see people who feel like failures, whose sincere efforts at sticking to extreme diets have been rewarded, in the end, with more weight gain. In the extreme, they see people who are so obsessed with losing weight that they hate their bodies, fear food, and get caught in vicious cycles of starving, bingeing, vomiting, self-hatred, and starving some more. They know that although every diet doesn't lead to an eating disorder, *almost every eating disorder begins with a diet.*

Garner has spent a great deal of time over the past two decades trying to persuade other researchers that dieting can be harmful not only for people with clinically diagnosed eating disorders, but for anyone, including fat people. Many obesity researchers believe that psychological problems cause many people to overeat and get fat. But Garner turns their world view upside down: It's *dieting*, he says—along with the social stigma against fat people—that causes the psychological problems that many fat people, chronic dieters, and people with eating disorders experience. The fat people who don't diet, and who have learned to challenge the culture that tells them they're worthless because of their weight, simply don't have those psychological problems. At professional conferences and in scientific journals, Garner's nay-saying has, for the most part, fallen on deaf ears. "I've learned not only that obesity is intractable," he says, "but that obesity researchers are intractable."

Obesity researchers are so obstinate, in fact, that they have ignored a half century's worth of studies proving that dieting can be useless and detrimental. Garner is one in a long line of researchers who have painstakingly detailed the problems with dieting. The first major study to demonstrate the ill effects of dieting dates back to World War II. In a classic, two-volume study on the effects of semi-starvation on conscientious objectors during the war, University of Minnesota researcher Ancel Keys clearly showed that people who are starved experience depression, anxiety, anger, and mood swings. Their psychological symptoms don't subside, he found, until their bodies rebound to their starting weight—which they almost always do.

In 1944, Keys (who was also the inventor of the U.S. Army K ration) recruited thirty-six young volunteers to participate in the study. The men, who responded to a Civilian Public Service pamphlet entitled *Will You Starve That They Be Better Fed?* were mainly Mennonites and members of the Church of the Brethren who had chosen alternative military service for religious reasons. They were physically and psychologically healthy, normal weight, brighter than average, and as religious people, highly motivated to participate in a study that they believed would help their fellow citizens. Like most dieters, they were determined to be good. For the first three months, the conscientious objectors ate a normal diet, did chores, exercised, and were fairly cheerful. Then they were put on a diet for six months that provided plenty of vitamins and minerals but restricted their caloric intake to half of normal. It was similar to the diet regime that is recommended every day to people who visit commercial weight-loss centers: semi-starvation.

The men lost weight rapidly, eventually shedding about half their body fat. They became cranky and quarrelsome, and stopped most of their activities in order to conserve energy. They were so lethargic they left their dorm rooms messy, began avoiding work, and became careless in their grooming and indifferent to their visitors. They lost all interest whatsoever in sex. One, overcome with guilt that he had broken the diet by eating several cookies, bananas, and some popcorn, vomited his food in order to "regain control." Another was so distressed he chopped off three of his fingers in an attempt to get out of the study. Most of the men became extremely preoccupied with food, spending what mental energy they had dreaming up fantastic concoctions they would eat when they finished the study; a couple made serious plans to become chefs.

All the men felt moody, listless, and blue. "The cumulative stresses of semi-starvation resulted in emotional instability," wrote Keys. "The men experienced transitory and sometimes protracted periods of depression. They became discouraged because of their relative ineffectiveness in daily living." Most had problems carrying on with their normal daily lives. "The persistent clamor of hunger distracted the subjects when they attempted to continue their cultural interests, manual activities, and studies."[1]

The men's psychological symptoms persisted even after they stopped dieting. Once they were able to eat what they wanted, they binged; their appetites were voracious, and they constantly reported feeling hungry, even though they were eating plenty of food. One recruit described how it took several weeks before his feelings of hunger, cold, weakness, and disinterest in social events subsided. He regained his weight, but like most of the other men, replaced a good deal of his former muscle with fat. "Now, eight months after the end of starvation, I am fat and healthy although my muscles have not yet returned to their former tone," he said. "I look back to those days in July and recall my feelings of apathy."

Even though the men in the conscientious objector study started out at normal weight and weren't looking to trim down, studies in later years would show that fat people who diet and are highly motivated to lose weight experience the same symptoms of depression, anxiety, food preoccupation, bingeing, and weight regain. "The effects of semi-starvation clearly apply to people who lose weight at *any* weight," says David Garner.

In 1957, Hilde Bruch criticized the widespread mania for dieting in the country, arguing in her book *The Importance of Overweight* that this obsession for slenderness was causing people far more psychological problems than being overweight. "Despite the handicap that overweight implies, there are people who function better when they are overweight," she wrote. "Some of them have made strenuous efforts to lose weight, practically giving up living in order to achieve it." Her patients who were formerly fat but dieted to thinness—"thin fat people"—lived with the constant strain and tension that Keys described in his semi-starvation study. Some of the college girls, she noted, regurgitated their meals to remain slim, so that while their figures improved, their lives deteriorated. "There are others who stay reduced but cannot relax; they seem to be as preoccupied with weight and dieting after they have become slim as they were before. Although they look slim, they not only continue to have the same adjustment problems as when they were fat, but they often seem to be more insecure, dissatisfied, and unproductive. In dealing with such people, one cannot help asking: 'What price slimness?' "

Bruch criticized obesity researchers for failing to recognize that dieting was not only psychologically debilitating but medically simpleminded. Most researchers, she believed, didn't acknowledge that obesity was not one simple disease, but any one of several conditions. It could be a variation of normal body build, a genetic condition, or an expression of a metabolic or neurophysiological disturbance. It could also be a response to stress or other psychological problems, Bruch felt, but it was a rather benign one compared with all the other possible agents of self-destruction one could choose from. To treat all types of obesity with a diet, she maintained, was quite unscientific.

"The current tendency to lump all cases of simple obesity together is at about the same level of scientific exactness that prevailed in medicine when 'a fever' and 'a headache' were considered adequate diagnoses," Bruch wrote. "In our approach to 'overweight' we still act like the old-time physician who put his hand on a patient and, finding his skin warm, would solemnly pronounce that he suffered from 'a fever' and would proceed to bleed, purge, or starve him. That we put a fat patient on a scale and register his weight accurately only obscures the issue, and covers up our ignorance with the appearance of objectivity and exactness."

Bruch believed that some people were better off fat, and others could only lose weight when underlying psychological issues that were causing them to overeat were resolved. She called most diet treatments ineffective and "primitive," and criticized researchers for blaming fat people when those treatments failed. "The obvious conclusion," she said, "is that the current approach and attitude are at fault, and not the patients whom we reproach for being 'uncooperative' in the face of unacceptable prescription and advice."[2]

In 1958, a psychiatrist and obesity researcher, Albert Stunkard of the University of Pennsylvania School of Medicine, reviewed all the hundreds of studies published on obesity treatments in the past thirty years and came to a similar conclusion. After he discarded the studies that cast the results in too favorable a light by ignoring dropouts, manipulating the numbers to make them look better, and failing to conduct any long-term follow-up, he was left with only eight. Of those, he found that only 4 percent of "grossly overweight" patients who entered weight-loss programs succeeded in losing as much as 40 pounds. Only 2 percent of patients had kept the weight off after two years. The often-quoted statistic that 90 to 95 percent of all diets fail dates clear back to this review by Stunkard, though no medical study since has been able to show a significantly higher long-term rate of success (the higher dieting success rate documented in the 1993 *Consumer Reports* survey was for people who lost weight on their own). Stunkard recommended that obesity researchers acknowledge that weight loss is a "terribly difficult business" and "fraught with danger." Fat patients, he said, shouldn't undertake obesity treatment lightly; some probably shouldn't try to lose weight at all. He added that researchers needed to stop hiding their failures—or blaming them on patients. "If we do not feel obliged to excuse our failures we may be able to investigate them."[3]

By the 1970s, a few women—dieters, feminists, and researchers—led the efforts to critique dieting and show how it may even contribute to overeating and eating disorders. It isn't surprising that it was mainly women who were instrumental in bringing the problems with dieting to light; after all, they were the ones who had experienced the endless cycles of failure that dieting provoked. Male medical researchers tended to consider women's experiences merely anecdotal, and tossed them in the trash heap of unscientific data. Women knew it was important to listen to women, and then to devise ways to translate those anecdotes into scientific theories, arguments, and data that couldn't be ignored.

In the early 1970s, a smart young fat woman named Lynn McAfee got a job at a medical library, retrieving books for physicians. She wasn't a researcher; she took the job because she had repeatedly tried and failed to lose weight ever since her pediatrician put her on amphetamines at the age of six. (She learned to tell time before the other kids in first grade because she had to know when to take her pills.) She desperately wanted to figure out what diet would work. McAfee asked everyone who worked in the library to flag articles on obesity for her, and she read them all. It didn't take long for her to realize that the studies her physicians had relied on to put her on diets and pills for the past fifteen years were seriously flawed. "I read them, and I was shocked," she recalls. "Over and over again, the studies showed huge failure rates. I sat back and thought, 'Well, I guess they'll be announcing this any day now.' "

"They" didn't announce anything. Finally, McAfee confronted her physician with the studies, and asked him why, if there's such a big failure rate, no one told their fat patients about it so they wouldn't feel so bad about themselves when they didn't lose weight. "Nobody wants to discourage people from dieting," he told her. McAfee, who is now a fat, stylish blonde in her forties with sparkling earrings and Marilyn Monroe–style hair, laughs. "Non sequitur alert! The message was, dieting doesn't work, but we don't want to discourage people from doing it." Women dieters, she realized, had been duped.

Angry, McAfee, along with a few friends who were involved in radical feminist therapy in Los Angeles, began to write pamphlets and tracts exposing the myths about dieting, photocopying them, and mailing them around the country. Radical feminist therapists believed at the time that most people weren't crazy, it was society that was mixed up, and people who seemed to have psychological problems were just trying to adjust. The same was true, they thought, about fat people: There's nothing intrinsically wrong with being fat; fat people feel bad about themselves because society makes them feel that way, and the stress of dieting makes them feel even worse. The women wrote a *Fat Manifesto*, denounced dieting and media standards of thinness, and named themselves the Fat Underground.

It wasn't until July 29, 1974, that the Fat Underground became visibly active. That was the day Mama Cass Elliott, lead singer with the rock group the Mamas and the Papas, died. The story going around Los Angeles was that Elliott, a fat woman, had died choking on a ham sandwich; it had turned into a sick joke. When McAfee heard about Elliott's death, she cried. "I was devastated," she remembers. "She was the only person on TV I ever saw who was my size." And when she heard the jokes, she was furious.

Because of all the research she'd read describing how people often died after crash dieting, McAfee wondered whether Elliott had suffered the same fate. She did a little digging. As she suspected, the ham sandwich story was false; the autopsy report showed that there was nothing in Elliott's mouth at all at the time of her death. The person who had told that story to the media had been in Los Angeles at the time of her death; Elliott had died in London. The singer had also, it turned out, recently been dieting. "The heart is a muscle, and if you continue to lose muscle tissue, it's going to affect your heart," McAfee explains. "It's the pattern we see over and over again, like with actor John Candy, people lose weight, start gaining it back, and die of heart attacks." A few days later, the Fat Underground members made a speech at a well-attended Women's Day rally in Los Angeles, accusing the diet industry of murdering Mama Cass, and telling the feminists there that they were guilty of ignoring their fat sisters. McAfee smiles at the memory. "This was West L.A., and these people thought they were radicals. You should've seen the stunned faces."

The Fat Underground then planned several guerrilla theater actions against the diet industry. They invaded Weight Watchers classes armed with scientific studies and demanded that the leaders explain why they were promoting diets if all the studies showed them to be useless. At a University of California at Los Angeles conference to train people in behavior modification techniques—how to use electric shocks and aversion therapy to get people to stop eating—they planted some thin friends in the audience who helped them block the exits and cut the telephone wires. With get-away cars waiting outside, the fat women stormed the microphone, pushed aside the presenter, and lectured the stunned audience on how foolish, paternalistic, and cruel their supposedly helpful techniques really were to fat women.

Their theatrics made a little splash at the time, after which the Fat Underground broke up. But in the short time they were together, the group educated many fat women and other feminists around the country about the myths of dieting. Their articles—which they distributed themselves, since most feminist newspapers wouldn't touch them—were well researched and soundly argued, written mainly by a brilliant young woman who called herself Aldebaron (now Vivian Mayer). A few of the Fat Underground members went on to work with NAAFA, helping the organization transform itself from mainly a social group for fat people to a group that also works strongly for their civil rights. Other Fat Underground members continued to promote the rights of fat people through theater and humor, in the Fat Lip Readers' Theatre, or through activism, with the Council Against Size Discrimination. Twenty years after Cass Elliott's death, in 1994, members of the Fat Underground reconvened for the first time at a NAAFA-sponsored feminist conference in Oakland. There, the group's lasting importance became clear. "You saved my life," said one fat woman from the audience. "The ripples from your work are why most of us are here," said another.

Around the time the Fat Underground was busy in Los Angeles, another young woman in Chicago made an observation which set off a series of studies that would eventually demonstrate the serious psychological damage caused by dieting. In 1973, Debbie Mack, a student at Northwestern University, noticed something strange about the sorority sisters she lived with. All of the young women were normal-sized, but worried about gaining a few stray pounds. During the day, they would diet, and complain about how fat they were. But in the evening, one of them would buy a big box of doughnuts, and no one could resist. Then they'd say, "I've blown my diet," and go ahead and eat them. But instead of having just one or two, they'd stuff themselves with doughnuts and then move on to ice cream or pizza. Afterward, they'd feel guilty and miserable and vow to diet again tomorrow.

Mack approached her psychology professor, Peter Herman, and told him she wanted to do a study to find out whether it was actually the dieting during the day that had caused her sorority sisters to binge at night. Herman was skeptical; as a student of the obesity psychologist Stanley Schacter, he had done many studies which showed that fat people were more likely to eat when they weren't hungry than were thin people. Instead of hunger, fat people were motivated by the clock, the hour, or the presence of food. That, he thought, was one of the things that made fat people different from thin people; they were more responsive to "external cues" than to their internal stomach rumblings. Herman thought normal-sized people, like the sorority sisters, would eat according to whether they were hungry, not to whether there were doughnuts around after they'd been dieting all day.

Mack and Herman devised a study in which they gave students a questionnaire to determine whether they restrained themselves from eating what they liked—whether they were dieters, that is—or whether they ate normally. They set up a test in which they gave students milkshakes, ostensibly to rate them on taste, before allowing them to eat freely afterward. The researchers measured how much food the students ate by weighing how much was left in the room after the students departed. The students who were not restrained eaters, according to their questionnaire, did what seems normal: They ate less lunch after drinking the milkshake. But the dieters acted strangely. The more of the milkshake they drank before lunch, the more lunch they ate afterward. They were like the sorority girls: Once they felt that they had broken their diet, the floodgates of their hunger opened up, and they binged.

Herman was surprised at the results. These dieters weren't eating according to whether they were hungry or full. They were eating, and overeating, based on whether they'd broken their diets. Now it seemed that like fat people, thin people who dieted were eating as a result of these "external cues." They were no longer able to regulate their eating based on their internal feelings of hunger or fullness.

Herman and a graduate student, Janet Polivy, continued to do studies on restrained eating. Eventually, they would show that it was only dieters who ate according to outside influences; fat people who didn't diet ate just like normal people. Their work cast an entirely new light on dieting, showing that dieting almost inevitably leads to bingeing, and to the numerous negative feelings that go along with bingeing—feeling out of control, depressed, fat, and like a failure. Dieting, it seemed, made people lose touch with their stomach's cues of hunger and satiety, and caused them to eat out of the feeling of whether or not they were being "good" or "bad"—and when they were "bad," as the nursery rhyme goes, they were very, very bad.

"It's a deprivation effect," says Polivy, who is now a professor of psychology at the University of Toronto. "If you're told you can't have something, then that's what you want. As soon as you tell yourself,

'I'm not going to eat any sweets,' you're going to crave sweets. As soon as you eat one, you think, 'I've broken my diet anyway, so I'll start over tomorrow or next week.'" Polivy, who up until then had always been a dieter, wanting to lose 10 or 20 pounds herself, found that when she stopped dieting and ate when she was hungry, she lost a little weight; but more importantly, she didn't worry so much about food.

In 1975, Polivy presented some of their findings to a research conference on obesity. She stood in front of the room, a young woman in a group of mainly middle-aged men, pointing to her slides and explaining matter-of-factly how instead of eating less at times when normal people eat less, chronic dieters each much more. "I concluded with some speculation that dieting might not be good for people, and maybe the obese shouldn't be encouraged to diet," she recalls. Her presentation didn't exactly go over well. Albert Stunkard showed some interest in her results, but others were outraged. One well-known obesity researcher jumped out of his seat, and in a rather unusual display of emotion for such a gathering, pointed at the young female scientist in the front of the room and screamed at her.

"You're killing people," he shouted. "You're telling fat people they shouldn't diet! This is wrong! You are *personally* responsible for killing them!"

"That gave me pause," says Polivy. "So I went and did more research."

For the next eight years, in numerous studies at the University of Toronto, Polivy and Herman found that, indeed, dieting disrupted people's physical sense of when and how much to eat, and led to overeating. Not only did dieters eat more than non-dieters in experiments where they had to eat a high-calorie snack, breaking their diet, but they ate more than non-dieters when they *believed* the snack was high-calorie, even when in fact it was low-calorie. In experiments where dieters thought they were being watched after breaking their diet, they ate like birds; afterward, when they thought they were alone, they would binge. Over and over, the researchers provided evidence for what they came to call the "what-the-hell effect" of overeating after breaking a diet. It wasn't only fattening food, they found, that prompted dieters to binge; dieters would also overeat, unlike non-dieters, in response to emotions, alcohol, anxieties, and anything else that disrupted their strict sense of being "good."

Dieting teaches people to ignore the physical feelings of hunger and satiety that regulate weight, and to ignore other feelings, too, the researchers found. Dieters stopped being able to handle other emotions—anxiety, disappointment, fear, stress—in a normal way, and used food instead to express their feelings. They wouldn't cry when they were upset; they'd eat. Some felt compelled to binge in order to deal with the stresses in their lives, and got caught in a cycle of disordered eating, bingeing, and purging. "The upshot of such misuse of food and weight seems to be not only losing touch with internal signals for behavior, but in some sense, with oneself," Polivy and Herman wrote. "Inner guides become increasingly unreliable and are abandoned for external ones in areas other than eating."[4]

Dieting, it seemed, led to disordered emotions as well as disordered eating, and in some cases—especially where young women had come from families that placed a lot of emphasis on weight and put them under strong pressure to be perfect and to control their emotions—it led to anorexia or bulimia. "Dieting leads to emotional and cognitive disturbances as well as to problems with eating; in severe cases, dieting contributes to eating disorders," as Polivy and Herman put it.[5] For those who did not purge their food, but overate after starving themselves, dieting also led to obesity.

In 1982, Dr. William Bennett and Joel Gurin (who is now the editorial director at *Consumer Reports*) wrote *The Dieter's Dilemma*. Their book, which was strongly influenced by the Fat Underground, as well as by the work of Janet Polivy, Peter Herman, David Garner, and Susan Wooley, brought anti-dieting research to the lay public. Bennett and Gurin argued that for most of us, our weight is genetically predetermined at a particular "setpoint." Studies in twins who were raised apart by fat and thin parents, for instance, show that they grew up to be the same weight regardless of the environment they were raised in. The body defends that setpoint vigorously, resisting attempts either to lose or—as one famous study of force-fed prisoners who quickly lost the weight they'd gained when they were allowed to eat normally showed—gain pounds. Citing numerous studies, Bennett and Gurin explained why dieters' attempt to overpower the body's setpoint are foiled: the body responds by lowering its metabolism, so it can achieve its weight on less food. The only way to change the setpoint, they argued, is to exercise. Even so, they said, people naturally come in a wide variety of sizes, and attempts to get below a weight that one can maintain comfortably without thinking about it are apt to be dangerous. "The endless quest for thinness," they wrote, "has done far more harm than good."[6]

In 1984, Susan Wooley of the University of Cincinnati challenged the nation's leading obesity researchers to rethink their approach to fatness. She presented a paper that she and her husband, fellow psychologist Orland W. Wooley, had written, entitled "Should Obesity Be Treated at All?" They answered the question in a way most physicians at the time considered wildly irresponsible: No. The Wooleys said that the research was clear that obesity treatment was harmful, and that the risks of obesity have been overstated in a society that is obsessed with thinness. Until researchers come up with a more successful approach to treating fat people, the conservative and prudent thing to do, they said, is nothing at all.

Wooley, a 200-something-pound woman who knew from experience that no amount of "willpower" would cause her to lose weight, made an elegant argument to the physicians present at the conference. Most obesity treatments, she said, started with the assumption that fatness was caused by abnormal behavior—overeating and underexercising— and could be treated by correcting that behavior, putting patients on diets and telling them to exercise. But the results of those treatments, she said, had been "frankly discouraging." Why? Wooley ran through numerous studies showing that obese people don't necessarily overeat—so there's no abnormal behavior to correct—and that there is strong physiological pressure to maintain a genetically predetermined weight.

Wooley argued that the assumption underlying obesity treatment, that the thinner you are the healthier you are, was also flawed, particularly for women. When Ancel Keys did a review of the major studies on obesity and mortality in 1980, he found that the risk of early death increased only at the extremes of over- and underweight, and that weight had no impact on the health of women in the middle 80 percent. Another long-term study, the Framingham Study, showed that being very thin was more dangerous than being fat, and that there was no relationship between fatness and mortality for women in the middle 60 percent of the weight range. Wooley said that while these findings don't negate the health problems, or simple discomfort, of the massively obese, they do call into question the rational basis for treating the great majority of patients who are mildly to moderately obese.

Wooley detailed the harms that can come from dieting, even when the dieter succeeds at losing weight. "Many treatment successes are in fact condemned to a life of weight obsession, semi-starvation, and all the symptoms produced by chronic hunger," she told the obesity researchers. People who are able to keep their weight off often have to be constantly vigilant, consuming as few as 800 calories per day, and struggling against losing control. Like the conscientious objectors in the Keys study, they become listless, depressed, and preoccupied with food. "Perceptible beneath the visible pride is often an unmistakable bitterness over the price they pay to have a socially acceptable body," she maintained.

As for the failures, Wooley said, their story is well known to anyone who treats obesity. "Again and again they have invested their time, money, and energy in treatments which fail, each time feeling less worthy." She stressed that physicians didn't take the psychological risks of dieting seriously. By treating obesity as a disease, rather than acknowledging it as a natural human variation, the medical establishment was contributing to the overwhelming cultural prejudice against fatness. That cultural obsession with weight, she said, was largely responsible for the current epidemic of eating disorders. "The development of these disorders is a perfectly predictable response to the social demand to maintain a body weight at which extreme hunger is to be expected. The truth is," she told the doctors, "that bulimia is probably the most effective method of weight control available today, and it should not surprise us that intelligent, young women seize upon it."

Wooley cautioned the obesity researchers not to take for granted the fact that it is women, especially, who worry about their weight, or dismiss weight obsession as an inevitable phase of female development. "Would things be different if our hospitals and clinics were filled with young men whose educations and careers were arrested by the onset of anorexia nervosa, bulimia, or the need to make dieting and body-shaping exercise a full-time pursuit?" she asked. She needed no answer.

Wooley concluded that it was hard to make a case for treating any but life-threatening obesity, where a person is basically too fat to move. She argued for conservatism in treatment: only those treatments that can be demonstrated to increase health and longevity, without making a person's life miserable, should be considered appropriate. Patients who are only trying to reach a socially acceptable weight shouldn't be treated, even if they are clamoring for diets, drugs, or surgery. "We should not try to solve social problems in operating rooms."[7]

When Wooley, who is a witty and vigorously persuasive speaker, finished, she received a big round of applause. Stunkard, who had asked her to speak, wrote to her later and praised her talk. But the enthusiastic reception Wooley got for her ideas didn't necessarily mean anyone had really accepted what she was saying. "People can simultaneously acknowledge the truth of what you're saying and be unfazed in their advancement of totally contradictory ideas," she says. "In general, the stuff I've written has been quite well received, but it just hasn't had any impact on what people do." Data alone, she says, is not enough to change even scientists, when they, too, see the world through the lenses of a culture that exaggerates the value of thinness.

Although there's been comparatively little change in the obesity field, Wooley says that feminists, consumers, and practitioners of alternative therapies are becoming more vocal. "Science will change its paradigm when new people coming into the field are persuaded by a different point of view. But I'll probably wait in vain to see people who've advocated dieting all these years say, 'Well, yes, you're right, all the data's in, we should stop.' It's just not going to happen that way."

During the 1980s, Janet Polivy and Peter Herman continued to test their belief that dieting causes psychological damage by studying what happens when people stop dieting. They developed an "undieting program," which was aimed at getting women to stop dieting and learn to eat normally. Their approach was similar to, and partly inspired, feminist writers of the era who were advocating an end to dieting. Polivy and Herman educated women about the potential risks of dieting, and helped them learn to accept themselves at their present body size. They believed that if people learned to eat according to their hunger, they would come to a "natural" weight—which wasn't necessarily thin—and possibly, if they were compulsive eaters, lose the excess weight they had gained from overeating.

The researchers led the participants through exercises to become reacquainted with their feelings of hunger and fullness, teaching them to distinguish between a growling stomach and a desire to eat just for the sensation or to stuff down emotions. They told the participants not to consider any foods forbidden, but to include in their normal diet small amounts of "bad" foods that previously would have triggered a binge. The psychologists also encouraged the participants to get regular exercise.[8]

Before the study, they tested the participants on their levels of depression, disordered eating behaviors, body dissatisfaction, self-esteem, and other psychological scores. After ten weeks, they retested the participants to determine how quitting dieting had affected them. "People who give up dieting are happier, they report less eating problems and eating concerns, and they feel better about themselves," Polivy says. "They like themselves better, they're less depressed, and they're willing to try things that they hadn't been willing or able to try previously to make some changes in their lives." The program didn't cause everyone to lose weight; about one-third lost weight, one-third gained weight, and one-third stayed the same, though all of the changes were minor.

Even after two decades of research, Polivy says most obesity researchers still refuse to acknowledge the problems with dieting. "They still believe that if you restrict calories, you'll lose weight, which is wrong," says Polivy. "You can't just indiscriminately tell everybody to lose weight. It doesn't work, they don't do it, and in fact, the weight may rebound and they'll gain weight instead."

But a few researchers who formerly supported dieting are coming around to her point of view. "People who used to be developing diet programs, like Kelly Brownell, Wayne Callaway, and John Foreyt, are now writing and speaking about how and why diets don't work," Polivy says. Brownell did pioneering research on the ill effects of yo-yo dieting. Callaway began to oppose dieting around 1980, when, following up on patients who were put on low-calorie diets, he found that their metabolic rates dropped and never came back up again. Foreyt, who wrote *Living Without Dieting* with Ken Goodrick in 1992, noticed the negative psychological effects of dieting around the same time. He now wraps up his lectures with a photo of a rare patient who lost 100 pounds and has kept it off for five years, but is obsessively devoted to maintaining that weight loss; Foreyt wonders whether, in terms of quality of life, she's really a success. Other traditional obesity researchers have become more broad-minded; some have asked Polivy to contribute scholarly articles to textbooks on obesity. And the one who stood up at the conference in 1975 and called her a murderess for telling fat people to stop dieting invited her to be one of the main speakers at another meeting two decades later.

In the fall of 1995, another researcher published a study that challenged obesity researchers to rethink many of their conclusions. Steven Blair, the epidemiologist and exercise physiologist, didn't criticize the treatment for obesity, as other anti-diet researchers had done. Instead, he took issue with the notion that being fat is bad for you at all. Obesity isn't the problem, he told researchers. It's inactivity. As long as you exercise, it really doesn't matter how fat you are.

Blair and his colleagues at the Cooper Institute for Aerobics Research in Dallas followed 25,389 men who had checkups at the clinic since 1974. He found—as researchers JoAnn Manson and Walter Willett had discovered in their studies on weight and mortality that led them to caution people against being even a few pounds over an ideal—that, yes, as a group, fat men were more likely to get sick and die early than thinner ones. Men who had a BMI of over 30 (that's 210 pounds for a five-foot-ten man) had a 28 percent higher chance of dying early than men who had a BMI of less than 27 (189 pounds for a five-foot-nine man). But then Blair added the men's physical fitness levels to the equation, and got a startlingly different result. Among the fit men (those who were able to stay on a treadmill a good long time), he found, the fat ones lived as long as the thinner ones. "For obese men who are at least moderately fit," says Blair, "their risk of mortality apparently is not increased at all."[9]

When Blair compared the death rates of the active fat men with those of the inactive thin men, it became even more clear how much more important exercise is than weight in determining health. In Manson and Willett's studies, lean people have the lowest death rates, and are most likely to live the longest. But in Blair's study, taking exercise into account, the thinner men who were out of shape were nearly *three* times more likely to die young than the fat men who exercised regularly.

The results were remarkable: The people who weighed average or below average lived no longer than the overweight ones—unless they exercised. And the chunky ones lived just as long—if they exercised. In other words, once Blair controlled for how much exercise the men did—and he's sure the same would go for women—their weight had *no bearing* on how long they lived.

What a bombshell, thought Blair, when he started seeing these results a few years back. It meant that the most influential obesity researchers in the country have spent years beckoning us to fret and obsess about something that may be totally irrelevant: how much we weigh.

As the author of stacks of articles on exercise published in prestigious medical journals, Blair has long been highly regarded by obesity researchers. But now he couldn't be more at odds with them. After all, he's found that as long as they get in good shape, someone who's overweight by 20, 30, or even 75 pounds is at no particular health risk. (And to those 100 million Americans credited with having healthy weights, Blair issues a warning: If you don't regularly work up a sweat—surveys show that two in three of us don't—being slim is no protection whatsoever.) Even people who have large amounts of belly fat, which most researchers agree can lead to insulin resistance and cardiovascular problems, can reverse those problems with regular exercise, says Blair. In his view, that leaves only those with a 40-plus BMI (more than 100 pounds over average weight), who in practical terms are often too fat to get out and walk, actually *needing* to lose weight. That's only 3 percent of Americans. Otherwise, the rest of us categorized as "overweight" or "obese" are committing no crime against our health prospects. We're just heavy.

"Across America, millions of women get on the scale every morning and have their day determined by the numbers they read," says Blair. "We need to forget about the scale and focus instead on regular activity."

To find his way to these conclusions, for the past ten years Blair has looked at results of checkups more than 100,000 people have taken at the Cooper Clinic, a colonial-style red brick building just down the jogging path from his institute. As part of that checkup, each subject climbed on the machine that's at the core of his research: the treadmill.

It's an innocent-looking gym machine, even when you're stepping up to it with electrodes attached to your chest to measure your heart rate. When I tried it, starting off, the pace seemed like an easy stroll; but after several minutes, with the incline increasing, it became a hike up Mount Everest. The longer you can stay on the treadmill without crying uncle, the fitter you are, Blair says. Gasping for air, I kept it up for twenty-one minutes, just long enough to get a "superior" fitness rating for a woman my age, in her thirties. Although the doctor who weighed me told me I could stand to lose a few pounds, to Blair, it's the number on the treadmill, not the one on the scale, that matters.

So far, no other study linking obesity to ill health has factored in the subjects' fitness level. And that leads to mistaken results, Blair says, because though excess weight is associated with cardiovascular disease, high blood pressure, diabetes, and colon cancer, those are exactly the problems regular exercise can prevent. "The kinds of diseases we see in overweight people are the same diseases we see in sedentary and unfit people of every weight," he says. Other researchers can always find a correlation between weight and early death because fewer heavy people than slender people exercise, he says. But that doesn't mean there are no fat exercisers (40 percent of the fat people he's studied are reasonably fit) or thin people who haven't worked up a sweat in years.

"The challenge that I like to throw out to obesity researchers is, 'How can you be so sure it's weight that kills?' " Blair says, and chuckles. "Maybe it's just inactivity."

Blair's conclusion that exercise (and also healthy eating, though he doesn't study nutritional factors) is far more important than weight in determining good health is based on more than his research. As with other anti-diet researchers, such as Susan Wooley, it's partly personal. Blair describes himself as "short, bald, and fat," and says there's not much he can do about any one of those traits. On the evidence of his own life, he says, "I am convinced that you can be fat and fit."

Blair's BMI of over 30 puts him well into the supposed danger zone for disease and early death. Yet he exercises as regularly as he flosses his teeth, running several miles a day, and eats a diet loaded with vegetables and grains and low in fat. So even if he followed the advice to adopt an even lower-fat, lower-calorie diet, he doubts he'd get healthier or be able to keep the weight off. He agrees with studies which show that obesity is mainly a matter of genetics, and that most dieters gain back what they lose.

Blair wonders if obesity researchers still focus on weight because of a bias against fatness. He points out that it would be almost impossible for him to get a study published in one of the leading medical journals that focused on the longevity benefits of exercise without taking weight into account. "Yet those journals publish papers on obesity that give very short shrift to physical activity and fitness."

Many people who published studies on the risks of obesity, he observes wryly, are themselves quite thin. "I may be biased, too, because I'm big," Blair says. But so far no obesity researcher has come up with data to contradict his view—which is shared by many anti-diet and eating disorders researchers—that it's exercise and healthy nutrition that matter for good health, and that weight just doesn't make a bit of difference. "I'd just like them to convince me I'm wrong."

Chapter 9

"Eat Your Vegetables and Go Outside and Play": Anti-Diet Health Strategies

I f researchers like Steve Blair, Janet Polivy, and Susan Wooley are right, and it turns out that dieting is indeed a waste of time, energy, and money, what then? We're still left with a situation where many people overeat compulsively, rarely get any exercise, and feel terrible about their bodies.

When you put aside the question of whether people should try to lose weight, and ask almost any obesity or anti-diet researcher what people can do to improve their health, you find a surprising amount of agreement. In fact, most of them will offer exactly the same advice: Exercise regularly, and eat a diet that is high in fruits, vegetables, and grains, and relatively low in fat. Put more simply, as Pat Lyons, who is a health educator for the Kaiser Permanent Health Maintenance Organization, points out, it's what our mothers told many of us when we were kids. "Eat your vegetables and go outside and play." This sensible advice goes for everyone, fat or thin. Beyond that, there isn't much you can do about your size, except learn to accept it, which is no easy task in this fat-phobic culture.

"If you're walking briskly five to seven days a week, working up a little sweat, and eating five or more servings of fruit and vegetables a day—well, what else can you do?" asks David Williamson, an epidemiologist and obesity expert at the Centers for Disease Control and

Prevention in Atlanta. "It isn't psychologically or spiritually good for people to be pounding on themselves because they can't be some ideal body size." Williamson knows this from experience: He grew up as a fat kid, teased for having to wear "husky"-sized boys' clothing. He says that though he'll always be more robust than the thin ideal, and he can't completely shake his negative childhood body image, he's been able to stay healthy and keep his weight stable by exercising every day. He thinks that the public health prescription about weight needs to likewise veer away from dieting—which he calls "unscientific and inhumane"—toward encouraging more activity and better nutrition. "Whatever your weight, you'll be healthier if you walk a little more and substitute some fruits and vegetables for fatty foods," he says. Most people who do those things, he says, probably won't gain any more weight, and some may lose a few pounds.

This prescription for a healthy lifestyle sounds simple enough, yet it's a lot easier said than done. How we eat and exercise have been the targets of so much negative criticism that it's hard to think about them in positive terms. Our weight obsessions have distorted our eating habits, to the point where many people can't imagine eating normally. Whether they overeat to relieve anxieties, binge in the wake of a diet, or keep detailed records of how many calories they eat and work off each day, such people don't trust themselves simply to enjoy food. Exercise, too, has been distorted by our focus on weight loss; it's "punishment" for the sin of eating too much and for not measuring up to the other hardbodies at the gym. Exercise isn't fun, but something we know we should do to lose some weight, and we haven't, so to hell with it. Underlying many people's resistance to eating healthy food and exercising is a negative body image, which makes it that much harder for them to feel like they deserve the pleasure of healthy meals or movement.

Anti-diet professionals, whose ranks are growing, have developed some strategies to encourage fat people and others who have weight obsessions or eating disorders to develop healthier habits. These professionals are a loose group of health educators, workshop leaders, nutritionists, psychologists, and dietitians who generally agree that people should stop dieting and work instead on accepting their size. They usually focus on one of three areas: normal eating; comfortable exercise; or improved body image. Unlike diet treatments, which are often negative and controlling, telling people exactly what they shouldn't eat and how they have to exercise, anti-diet strategies are more positive, encouraging people to trust their own appetites and desires and to experiment with healthier lifestyle choices. Most anti-diet professionals recognize that not all fat people are the same—or necessarily have any problems to begin with—and that treatments should be individualized. Most also realize that their programs or suggestions may not be enough for some people, whose physical or psychological problems are such that they need the care of physicians or therapists instead.

Like any other group of people, anti-diet professionals are a mixed bunch, so beware. Many are well trained, experienced, and flexible in their approaches; but others are not. Some think it's important to collect data on their programs, and others don't. A few get so caught up in the rightness of their own methods that they run the risk of becoming as prescriptive and controlling as the diets they criticize. Others, gurulike, hint that if you follow their plan, you'll lose weight; some might as well open a franchise and start weighing people in at the door.

Whatever the program, the point of anti-diet strategies is not to tell people exactly how to eat and exercise, as a diet program would; rather, it is to encourage them to figure out for themselves how to develop habits that are not only healthy but will make them feel the most relaxed, happy, and comfortable in their bodies.

Healthy Eating Strategies

The idea behind many anti-diet programs designed to help people learn to eat normally is that dieting has messed up people's natural abilities to eat right. To learn how to eat calmly, without overeating or constantly fearing that every morsel will make them fat, people first have to stop dieting. After that, say anti-dieters, they can begin experimenting with more nutritious food choices.

Janet Polivy and Peter Herman's research on "undieting" has served as a model for many professionals who treat compulsive eating. While they recognize that some fat people don't have eating problems, and therefore don't need any treatment, others may have been systematically overstuffing themselves for years, out of family habit, stress, or as a reaction to dieting. On diets, according to Polivy and

Herman, people learn to rely on *external* rules to control their eating, and they inevitably break those rules. Dieting usually makes people feel deprived, and they respond by overeating. Telling people what and how to eat, something every child wants to have the power to decide for themselves, is not only emotionally disempowering but causes people to lose the eating skills they were born with. But if people can stop dieting and relearn how to follow their *internal* eating signals instead—listening to when their body tells them they're hungry or full—they can eventually build up their normal eating skills and feel better about themselves.

The question is how to teach people to make that shift, to learn to eat normally. Children know how. Research on children's eating habits shows that they naturally regulate how much they eat. Youngsters will refuse one bite too many, even if it's flying toward them accompanied by airplane sounds. Leann L. Birch, a Pennsylvania State University psychologist, has done studies showing that kids, given a variety of foods and the freedom to select whatever they like, will systematically keep their caloric intake consistent. This is called "demand feeding." But, she says, parents begin interfering with children's internal eating cues as early as age three or four by controlling how much they eat. Once food becomes loaded with emotional meaning, offered as a reward or withheld as punishment, those cues get skewed.[1]

How can someone relearn to eat like a child? Anyone who has spent her life eating according to a thousand external considerations— Do I get another bread exchange today? How many fat grams should I count for the marinade if the fish is grilled? Will this cheesecake go straight to my thighs?—is unlikely suddenly to be able to stop and feel free to eat whatever she likes when she's hungry and quit when she's full. The question of good nutrition also raises its head; people who don't diet still need to be aware of making healthy food choices. Even if you learn to eat normally, according to your hungers and desires, you're going to be in big trouble if you don't eat plenty of grains, fruits, and cancer-fighting vegetables, for a lot of health reasons that have nothing to do with weight.

Several techniques have been developed to teach demand feeding to adults, to help them stop dieting and learn to eat normally. Many of them are described in popular books, including *Fat Is a Feminist Issue*, by Susie Orbach; *Overcoming Overeating*, by Carol Munter and Jane Hirschmann; *Making Peace with Food*, by Susan Kano; and

Breaking Free from Compulsive Eating, by Geneen Roth. Other programs are based on clinical research and used in professional practices. These too are described in books, including *Hugs Plan for Better Health*, by the dietitian Linda Omichinski; and *Beyond Dieting*, by Donna Ciliska; as well as a training method, "Treating the Dieting Casualty," developed by the dietitian and therapist Ellyn Satter.

All of these programs teach people to stop dieting and eating compulsively, but there are differences among the methods. Any one of them may have something to offer an individual, depending on what seems most sensible to her. "There are a lot of causes to compulsive eating, so there are a lot of approaches to working it out," says Joe McVoy, the eating disorders specialist who founded the Association for the Health Enrichment of Large People (AHELP). "For those who have emotional trauma such as sexual abuse, Geneen Roth's program may be helpful. For others who have dieted for years and are compulsive overeaters, Jane Hirschmann and Carol Munter's approach may help. It depends entirely on the individual." People who feel that their eating is seriously out of control might need more help than books can offer, he says, and should consider seeing a dietitian or therapist who is experienced in treating compulsive eating and is knowledgeable about anti-diet research and methods.

One of the most popular anti-diet programs is Overcoming Overeating, based on the book by that name by Carol Munter and Jane Hirschmann, which has sold more than 200,000 copies. There are Overcoming Overeating centers in several cities, including New York, Chicago, and Houston, and other independent practitioners follow the tenets of the book. A couple of years ago, I attended an Overcoming Overeating workshop in Colorado; later, I went to an advanced Overcoming Overeating workshop in San Francisco.

The first thing that struck me in Denver was that the caterer for the workshop must have been confused. It didn't make sense that at a seminar to help people stop eating compulsively, the refreshment table was heavy with buttercream mints, animal crackers, and jelly beans. It was early morning; I wanted a bagel or something resembling breakfast. Nevertheless, dozens of women in their thirties, forties, and fifties seemed pleased to be given such outright permission to eat "bad" foods if they wanted to, and were busy filling napkin bundles with sweets.

Soon, about a hundred people—almost all women—were seated in the high school cafeteria, their comfy Saturday clothes overflowing the bright plastic chairs. They had each paid $85 to be there; some of them to try one more way to lose weight; others just to try to bring some semblance of sanity to their eating habits. Most of them, no matter whether they were heavy or not, had spent their lives dieting and feeling too fat.

"It's a kind of madness," says Barbara Jensen, an attorney sitting near me who is tall—six feet—doesn't look fat but says she has felt fat for as long as she can remember. She's lost and gained the same 20 pounds more times than she cares to count. And each time she puts the weight back on, she blames herself. "I know it's a waste of energy," she says. "I know society makes women feel bad about their bodies. But that doesn't help. I'm just tired of feeling huge."

Laurie Capelli says she's been dieting since second grade. A large woman, she's tried fat farms, acupuncture, and commercial weight-loss programs. "I want to lose weight more than anything in the world, and I can't do that," she says. "I've been a failure. When I feel bad, I eat." Next to her, Shanan Campbell, a gamine woman in her early twenties who first went to a commercial diet center at the age of six-teen, says her weight has been fluctuating by as much as 50 pounds ever since. "It feels like I've been dieting or bingeing every day of my life," she says. "I'm a wreck." The women here are willing to try any-thing new, no matter how extreme, to eat normally, and, most hope, to get rid of those extra pounds for good.

Anything, that is, except perhaps the radical technique that Carol Munter is suggesting. What the tall, sophisticated New Yorker has already told the group has made sense enough: You need to accept and love your body the way it is, stop berating yourself for not meeting a nearly anorectic societal ideal, throw away the calorie counters and scales, get rid of all the clothes in your closet that don't fit, and get off the endlessly self-defeating cycle of dieting and overeating. Diets have made you feel terrible about yourself, Munter tells the group, and probably made you fatter than ever. Only after you accept your size and improve your self-esteem can you begin to understand why you overeat—if you do—and then make positive changes in your eating or exercise habits.

Fine, so far. But then Munter goes over the edge, sounding like a Weight Watchers leader gone berserk. You can't just stop dieting, she says. You have to prove to yourself you've stopped. How? "You have to go out and buy large quantities of food. Stock up on more of everything you desire than you can possibly eat." There's a stunned silence. Hands dipping into snacks stop in midair. "She's joking," one woman whispers audibly. She is not. Nor is she talking about just stocking up on "good" diet foods—rice cakes and bok choy, say—to have on hand when the urge for fudge brownies hits. Munter is talking about buying the brownies, and none of the low-fat versions, either. She tells the group, almost wickedly, to "legalize" all foods, no matter what their gooey, caloric, fatty content. "Ice cream equals lettuce," she says. "Candy equals fish."

Ignoring the nervous laughter, Munter presses on. "Two boxes of cookies are not stocking up," she says. "If cookies are a problem for you, but twenty boxes. When you get down to fifteen, buy five more." One client, Munter tells the rapt group, filled her bathtub with M&Ms. Another went to the bakery warehouse, loaded her car, and created a pastry sculpture in the middle of her kitchen. And the really successful ones, Munter says, carry a large food bag with them wherever they go—filled with muffins, Chinese noodles, cashews, chocolate, whatever—approximately a well-stocked pantry on the move.

The idea behind this free-for-all, Munter explains, is to counter the feeling of deprivation that goes along with dieting. By Munter's logic, if you keep an abundance of food around and stop investing what you eat with "bad" and "good" labels, you're less likely to feel deprived, less likely to feel bad about yourself for eating "bad" foods, less likely to despair, and less likely to overeat. "The cookies get a lot less interesting when they aren't off-limits," Munter says. "When people legalize food, they end up eating less." And when they eat less, she adds cautiously (and here's where the audience pricks up its ears), you may even lose weight—"if it's in the genetic cards for you."

Munter lets this sink in a moment. "Eat everything you've been deprived of?" asks Gerri Hanwell, a retired systems analyst. "It sounds crazy."

Indeed it does, to someone who has dieted all her life. But for Carol Munter, and many other women, this dramatic technique has worked. Munter, who used to be about 60 pounds heavier, gave up dieting in 1970, at the height of the women's movement. She and several other Manhattan women, frustrated by their repeated failed attempts to lose weight, started a self-help class. "We were all expert dieters, and fatter than we'd ever been in our lives," says Munter. She proposed that they try something radical: Stop dieting and—against all advice of popular culture—focus instead on accepting their bodies. They covered a room with mirrors and practiced looking at themselves, whatever shape they were in, without sucking in their stomachs or making self-critical remarks. They tossed away their diet books and tried instead to eat according to their bodies' own advice: hunger and cravings. They talked about the emotional reasons that caused them to overeat, the times when food quieted their anxieties and soothed their frustrations, and when extra pounds protected them if they felt powerless and sexually vulnerable.

One of the women in the group, Susie Orbach, was so taken with the idea of losing weight without dieting that she published the first widely popular anti-diet book, *Fat Is a Feminist Issue*, in 1978: "We turned our strongly held ideas about dieting and thinness upside down. Nothing terrible happened." The funny thing was, she said, over time, most of the women lost weight.

Over the years, Carol Munter and, later, Jane Hirschmann expanded on the ideas the women in this group came up with. In addition to the stocking-up technique they developed to give people a handle on their compulsive eating, they teach them how to figure out when they're really hungry. In her workshops, Munter tries to teach people to recognize the difference between what Orbach calls "mouth hunger"—cravings brought on by thoughts and emotions ranging from boredom to anger—and "stomach hunger," unmistakable for its hollow grumbling.

"But how do you *know* you're hungry?" asks a woman at the workshop, her pile of animal crackers and jellybeans fast disappearing. Munter suggests a few exercises, such as pausing before eating to ask whether your stomach really feels empty. "When you wake up, the question is not, 'What's for breakfast?'" she says, "it's, 'Am I hungry?'" If you *are* hungry, then fine: consider what you really crave. If it's chocolate ice cream, imagine it sliding down your throat first thing in the morning. Too cold? Maybe something warmer. Oatmeal? Nah, too gooey. Warm up a slice of last night's pizza? If it sounds good, go right ahead. Eat all you want, until you're full.

"But how do you know . . . ?" Munter anticipates the next question: It's even more difficult for ex-dieters to know when they're full than when they're hungry, she says. A start is to ignore the old Depression-era paternal messages about cleaning your plate. Experiment with pushing back from the table before you feel stuffed. "People are amazed to find that it doesn't take that much to feel full," she says.

If you're not hungry but still want to eat, Munter tells the group, that's not terrible. It's just an opportunity to try to figure out what's bothering you. Too often, she says, compulsive eaters use food to stuff down their anxious feelings, never allowing them to surface. "Sit with it awhile before you eat," she says. "Find out what's eating you."

Munter admits it takes a long time for people to start eating out of real hunger. Some go through weeks of eating great quantities of potato chips or ice-cream sandwiches before the forbidden foods lose their allure. But then, she claims, they learn to pick and choose what they really want to eat. "You'll discover that underneath your craving for hot fudge sundaes is a craving for vegetables." Only after a person has stopped overeating, says Munter, can they begin to take nutrition into account when they ask themselves, "What am I hungry for?" Karen Carrier, a nutritionist who works with the method in Texas, says it's similar to the situation when a person is drowning: First you throw them a life preserver, then later you can teach them to swim.

But it isn't easy. In the first months following the workshop, Barbara Jensen found that dumping her dieting regime, accepting her body, throwing out her scales, and eating according to hunger signals was a lot harder than it sounded. After Munter's pep talk, Jensen went to a late-night grocery and bought $240 worth of ice cream, candy, *chili con queso*, and pastries. Every day for the first few weeks—in response to her cravings—she ate three or four Pop-Tarts smothered in vanilla almond ice cream for breakfast. She threw away her scale, but suspects she gained 5 to 10 pounds.

When her first eight boxes of pastries ran out, Jensen wanted to go back on a diet. She couldn't tell when she was hungry, and she was afraid she'd never stop gaining weight. But she followed instructions, bought eight more boxes of pastries, and found several weeks later that most were still in her cupboard, untouched. She began to crave tuna salads for lunch, and noticed she felt like stopping a quarter of the way through a pint of ice cream, rather than eating the whole thing. Slowly, she began to stock her house with fruits and vegetables.

"It turns out it feels good to eat vegetables, and to exercise," she says. "I'm not doing those things out of some sort of punishment to myself for being fat."

Jensen says she isn't sure whether she'll ever be as thin as she once dreamed of when she was dieting. "If the only thing that comes out of this is that I feel good about myself," she says, "well, that's better than losing thirty pounds."

Overcoming Overeating may be a powerful way for some women to break a long habit of compulsive eating. But for others, it may be too dramatic or raise too many expectations about weight loss. Munter and Hirschmann say they have a few clients who have lost over 100 pounds, while some lose 10 or 20, and some stabilize at a weight most people in society would consider too high. But for women who are never going to lose weight, because of genetics or a long history of dieting, even the slightest hint of losing weight that Orbach, Munter and Hirschmann, and other anti-dieters like Geneen Roth make can be a setup for yet another failure. They can't promise anyone they'll lose weight and keep it off, any more than Richard Simmons, Susan Powter, or Jenny Craig can.

Munter and Hirschmann don't overtly emphasize weight loss, and they tell workshop participants that if they do lose weight, and people compliment them, they shouldn't get sucked into feeling that somehow they're better people for being thinner. "When people compliment you, just say, 'That's interesting,'" advises Munter. Some people do lose weight when they normalize their eating, but not everyone. But the fact that the topic of How to Handle Weight Loss takes up so much time in their workshops, and that they frequently mention clients who have lost weight, does more than hint, despite their intentions, that this may be another way to "lose pounds fast." (Geneen Roth, whose workshops are held in giant hotel conference rooms where people engage in group visualizations and therapists roam the perimeter with tissues for tears, places much more emphasis on losing weight than Munter and Hirschmann. A large chunk of one session of Roth's "Breaking Free" workshop that I visited was devoted to testimony from a woman who lost 300 pounds; the winking promise was that you'll lose weight, too, with her method.)

For other people who try Munter and Hirschmann's method, the permission to stock up on everything may be too much to handle. It gives some women a license for their compulsion, with no boundaries, and they end up gaining lots of weight. "It was overwhelming," says one Palo Alto, California, woman who gained 50 pounds after trying Overcoming Overeating. "Stocking my house up with so much food after all those years of being afraid that anything I ate would make me fat was just too scary, too much for me."

Emily Fox Kales, an eating disorder specialist at Harvard University, agrees. "Telling people right off the bat to go home and stock their refrigerator with every forbidden food and suddenly have to coexist with it is a little premature," she says. "Many people need to do this in a more systematic way, slowly learning to trust themselves with foods." She will often have clients bring a "forbidden" food into a session and slowly guide them through the consumption of the food in a conscious and focused way. They become aware of that food, slowly begin to feel safe eating it, and might try one or two more during the week.

After attending an "advanced" Overcoming Overeating workshop in San Francisco, I realized that the practice of always asking yourself whether you're hungry and what the perfect thing to eat would be could lead, for some people, to another kind of compulsive eating. At the very least, it could make for some over-particular eating habits. Carol Munter mentioned in San Francisco that before her flight she made a special trip to her favorite bakery in New York to buy her favorite muffins, in case there weren't any *really* good muffins in San Francisco (believe me, there are); she also mentioned she only eats the muffin *tops*. Another anti-diet workshop leader who advocates a similar technique of eating exactly when and what you desire is known for ordering several desserts at once at a restaurant, so she'll have the perfect dessert experience. It's fine to be so particular about food, I guess, if you can afford it, but at some point your fellow diners are going to start thinking you're a little neurotic.

In the "advanced" Overcoming Overeating workshop, held one afternoon, a few participants lugged along large insulated food containers to show to the rest of the people in the workshop. Each three-foot container had several separate compartments for both hot and cold food items, to satisfy any foreseeable craving that could hit at any moment during the day. Next, I expected someone to wheel in a mini-fridge. Carrying food bags may be a good solution for some women, but it seems to me it can take away a good deal of the satisfaction and ritual of waiting for meals, getting good and hungry for them, mulling over what to cook, then preparing and eating them with some ceremony with family or friends.

Finally, the desire to eat something when you aren't hungry

doesn't necessarily signal that you're always responding to some sort of emotional problem, as the Overcoming Overeating technique suggests. Sure, the impulse to reach for a bag of goldfish crackers after you've just finished lunch and are faced with a difficult task may be a sign of anxiety, worth paying attention to. But wanting to eat a piece of warm strawberry rhubarb pie that a friend brought over under the same circumstances could mean something else. It could be a sign that the pie looks incredibly delicious, you want a piece, and you'll probably end up eating less for dinner later on. No big deal. Sometimes the desire for food, even when you're not hungry, comes from pure lustful pleasure, and there's nothing wrong with that.

Another model for treating compulsive eating comes from Ellyn Satter, the dietitian and therapist from Madison, Wisconsin, who has worked with eating-disordered clients for three decades. Author of *Child of Mine: Feeding with Love and Good Sense* and *How to Get Your Kid to Eat . . . But Not Too Much,* Satter is best known for her work dealing with children's eating habits. Because her books show parents how to create a healthy eating environment in which their children can be trusted to be in charge of eating what they want, developing normal eating habits, many women with eating disorders and compulsive eating problems have used her books as a resource to relearn for themselves how to eat normally, as children do.

Satter now trains dietitians to treat compulsive eaters directly with her "Treating the Dieting Casualty" program. Her method is different in many ways from Overcoming Overeating, Geneen Roth's "Breaking Free," and other programs. Like them, she believes that people have the ability within themselves to regulate their own food intake, and that compulsive eaters need strong permission to eat what they want and discover when they're really hungry, and for what. But her style is much more structured, individually oriented, and careful than the others. "Hirschmann and Munter are from New York, and their method is a reflection of who they are as people—rather flamboyant," says Satter. "I'm from the Midwest, South Dakota Norwegian, so my method is much more moderate, systematic, and gradual." She believes that along with permission to eat what they like, many compulsive eaters need to feel a sense of safety, so they won't feel wildly out of control.

What makes Satter's method appealing is that she starts from the point of view that eating should be one of life's great pleasures. The pleasure in eating has been spoiled for so many people—particularly large people—by conflict and anxiety, which stem from the very negative, overcontrolling, diet-obsessed environment we live in. People who have dieted all their lives feel extremely negative about food and about themselves, distrusting themselves to make any choices about what they want to eat. Even though diets are becoming less popular, and the trend is toward prescribing low-fat healthy eating and exercise instead, that new prescription, says Satter, can become just another type of external control. She believes there needs to be a whole shift in thinking, toward people trusting themselves. "They need to be able to eat and exercise in a way that feels comfortable and positive," she says, "and accept whatever weight comes out of that process."

Satter trains dietitians to work individually with compulsive eaters who are burned out on dieting, who don't know how to eat normally, and who have lost touch with their internal regulators of hunger and appetite. Some of these "dieting casualties" might resort to crude methods of regulating their eating, such as occasional vomiting. Satter's method isn't directed at people with full-blown eating disorders, for whom she usually recommends psychotherapy. But not everyone who purges, she says, has an eating disorder; she defines an eating-disordered person as someone who is unwilling to take a risk with her weight to stop eating compulsively.

The work she does is individual, partly to give support and partly because each person's compulsive eating problem is different, and each person needs to find out how to eat according to no one but herself. There are many different kinds of compulsive eaters, Satter says. Some people have been overfed since childhood, because their parents encouraged them to overeat, and they continue to stuff themselves as adults. Others learned to overeat as a response to a stressful event; Dad dies, so Grandma overfeeds the kids to make them feel better, and they overeat to make her feel better. Many people overeat both as a reaction to a parent's attempts to restrict their food, and later, to dieting. Kids who already have a genetic tendency to be fat have their problem exaggerated when parents put them on a diet, and they respond by overeating. Some people have structured their eating in chaotic ways, skipping breakfast, eating lightly in front of others, and then bingeing alone at night. The goal of all the treatments, Satter says, is to help each person figure out orderly, positive eating habits for themselves: Normal eating.

What is normal eating? Satter has a nice definition she uses in her books and training materials:

> Normal eating is being able to eat when you are hungry and continue eating until you are satisfied. It is being able to choose food you like and eat it and truly get enough of it—not just stop eating because you think you should. Normal eating is being able to use some moderate constraint on your food selection to get the right food, but not being *so* restrictive that you miss out on pleasurable foods. Normal eating is giving yourself permission to eat sometimes because you are happy, sad, or bored, or just because it feels good. Normal eating is three meals a day, or four or five, or it can be choosing to munch along the way. It is leaving some cookies on the plate because you know you can have some again tomorrow, or it is eating more now because they taste so wonderful. Normal eating is overeating at times; feeling stuffed and uncomfortable. It is also undereating at times and wishing you had more. Normal eating is trusting your body to make up for your mistakes in eating. Normal eating takes up some of your time and attention, but keeps its place as only one important area of your life.
>
> In short, normal eating is flexible. It varies in response to your hunger, your schedule, your proximity to food, and your feelings.[2]

Satter trains dietitians to teach people to eat normally over a period of eight to ten weeks, introducing clients to foods, using exercises to calm them, and letting them become aware of their feelings about food. Eventually they become more relaxed about eating, and trust themselves more and more to eat with confidence and pleasure. She will, for instance, do an exercise involving Wheat Thins (a type of cracker, any compulsive eater will tell you, that is easily consumed by the box). After using breathing and relaxation techniques to help the client feel calm, Satter will then show them the crackers. Confronted with the food, their tension goes up, and they can begin to sort out why they feel tense. "Many times it's anxiety, because food is pretty fearsome, and sometimes it's excitement, because eating is exciting business, and often it is shame, because they feel they shouldn't be excited about food." Experiencing and understanding their ambivalent and frightening feelings about food helps people learn to tolerate those feelings, and gradually they can get to the point where they can remain calm, focused, and positive while they eat.

Through a series of self-awareness exercises, clients begin to feel more entitled to eat, and more confident in their ability to decide what they want to eat and when. Over time, they build up skills that make them competent, orderly eaters. They become aware of their hunger and fullness, and make choices about how to manage those feelings. If they're a little hungry, but eating lunch with a friend in an hour, then they learn it makes sense to wait. But if dinner's in two hours, they may have a little snack to tide them over. Satter doesn't advocate toting around big bags of food, or being prepared to eat anything at any moment. A little structure, she believes, helps make eating more pleasurable for clients. "At some point they realize that their eating is more enjoyable to them if they come to a meal or a snack hungry and interested in the food there. Then they begin to realize that pragmatically it works better if they have a particular time and place to eat, because then they can round up their food, set aside the time for it, and it can be an event. They devote attention and time to that event and then afterwards they can forget about it."

It isn't until late in the process that Satter introduces the idea of nutrition. Most people, she says, know a fair amount about nutrition already, but think in terms of shoulds and shouldn'ts: should eat celery sticks, shouldn't eat banana cream pie. Satter emphasizes moderation, varying meals, and coming up with strategies for a nutritious diet. "It's kind of like Home Ec. class. You think about different food groups in terms of what makes a meal satisfying," she says. "Carbohydrate is bulky and will fill you up fast, protein is generally more chewy, and fat will stay with you awhile, so you put together a meal that has a little of each." Pretty soon you can work in vegetables and fruits as things that will make meals tastier and more exciting—not as "diet foods" that seem like a bland alternative to something you really desire.

Unlike other anti-diet program leaders, Satter doesn't mention weight change much; she doesn't even suggest that some people will lose weight. She feels strongly that weight is the wrong thing to focus on, period. It's only possible to overcome compulsive eating if you cannot only trust yourself to decide what to eat but trust the weight that naturally comes out of that process. "I acknowledge the longing my patients have to be thin, and I don't criticize them for that longing, but

I don't encourage them to try for thinness," she says. "The minute they do, they get back into that same old struggle and start to ignore their internal regulators, and begin to eat fanatically again."

Satter's method, like other anti-dieters' techniques, may be more helpful to some people than others. It makes good sense to me for several reasons. For one, it is grounded in solid research and theory. Satter's method has evolved over her years of experience dealing with individual clients. She has collected data on her clients, using standard psychological tests, to be able to present it to other professionals in the field and substantiate her theories. Unlike most anti-diet self-help authors, who tend to dismiss the medical and scientific establishment as a bunch of bad guys, Satter and others like her read the literature and attempt to communicate with and change the prevailing establishment, which in the long run will have more impact.

Most importantly, her technique emphasizes pleasure, self-trust, and competence, and doesn't make recovering from compulsive eating take as big a place in your life as compulsive eating did. At some point, she recognizes, compulsive eaters simply need to learn positive skills for healthy eating and get on with their lives. Eating can stop being a huge issue and just be eating. Eating is wonderful while it lasts, but a lot of other things go on in life between meals.

Exercising for Enjoyment

If there's one thing that everyone agrees on, it's the positive benefits of exercise. There may be quarrels over how much exercise is necessary, and what kind of exercise is most beneficial, but no one questions that activity is good for you. Physical activity can get out of hand with some dieters, becoming "exercise bulimia," getting in the way of the rest of their lives, but for most people, it's overwhelmingly positive. If you want to live longer, reduce the stress in your life, and lower your blood pressure, cholesterol, and risk of disease, you should get moving. "Exercise," as one obesity researcher told me, "is a no-brainer."

Yet for all the time, concern, and money spent on weight loss in this country, relatively little attention is paid to exercise. There are millions of gimmicks and plans for how to make fat people thin, but little focus on how to make inactive people active. There's more money to be made, of course, in getting people to sign up for Jenny Craig than in getting them to take a walk around the neighborhood every day. So there's more focus on eating than exercise. When researchers discuss the fact that Americans have gained, on average, 8 pounds in the last decade, they emphasize how we all overeat. They don't talk so much about how fewer of us get regular exercise. But the real problem isn't just that we're eating more, it's that we're moving less.

According to Michael Pratt, physical activity coordinator for the Centers for Disease Control and Prevention, fewer than one-third of all Americans exercise regularly. By "regular," he means the amount of exercise the CDC and the American Council on Sports Medicine recommend for good health, which is less than people might imagine. "Everyone should get about thirty minutes of moderate exercise on most days of the week," says Pratt. That exercise, he says, doesn't have to be exhausting to be beneficial, nor does it have to be done, as people have believed in the past, with an aerobic workout, hitting a target heart rate. People who exercise vigorously and almost daily are probably healthiest. But there is quite a bit of evidence, he said, that people who simply accumulate half an hour of activity on most days, even in short spurts—walking, gardening, bicycling, chasing after children—are doing just fine.

Why, then, are so many people in the United States so reluctant to get even a modest amount of exercise? Unlike dieting, exercise doesn't make you feel bad or deprived. It not only makes you look better and improves your health profile, as dieting is supposed to do, it makes you feel wonderful. Pleasurable exercise builds up strength and self-confidence; it clears your head, brightens your outlook, and livens up your libido. The benefits are immediate and lasting. "If you go out for a walk," says Cinder Ernst, a fitness trainer for large women in San Francisco, "you're a winner; you feel better right away."

But for many people, it just seems so hard to get started. Our society is set up to be as sedentary as possible, so that getting regular exercise can require a big effort and a shift in priorities. Exercise isn't built into life, as it used to be. Most of our cities are designed around the automobile; in some towns, it's difficult to walk from place to place because there aren't even any sidewalks. Many of us could get plenty of exercise just by propelling ourselves, by our feet or bicycles, to where we need to go. But often the streets aren't safe and bicycles are discouraged. Few companies, no matter how much they promote "wellness" programs for their employees, are willing to install showers and bike lockers so people can ride to work. We have more and more labor-saving devices designed to make us more and more sedentary—remote controls, garage door openers, computers, leaf blowers, power lawn mowers, drive-up fast food. "If you start tabulating all of the little devices that have become automated, and all of the opportunities for being active that are disappearing, these little things add up," said Pratt.

The images of super-bodied athletes with high-performance gear that we see in fitness ads and magazines deter us even more. If that's what it takes to be fit, we think, sitting there in our ratty old sneakers and shorts that keep hiking up in back, then we might as will give it up right now. For one thing, it seems like you need lots of expensive equipment to exercise. There are gear-heads in every sport who'd like to convince the rest of us that if we don't have the cool $1,000 mountain bike with shocks, endbars, and an aluminum frame, we might as well stay home. It isn't good enough, we think, to tune up the old Schwinn and ride it around the park. We can't do aerobics, it seems, without shiny leggings, a thong-bottomed leotard, and strap-on arm and ankle weights. And shoes: we think special shoes are required for each sport, whether we want to walk, run, hike, play tennis, bike, or do step-aerobics—at around $75 a pair. Otherwise, we figure we'll either injure ourselves or somehow be doing the sport wrong.

We don't realize that almost none of that equipment is necessary just to get started; special gear is only a good investment when you've been doing something long enough for the equipment to really make a difference. A good pair of all-around cross-training shoes and some sweats are all anyone needs to get started walking or going to the gym, or a comfortable swimsuit and goggles if you're heading for a pool, but that's about it.

We also think we need a top-of-the-line body even to begin to exercise. Unless you already look great in stretchy black shorts, it's difficult to contemplate bicycling or in-line skating in public. Fat is the enemy in the gym, and so it's no wonder that people who don't look great in lycra avoid going there. The atmosphere in a gym, where people see exercise as not only physically but morally competitive, can be toxic. In an environment where model-thin women complain about their bodies in the locker room, and instructors emphasize that hard bodies only come to the disciplined and deserving, someone who's not in great shape gets the strong message that they don't fit in. Teachers don't modify routines for them in class, or worse, single them out. Other students look at them askance, step in front of them in aerobics class, and generally give them you're-a-slob vibes. "The last place you want to go if you're heavy is to a gym where everyone's in a leotard, checking each other out," says David Williamson. "People are not only heavy because they don't exercise, but they don't exercise because they're heavy, which is sad."

Even people who might try exercising by themselves, in a safe, nonjudgmental environment, fear failure. That's mainly because exercise in this culture seems like a means to only one end: weight loss. For many people who struggle with their weight, exercise is like a diet. They figure if Oprah can do it, they can do it. The myth that the exercise diet will make you thin has become more widespread since it's sunk in, to many people, that dieting won't do the trick. Many exercise ads look like ads for weight-loss products. They feature super-aerobicized hard bodies in midriffs and thongs, promising quick results. "Burn fat, lose weight, keep it off," says one typical newspaper ad for a fitness machine, featuring a genetically thin model with implants. Fitness gurus like Susan Powter, and TV host Oprah Winfrey, spread the myth that if everyone just exercises—even though they, unlike celebrities, can't spend most of their waking hours working out with a personal trainer—they'll lose weight. We come to admire the exercise-obsessed rather than to wonder whether they should get a life. *Vanity Fair*, for instance, praised actress Demi Moore for taking a twenty-four-mile bike ride and going dancing on the day her waters broke with her daughter. She had taken a two-and-a-half-hour hike the day before. Soon after the birth, she went back to work, "holding herself to a ferocious discipline." Moore, we learn, jogs at three in the morning with her trainer, wearing a miner's headlamp, and was able to pose in body paint for the *Vanity Fair* cover two months later. *Vanity Fair* assures us, "there wasn't an ounce of flab on that chiseled torso."

Convinced they can do it too, people go on a crash exercise program for a few days, wearing themselves out, and then give it up. The Nordic Track sits in the basement collecting dust when they don't burn off all the fat the ad promised; the new aerobic shoes get kicked under the bed; and people feel worse for trying. The exercise diet isn't fun, but a necessary chore to suffer through to lose a few pounds. You see people on the exercise diet in gyms, grimly riding bicycles to nowhere, suffering until they've burned the right number of calories or hit the requisite target heart rate. If, after all that misery, they don't see results right away on the scale, they figure it isn't working, and they stop.

When weight loss is the motivation for exercise, it's doomed from the start. For one thing, studies show that people don't lose that much weight exercising—an average of 4 to 7 pounds. If people have been quite inactive, exercise can make more of a difference in their weight; it can help other people stabilize their weight, and keep them from gaining more. Exercise also makes people feel more in touch with their bodies, and can sometimes help them stop overeating. But not everyone gets thin exercising, although they can get fit. Cinder Ernst says that the people who come to her aerobics classes to lose weight are the ones who are least likely to keep it up. "They're gung-ho in the beginning," she says. "After three weeks, when they haven't lost a lot of weight, they stop coming. Then they lose all the other benefits of exercising—flexibility, strength, mobility, stress reduction, and self-confidence."

The main goal of fitness instructors who are involved in the anti-diet movement is to help people get off the exercise diet and learn more pleasurable and sustainable ways of incorporating movement into their lives. "People have in their heads that they're either on the exercise plan or they're not," says Pat Lyons, the health educator for Kaiser Permanente, who wrote a fitness book for large women, *Great Shape* (1990), with Debbie Burgard. "The either/or mentality is just like dieting. They figure to do it right they have to do it a certain number of times. Then they don't lose a lot of weight, they don't get the big pay-off, so they figure, 'Why bother?' " Even when they notice that they feel better, have more energy, sleep better, feel stronger, and are in a better mood most of the time, says Lyons, it's hard to convince people that you can be healthier if you're active even if you don't lose a lot of weight.

Lyons, who at five-foot-eight and 260 pounds looks like someone who hikes and swims regularly (which she does), tries to get women to stop thinking of exercise in terms of weight loss. "If your goal is to fit into size eight jeans, you're setting yourself up for failure," she says. "But if you do it to improve the quality of your life, to get in shape and feel more coordinated, you'll feel satisfied with yourself." Lyons says she takes long walks every day, even though she hasn't lost any weight, because she loves to be outdoors and stay strong.

Lyons developed "Great Shape" exercise classes for the Kaiser Permanente HMO in California, inviting women sized 16 and up to come dance for an hour a week. Unlike Richard Simmons's class, the participants were not encouraged to diet; just be active and have a good time. Each week, they did movements that were easy and appropriate for their large bodies, and worked on a sense of camaraderie, not competition. With a large-sized instructor, no one felt out of place or too fat. Even after eight weeks, the results, in terms of health and outlook, were tangible. "If you aren't exercising for weight loss, and just doing it to be doing it, that changes everything," says Lyons. "The 'Why bother?' becomes a question about the quality of your life." When they stopped worrying about losing weight, the women in the Great Shape classes discovered that dancing made them feel great, and gave them a sense that they could successfully accomplish the movements, and that they had grace, rhythm, and style, too. Their bodies, they found, *enjoyed* moving.

And their health improved. Before each series of classes Lyons took a survey, asking questions about the women's health and activity habits. At the end of the class she repeated the survey, and found that nearly two-thirds of the women reported health improvements, including lowered blood pressure, lowered blood sugar, fewer aches and pains, more energy, less depression, and more optimism. The percentage of those who considered themselves in very good or excellent health, and who said they felt good about themselves, also increased by two-thirds.

In one Great Shape class in Vallejo, California, most of the women are still fat after a year of exercising once or twice a week, but they don't move with the kind of timidity and shame that characterizes the way many heavy women carry themselves. Vanessa Espinoza, the instructor—a large woman with big, muscular calves and a very flexible body—encourages them through sock-hop moves, Virginia Reel twirls, and grapevine steps. The mood, as they go through the dance routines, is very upbeat. One woman, who is in her fifties and perhaps 250 pounds, tells the group at the end of class that she used to be afraid to even walk around the block for fear of ridicule. Now she not only dances twice a week but swims on four other mornings. "I have more energy, mentally as well as physically," she says. Another says, "I'm the classic yo-yo with my weight, and it's nice for a chance to feel good about my body the way it is." A third describes the humiliation she felt walking into a gym, where people wouldn't show her the machines and were rude to her, and how good it feels to be welcome in an exercise class.

Lisa Tealer, another Great Shape instructor who also works as a large-size model, says the changes she's seen in her students are remarkable. "Some people have completely come out of their shells, feeling more comfortable about their bodies, challenging themselves in their classes and outside," she says. Many people she sees are more mobile, muscular, and relaxed. But the biggest change is in their self-esteem. Exercise gives women a chance to appreciate their bodies for what they do, not to denigrate them for how they look or what they weigh. "It's wonderful," Tealer says, "to see fat women build up self-confidence along with their muscles."

Unfortunately, programs like Great Shape are few and far between. Some individual gyms offer classes for large women, but many of them—like Richard Simmons'—make it part of a weight-loss program. A few large women have taken it upon themselves to become certified as instructors to open their own classes. In San Diego, Marty Lipton, who is five-foot-two and weighs 240 pounds, teaches five classes a week for large women. After thirty years of trying to be thin, dieting up and down, Lipton, who is active in NAAFA, decided she'd be better off making the body she had more fit. "The more I read, the more I realized that the problems associated with fat are problems associated with being sedentary and thinking that if you're fat, it doesn't matter what else you do." She began exercising and teaching fitness classes, and her mobility improved. "I didn't lose any weight, but my back didn't hurt." Her body composition changed, dropping from 45 percent to 38 percent fat. Her cholesterol numbers dipped from 180 to 135. Now, she swims, walks, does in-line skating, or teaches aerobics every day. "I've gotten past thinking, 'Gee, I'm fat, so I can't do anything.' " she says. "I try to teach other women who are forty to eighty pounds above the ideal that they can feel good in their bodies, too."

In New York, Dee Hakala, a 200-pound fitness instructor, teaches fifteen classes a week for women of all sizes in her "New Face of Fitness" program, which is expanding to several YMCAs around the country. Hakala used to weigh 100 pounds more and was, as she calls it, "a medical nightmare couch potato." She had diabetes, high blood pressure, and couldn't move well. She began exercising; though she lost a lot of weight, she is still a large woman. In her classes, she tries to make everyone feel comfortable, no matter what their size. She provides modifications of moves, and she doesn't let the super-fit front line in a class dominate the class—often moving them to the back. "Exercise is for health, not for the physical sideshow that goes along with it," she says. "We need to reopen the doors to the gyms, and redefine fitness."

Still, many people who feel fat and out of shape are more likely to start exercising privately than go to a gym. A few things, according to Pay Lyons, can make it easier to become fit. One is to get an exercise buddy, who will help you feel comfortable in exercise classes, make walks more enjoyable, and help you develop a routine. If you schedule time for exercise, too—alone or with a friend—you'll be more apt to do it by the end of a busy day.

Another suggestion, says Lyons, is to find a type of movement you really like; if you hate to run, there's no sense making a firm resolution that this Monday, you'll start running three miles a day. Everyone has different types of movement they like best. Walking, bicycling, dancing, swimming, tennis, yoga: find whatever makes your body feel good. Above all, movement should be pleasurable. Everyone, says Lyons, needs a chance to become accustomed to a new movement, and might consider trying it a few times before deciding they don't like it.

Whatever movement people try, it helps to start going at it slowly. People can set themselves up for small successes by taking it easy at first, then adding more exercise when they feel comfortable. Lyons started exercising by running around the block once in her jeans and tennis shoes, then sitting down for a cigarette. The second day she went two blocks; after a few weeks she quit smoking; and soon she was strong enough to run San Francisco's seven-mile Bay to Breakers race. If all a person can do is walk around the block, says Lyons, that's a start. She cautions that large people should only do movements that are appropriate for their bodies; watch Richard Simmons' exercise videos, not Cindy Crawford's. Other fitness experts say it's important to respect your body's limits and stop when you're tired. Challenge yourself, but don't try anything too scary. As the women's mountain-biking champ Jacquie Phelan says, "Respect your inner chicken."

It also helps, when starting up, to get some training. People aren't born knowing how to do sports, Lyons points out. Taking classes, asking the activities director at the gym to show you how to work the machines, or hiring a personal trainer for a few sessions can improve performance fast. Having someone show you how to improve your swimming stroke, for instance, can make an enormous difference.

Exercise, according to researcher Steve Blair, doesn't have to be done in one hour-long bout every day, either. He suggests looking for opportunities throughout the day when you can move instead of sitting or standing still, such as taking the stairs instead of the elevator, getting off the bus a few blocks before your stop, pulling some weeds in the garden, getting up from the computer and pacing around the room, and using a push-mower instead of a power lawn mower. ("I bought a push-mower," he says, "and now my wife is in really good shape.") If possible, he suggests, walk or ride your bike to work or do errands. With exercise, Blair says, "everything counts."

Building a Better Body Image

Developing positive eating and exercise habits go a long way toward making former dieters feel better about themselves. But after years of worrying about their weight, convinced that they're not all right the size they are, the thing that is most difficult for many people to change is their body image.

Most women, regardless of their weight, feel uncomfortable about their size. They feel fat. Their legs are too big, their breasts too small, their stomachs too round. They dislike the bodies they live in, and as a result, end up disliking the person who lives there.

There are plenty of reasons why we hate our bodies; we're bombarded with images of thinness and perfection, and we live with the myth that through dieting, exercise, makeup, and plastic surgery we can all achieve that perfect image. We feel we have to look good to be successful, and in this increasingly image-conscious society, that's at least partly true. To others, how we look is, to a great degree, who we are. "Our body image is at the very core of our identity," writes the psychologist Judith Rodin, author of *Body Traps*. "Our bodies shape our identity because they are the form and substance of our persona to the outside world."[3]

That doesn't mean that body image can't be improved—

particularly after people become aware of how poorly they treat their bodies and why. Many women feel terrible about their bodies, but don't want to admit they do because it seems so vain. We're caught in a double-bind: We're almost forced to be negatively preoccupied with our bodies, but if we acknowledge how much we worry about our weight and shape, it makes us seem like we're the stereotype of a shallow, ditzy, looks-obsessed woman. Most psychologists who treat body image say that the first step is recognizing the problem, and acknowledging that it comes from a society that places ridiculous demands on women to fit an impossible mold. The next step is trying to give your body more good, positive care. "If you treat your body with more respect, you will like it better," says Rodin. "What your body really needs is moderate exercise, healthy foods, sensual pleasures, and relaxation. Give it those, and it will respond by treating you better."

Given how much some women hate their bodies, that's difficult to do. There are other complicated reasons why some women hang on to a poor body image, says another psychologist, Marcia Hutchinson, author of *Transforming Body Image*. Some people make their bodies a Big Problem because this allows them to have the fantasy that if their bodies were different, everything else in their lives would be different, too. If they had a perfect body, they'd have a man, a good-paying job, and sky-high self-esteem, too. A bad body image shields them from failure, and in many cases, keeps them from success. It keeps them from confronting whatever fears of power, intimacy, rejection, sexuality, or success are between them and their fantasy.

But psychologists who treat body image problems say it's possible to at least make *some* improvement in the relationship between a woman and her body. I sat in on one workshop Marcia Hutchinson gave on transforming body image in a rural conference center in New Hampshire.

One of the first women I met in the group, sitting in a circle on the floor, was Elizabeth Beale.* I was surprised that a woman who looked like her was at the workshop: If you saw her walking down the street, you wouldn't think she had reason to hate her body. The forty-seven-year-old librarian, who is five-foot-six and weighs 145 pounds, looks healthy and fit for her age. But that's not how she sees herself, she says. She is so ashamed of the size of her hips and thighs that she wears loose, dark clothes, avoids mirrors, and tries never to draw attention to herself. "I don't want to wear anything that says, 'Hey, look at me.' I'm just hiding."

Hutchinson, a graceful fat woman who sits cross-legged in the circle like a Buddha, asks the ten women in the room to lie on the floor for an exercise. So many of us, she says, have a mental picture of ourselves—our body image—that doesn't fit our actual size. She tells us to close our eyes, stretch our arms in front of us, and place our hands as far apart as we think our hips are wide. I peek: Beale, for one, looks as if she's trying to encircle a redwood tree. "No one in this room thinks she can get through a doorway," says Hutchinson.

We're not so unusual. Most women can't accurately guess how wide they are. It's well known that women with anorexia can look at their gaunt reflections in the mirror and point out huge pads of fat. But a few years ago, psychologists who looked at how such women distort their size and compared them with normal women got a surprise: The normal women also viewed themselves as much larger then they really were.[4] More than half of all American women, it turns out, overestimate the size of their bodies. Most women who stand in front of their full-length mirrors asking, "Who's the fattest of them all?" get a stern reply: "You are, you pig."

And it isn't that women are generally bad at judging size. When psychologists at St. George's Hospital Medical School in London asked fifty normal-sized women to estimate the width of a box, the women were dead on target. But when asked to estimate their body widths, they exaggerated the sizes of their waists by about 25 percent and their hips by 16 percent. More than half the women criticized their hips as the part of their bodies they hated most; the only ones who were content with their size were those who were 10 pounds underweight.[5]

Being thin doesn't mean always guarantee satisfaction, though. Nor does being fat always result in a poor self-image. As with compulsive eating, it isn't the size of a person that matters so much as the weight of her discontent. One thing that contributes to the difference among women in the amount of uneasiness they feel about their bodies, several studies show, is how much their parents and friends emphasized their appearance as a child.

Chubby, awkward kids who are teased about their bodies are apt to grow up with poor body images, as are pretty girls whose sense of self-worth is strongly tied to their looks. Whenever body shape is given undue importance, positively or negatively, it becomes a focus for future problems. Elizabeth Beale, for instance, says she was self-conscious about her size from the time she was five, when her parents first put her on a diet and discouraged her from wearing clothes they said made her look plump. She remembers refusing to color in the brides in her coloring books, thinking she was too fat and ugly ever to marry. Yet today, when she looks back at photos of herself, she's surprised. "There were times when I wasn't overweight at all," she says. "But that's how I always felt."

She wasn't much different from most girls who grew up in a culture where it was hard to fit the image of the coloring-book brides, hard not to color outside the lines. The ideal body today is, after all, several sizes smaller than what nature intended for most women. "We live in a culture where it's normal for women to feel we should be thinner, prettier, firmer, and younger," says Hutchinson. "So it's normal for us to have body image problems."

Men, too, are sometimes troubled by body flaws—particularly, studies show, a balding pate.[6] But women judge their bodies much more harshly. If you've ever changed your outfit six times before going out, relentlessly shopped for clothes that never seem right at home, or obsessively checked out your rear view in the mirror, you know how body image concerns can infiltrate daily life.

When it comes to body size, even in this fat-obsessed culture, women view themselves much more harshly than others view them. "Women aren't scrutinized nearly as much as they think they are," says April Fallon, a psychologist at the Medical College of Pennsylvania. When she asked 291 men and women to rate sketches of a range of women's body types, the women predicted men would prefer much thinner bodies than the ones the men actually picked as their favorites.[7] "If a woman is twenty pounds over the ideal, that doesn't actually have a big impact on people's interest level," says Fallon. More likely, she says, a poor body image gives a person an air of resignation and unhappiness. "That," says Fallon, "is something people notice."

People whose body images are so poor they're reluctant to go out, meet people, or find a job may be suffering from what psychologists call "body dysmorphic disorder," and could benefit from therapy. But there are a few techniques that body image experts practice which they say can be helpful to start working on a positive relationship with your body.

In her workshop, and in her book, Hutchinson proposes visualization exercises for improving how people see themselves. In one of her exercises, she recommends recalling the times parents, lovers, or friends attached names to your body—"Fat Face," "Baby Whale," "Bertha Big Butt"—and feeling the weight of those labels. Then imagine stripping off the labels, one by one. "You have to peel away the obstacles to seeing your body as an acceptable, comfortable home," she says.

Movement, along with all the other ways it makes you feel good, can also do wonders for body image. Hutchinson also uses a technique called the Feldenkrais Method, a series of gentle floor exercises intended to increase a person's awareness of how her body parts move and are connected. Almost any kind of movement will help. When the psychologist Rita Freedman, author of *BodyLove*, surveyed 200 women, 87 percent of them said exercise had improved the way they felt about their bodies. For women who were not athletic as children, exercise often prompts an epiphany: They realize for the first time that their bodies are valuable not only for the way they look but also for what they can do. Freedman suggests forms of exercise, such as dance, yoga, and walking, that are relaxing and directed toward making you feel better about your body at its present size.

Freedman also suggests that people accentuate what they like about themselves. Even the toughest self-critics take pride in their eyes, hair, hands, or some other body part, she says. She tells clients to use a mirror constructively to zero in on the parts they like, rather than the parts they hate, and encourages them not to be afraid to play up the parts they like about themselves, learning to enjoy their bodies by indulging in small, sensual pleasures such as soaking in a scented bath, slathering on lotion, getting a massage, or wearing silk. Buying clothes that really fit and are flattering—and giving away ones that are too small—can make people feel better about their bodies, too. Freedman points out that transforming the way you feel about your body, like changing your eating habits, is a slow process. But like those, once started, it is a series of small, positive changes.

After the workshop, Elizabeth Beale still felt fat, but even a few weeks later, she noticed a difference. She got up the nerve to wear a hand-painted silk scarf—a real attention-grabber—and relished the compliments. She's learning to catch herself before she starts criticizing her body flaws. And she's taken up figure skating.

"I've just stopped thinking so much about my body," she says. "It gives me time for more important things in my life."

The goal of all anti-diet treatments, for normal eating, exercise, or body image, is just that: To allow women who have spent huge portions of their lives being obsessed about their weight, eating, and bodies, to get on with more important things in their lives.

Chapter 10

The Anti-Diet

Ten Steps to a Healthier Body—and Attitude

If you don't diet, then what? The prospect of continuing to gain weight is frightening and depressing to many people. But there are alternatives to starving yourself. The focus needs to be on becoming healthier at any weight, not trying to reach an ideal size. Some people who adopt a healthier lifestyle may in fact lose weight, others may become more fit, and others may stabilize. All are better than continuing on endless cycles of starving, bingeing, and gaining weight.

A prescriptive "anti-diet" is something of a contradiction in terms. These are merely suggestions I've compiled from many people who have successfuly come to peace with their food and eating, and are healthier as a result.

1. Stop Dieting

Stop eating according to anyone' else's rules. Stop counting calories, food exchanges, fat grams, or carbohydrates. Don't bother reading best-selling diet books or eating plans. Don't take diet pills or herbal diet aids, and don't eat any low-fat or diet foods that you don't absolutely prefer to the higher-calorie versions. Don't restrain yourself from eating what you like, and don't deprive yourself. Boycott the diet industry entirely.

Do not weigh yourself. Weighing yourself is bad for your mood. Throw away your scales and quit putting things off until the day you're finally thin.

Slowly give yourself permission to eat what you like and tell yourself you deserve to enjoy good food. Quitting dieting doesn't mean to go wild eating junk food, however. Overeating is often a reaction to dieting, and once you stop dieting, it's usually a temporary phase. Strive to eat consciously and intelligently. Everyone knows that a diet filled with vegetables, fruits, and grains—real, whole foods, in other words—is apt to keep you healthy. Saturated fats, hard artificial fats like margarine, and processed foods are not going to make your heart happy in the long run. Enjoy some formerly forbidden foods now and then, whether it's cookies, rich desserts, creamy cheeses, or chocolate, but eat those things consciously, in full sight of others, with a sense of entitlement, and see if a little will go a long way. Experiment to find good, nourishing foods that really satisfy you.

When you stop dieting, it's likely that over time your eating will become more normal, less anxiety-ridden, and above all, more pleasurable.

2. Get Moving

Many studies show that it's inactivity, not weight, that causes many of the problems we associate with being fat. Moderate exercise is the closest thing we have to an elixir of youth—it makes you feel healthy, strong, agile, coordinated, refreshed, and confident.

The trick is discovering what kinds of exercise you truly enjoy, or you'll never keep doing it. Don't go on an "exercise diet," putting yourself on a crash program of running or going to the gym if you hate those activities. What do you really like to do? Put on some loud music and dance around your living room? Garden? Hike? Take long walks with a friend? Experiment with different types of movement, like walking, swimming, yoga, bicycling, or dance. Give it some time, be easy on yourself, and find which types of exercise you can not only sustain, but look forward to every day.

If you can incorporate more movement into your day-to-day activities, you'll be a lot healthier. Walk to work if you can, or at least to the bus stop. Take the stairs, mow your lawn, ride your bike to work, do stretches in your office—find little ways to be more active all day long.

3. Eat Like an Italian

Many Italians eat with a great deal of pleasure, don't gain weight, and don't obsess about their size. Our stereotype of Italian cuisine is an Americanized version—heaping plates of lasagna or fettucine alfredo, cream-filled pastries and tiramisu. Italians, instead, are much more moderate in their eating habits, savoring smaller portions of food, rarely eating desserts. They don't stuff themselves because they know that good food will be waiting for them at the next meal.

Italians, traditionally, take pride in eating fresh, local ingredients. They buy fruits and vegetables that are in season, and are very fussy about the quality of their bread, olive oil, and wine. They don't eat a lot of processed, packaged food, because it doesn't appeal to them. Nor do many of them eat between meals, because it would spoil the pleasurable experience of being good and hungry when mealtime comes.

Italians eat with a sense of ritual and community that is often lost in American culture. Many go home for lunch, eat something hot and well prepared, and sit down with a nice place setting. The idea of grabbing a sandwich and eating at the desk would be impossible to many of them. Lunch should be a nice, relaxing meal, finished off with a good espresso. The evening meal is something to share with friends and family, not something to throw in the microwave and eat in front of the TV.

We often think of Americans' eating habits as being too indulgent, but in fact our eating is often filled with shame and guilt, and we don't relish the pleasure of our meals enough. If we focused more on eating with true delight, with wonderful, seasonal ingredients and a sense of ceremony, we would end up eating less—and enjoying it more.

Part of taking the time to enjoy food is learning to cook. If you know how to prepare simple, healthy meals confidently—sauteeing some onions or garlic in olive oil, for instance, adding some sliced vegetables, maybe some anchovies or capers, throw in a few white beans, serve it on pasta, top it with a little freshly grated cheese, improvising—it becomes a lot more fun to eat good food. Buy a couple of Mediterranean cookbooks and have a good time.

It's also important to have access to good-quality vegetables. One way is to go to local farmer's markets, where you can interact with the people who grow your food, and have a nice Saturday morning outing. In many areas you can subscribe to a farm through a Community Supported Agriculture program, where a box of freshly picked organic vegetables is delivered to your neighborhood every week, saving a trip to the store. The surprising mix of vegetables that arrives can inspire you to cook new dishes and eat more vegetables.

4. Everything in Moderation, Including Moderation

In the United States, we overeat, overdiet, overwork, and over-relax. We do everything in extremes. We panic at news that fat is bad for us, and so we eat no fat and then load up on sugary carbohydrates. Then we fret that carbohydrates are killing us and we start eating quantities of protein. We have a hard time finding the middle ground.

Moderation, instead, would make us a lot happier. Like chocolate? Eat it sometimes. Don't feel like exercising? Take a day off. Feel like going for a 40-mile bike ride and exhausting yourself? Enjoy it. Moderation doesn't mean always achieving a perfect balance in your life, always eating the right amount of the right foods every day, getting the perfect amount of exercise. You can eat eight servings of vegetables today and two tomorrow, and everything will average out. Moderation means that you don't deny yourself all the time, don't indulge yourself all the time, and figure that all in all, it will work out.

Moderation also means going wild sometimes. Every once in a while, stay up too late, drink too much, eat too much, exercise too hard, push things to the extreme, really live. *That* keeps you in balance.

5. Listen to Your Body

Dieting wreaks havoc with your natural sensations of hunger and fullness. Eating normally requires relearning how to tune in to your body, as a child does, knowing when you really want to eat and when you're full, then managing your hunger like a grown-up, waiting to enjoy mealtimes. Your body knows how much food it needs—you just need to listen to it. Taking the time to eat consciously helps, stopping to really experience the smells, tastes, textures and shapes of the food you eat. Pause while eating to decide whether you're full, and don't be afraid to put down your fork midway through your meal—you can always save leftovers.

Developing more quiet awareness of how your body moves, and how your breath and energy circulate through yourself, can also help you relax about your body size and image. Yoga, Feldenkreis, tai chi, tai kwon do, dance, and other meditative-movement disciplines can help you develop a more centered sense of your body. You become more aware of your body as a moving, breathing extension of yourself, not a big blob that you're always hating and trying to change. You begin to appreciate your body for qualities other than its size—its grace, agility, suppleness, sensuality, and strength. Eventually, you begin to take better care of your body, giving it the movement and nourishment it needs.

6. Make the Time to Treat Yourself Well

Exercising, cooking, sitting down to meals, going to the farmer's market—a healthy lifestyle requires a lot of time and planning. With jobs, kids, commuting, and family responsibilities, that time just doesn't seem to exist. We're all too busy. So we let exercise go and we eat on the run.

Achieving a healthier lifestyle may mean shifting priorities a bit, toward yourself. So many women, in particular, are so busy taking care of the rest of the world—their family, people at work, friends—that they don't make time for themselves. Eating can become a quick way to try to do something nice for yourself when you don't have the time to really take care of yourself. When you're overwhelmed by other people's demands, it seems like a care-taking gesture to give yourself a little treat. But often so much guilt is attached to eating—we feel we don't really deserve it—that we feel bad, overeat, and end up not accomplishing what we desired, which was to take care of ourselves. The impulse to do something to nourish yourself is positive, but many people don't use food to truly comfort or treat themselves. A more conscious effort to really treat yourself and your body well—sitting down to a satisfying meal instead of eating by the light of the fridge, or going out and taking a walk to clear your head—would make you happier and healthier in the long run, and keep your weight more stable.

A little selfishness may be in order to achieve a healthier lifestyle.

Other people in your family may have to work around your schedule for a change. You need to go to your yoga class on Tuesday nights, and that's that. You need to take the time to leave the office for lunch, maybe even take a little walk, and not just work on through, eating at your desk. You'd like to prepare a nice meal and sit down for a pleasant dinner, so the telephone can just wait. Other people will eat up as much of your time as you let them, so you have to be tough about carving out time for yourself.

Planning is essential. If you don't wake up in the morning and figure out when you're going to get some exercise that day, it likely won't happen. If you don't schedule a trip to the farmer's market on Saturday morning, you'll never get there. Once healthy routines become established in your life, you may find they don't take so much time and effort. You may find, in fact, they're what you enjoy most about your day.

7. Stop Talking about Weight All the Time

Weight has become an all-consuming topic of conversation for many women. Beyond discussions bemoaning their size or weight, some women can tie themselves up into endless intellectual knots talking about the meaning of food, why they eat, why they gain weight, etc., etc. They can go into mind-numbing detail about what they ate yesterday and how they feel about it. They may read every book available with every new theory about food as love, as sex, as comfort, as sublimation; they become experts on eating disorders and food neuroses. All this diet chat may be useful to a point—but then it borders on obsession, not to mention utter boredom.

If we stopped talking about eating and weight all the time, it might cease to be such an important and debilitating issue in our lives. We might also find a lot more interesting things to talk about. A few suggestions:

• Don't compliment friends when they look like they've lost weight.

• Don't complain about feeling fat, or fish for compliments from friends who'll tell you that you don't look fat.

• Don't judge other women by their weight.

• When the conversation turns to weight and eating habits, start talking about a film you saw recently, a book you read, politics—anything else.

• Substitute negative, guilt-ridden comments about food ("I ate too much last night") with more positive ones ("I found the most beautiful golden beets yesterday, roasted them for dinner, and they were wonderful.")

• Don't just stop making negative comments about weight and food to your friends—stop talking that way to yourself. Try to catch yourself every time you berate yourself for being fat or eating too much, and shift the topic. You don't need to bore yourself, either—or make yourself feel bad.

8. Develop Your Physical Personality

Many of us think about our bodies only in terms of weight. If we're fatter than usual, it's bad, and if we're thinner, it's good. But that's a very two-dimensional way to look at a multidimensional body.

All of us have physical personalities. When you watch people walk, some are stiff, some are loose, some sway, some have a lot of attitude. Some people gesture widely, some sharply, some elegantly. We all learn a great deal about other people by their body language—do they seem to shrink up inside themselves, slump over, or stand up tall and inhabit their body with grace and vitality?

Recognize the positive aspects of your physical personality, and appreciate them. Exercise can help you develop the physical sense to move with more grace and confidence; yoga, in particular, can help with good, upright posture. You may not be light and quick, but you may have good endurance. You may be a good dancer, a lively walker, a strong swimmer. You probably have a long list of other physical attributes you like about yourself—your hair, your hands, your flexibility, your quick reflexes. If you acknowledge your physical abilities and play them up, you may find new confidence in your body.

Learn to love your curves, too. For most of human history people adored women's curves. Take a walk through a museum and notice how many of the beautiful women in paintings have bodies like yours. You'll be pleasantly surprised.

Traveling is another way to get perspective on how unnatural America's obsession with thinness really is. In many other countries women are considered sexiest if they have a good amount of meat.

Women who might cover themselves up completely at the beach in the United States wander around in bikinis on beaches in the southern Mediterranean, feeling completely comfortable.

Even in the United States, more men like curvy women than they let on. The problem is that thinness has become a mark of virtue and discipline in this culture. As one man in his fifties explained to me, when he was young, the most important thing for a successful man to have was a virtuous wife—a virgin when they married. Now the most important thing is for a wife to be thin. Both, of course, put women in a position of powerlessness, of being controlled, of being a trophy.

How much you weigh is not a reflection of your character. Curves can be soft, sexy, squeezable, and alluring. They're what men have liked most about women for a long time. If you've got them, you might as well flaunt them.

9. Carry It Off with Style

Part of developing your physical personality is learning to express it. Many women who have spent years feeling self-conscious about their weight have concentrated on trying to hide their bodies. Others feel that they don't deserve to dress up and feel good about what they're wearing. They put off buying something flattering until that magic day when they can fit into pants that are two sizes smaller than the baggy ones they're wearing.

This is the wrong strategy.

Start by going through your closet, perhaps with a ruthlessly honest friend, try on everything, and get rid of any garment you own that doesn't make you feel good when you wear it. Also get rid of anything that doesn't fit right now. You don't want a skirt in the back of your closet screaming that you used to be thinner. Toss it. You can feel good about donating your clothes to charity or to a battered-women's shelter, giving some away to friends, or selling the good-quality ones to a consignment shop.

Once you have all that luxurious space in your closet, start *wearing* the clothes that make you feel good, even if you previously reserved them for dress-up occasions. Then gradually buy a few pieces you really love to add to your wardrobe. Finally, some companies, like Liz Claiborne's Elisabeth line, are starting to cater to larger women with really fashionable clothes. Think about buying clothes the way Europeans do—buy only a few things, but good quality, and wear them all the time.

Forget all the advice about how you can't wear bright colors, stripes, or prints if you're big. Wear whatever you really enjoy wearing. I have a friend who is about 250 pounds, and she manages to pull off lacey black skirts, boots, and bright red hair—she looks gorgeous. And who says miniskirts are only for people with coltlike legs? Don't be timid. Express your personal style.

10. Rebel Against the Diet Culture

Our great-grandmothers wore painful and debilitating corsets to make their bodies fit the fashions of the times. We're still trying to mold ourselves into an impossible shape. The inner corset we wear is one of the strongest and most insidious remnants of oppression against women that we still put up with.

We need to begin to resist and change the diet culture—to undo the ties to our inner corsets. The first steps have to be personal, learning to eat healthfully and normally again, silencing the dieter in our heads. But it's hard to say no to dieting if you think losing weight will get you a lover or a better job—and in this culture it does improve your chances. It's also difficult not to size yourself up against other women, to feel relieved you're not as fat as some and jealous you're not as thin as others. No matter how many times you tell yourself you're just fine the way you are, there's still going to be a little voice inside that says, "If only my stomach were flatter . . ." That voice is the sound of our culture, and we can't turn it off by ourselves.

That's why we need a widespread rebellion of women who understand that weight is not a matter of health or discipline but is a weapon used to keep us in our place and make us feel small. We need to start throwing our weight around:

• *Stop apologizing for your size.* Women are accustomed to feeling inferior because of our size. We've learned from an early age that our worth can be measured on a scale, and we've internalized the belief that there's something wrong with us for being our natural size. We think it's our fault, and collude with the culture that tells us we should be ridiculously thin to be worthwhile. But we don't go around apologizing for our height or the color of our hair. If someone doesn't like our physical attributes, it's really their problem, isn't it?

• *Stop reading and watching media that make you feel bad about yourself.* It's ironic that women's magazines, which spend so much time and effort telling women how to improve their health and self-esteem, keep on promoting a dangerously thin body ideal. To some extent, they can't help the images in the ads they run; the cosmetics and clothing companies send those in. But they are responsible for the extremely thin models they use in their fashion and editorial photos. Some magazines, such as *Glamour,* have started occasionally featuring larger women in fashion spreads. *Mode,* a glossy magazine for women size 12 and up, has been very successful, proving that it's a myth that all we want to see are fantasy images of waiflike women. Larger women love to see someone who looks great and still has some meat on her bones.

Like fashion magazines, most of everything on TV features perfect-bodies bimbos. Only watch shows that don't make you feel miserable. Or spend the time you'd be watching television doing some dance or yoga videos instead.

• *Don't buy products whose ads promote extreme thinness.* This can be tricky. If, for instance, you decide never to buy any clothes that are only advertised on skinny women, you wouldn't even be able to shop at Lane Bryant. (Lane Bryant, which makes clothing for women sizes 14 and up, has a particularly ironic ad featuring models who are as thin as any others, captioned "What real women wear.") But you have to draw the line somewhere. Personally, I don't buy anything made by Calvin Klein, who is one of the worst offenders in the category of Glorifying Emaciation. Nor do I shop at stores where the saleswomen act like I don't exist because I'm not thin.

Buy products that don't make you feel terrible when you look at their ads. When a company like the Body Shop shows a pretty plump doll—Ruby—with the headline, "There are 3 billion women who don't look like supermodels and only 8 who do," it may be time to stock up on moisturizer.

• *Protest the public health focus on the "epidemic of obesity."* Former Surgeon General C. Everett Koop's Shape Up America! campaign has focused on the need for Americans to lose weight by dieting. More reasonably, we should promote programs that encourage people to eat better and exercise more. According to a 1995 survey of 1,599 urban residents, many people would like to eat better and exercise more, but they don't have the resources they need to follow through. Safer parks, more community recreation facilities, gardening projects, farmer's markets and full-size grocery stores in low-income neighborhoods could greatly improve public health. So could school-based nutrition and exercise programs.

• *Protect children from weight obsession.* Let children know that their body size is perfectly fine the way it is. Putting children on diets should be considered something close to abuse. Don't support athletic subcultures—ballet, gymnastics, ice skating—that insist that girls be extremely thin. Encourage school programs that promote positive attitudes toward eating, exercise, and diverse body sizes. Programs to help prevent dieting and eating disorders before they start, giving girls the skills to resist the pervasive negative body size messages that attack them at an early age, are essential.

• *Organize.* It helps, when standing up to the diet culture, to do it in groups. The National Association to Advance Fat Acceptance (NAAFA), a 4,500-member organization based in Sacramento, California, works to educate people about the myths of obesity, and to protect the civil rights of fat people. The group keeps up on obesity research and attempts to participate in policy-making conferences about weight. NAAFA also provides a rare social atmosphere where fat people can enjoy themselves in an atmosphere where no one will humiliate them for their weight. Most important, NAAFA members are role models of people who don't hide, ashamed, because of their size, but are proudly big and bright, and engaged with the world. In this culture, that takes a lot of courage. There are several other groups that promote size acceptance nationwide, many accessible on the Internet or in magazines for large-sized women.

• *Make dieting a feminist issue.* Women's groups need to acknowledge that weight obsession, eating disorders, and bias against fat people are not trivial. What have the major national women's organizations done to help the epidemic of eating disorders in this country recently? Why haven't the women's health organizations strongly challenged the diet industry, diet products, and obesity research that places too much emphasis on weight? The feminist movement in this country has ignored the damage done to women by the diet culture for far too long. Despite all the gains that women as a group have accomplished in the past century, individually many of us feel inferior, ashamed of our size. We need to acknowledge that real freedom, choice, and respect for ourselves would mean accepting our bodies the way they are.

- *Celebrate International No Diet Day, May 5.*
- *Be rebellious.* The best defense against the diet culture, of course, is a good offense. Show the world how great it is to live large. Be proud, sexy, and strong at your size. Be cheerful in your body. What have you got to lose?

Acknowledgments

When I first began thinking about this book, Lacey Fosburgh, a wonderful teacher, writer, and friend, nudged me along. She died in 1993 from complications that arose during treatment for breast cancer. I am forever grateful to her for passing along so much to me during her last difficult years.

Many other people offered me support and encouragement along the way. My agent, Sarah Lazin, took me out to lunch every year since I was nineteen to talk about writing a book; it wouldn't have happened without her persistence and ever-sensible advice. Lisa Margonelli spent long days in the library doing research for this book, emerging with some unexpected gems. I'm grateful to Susan West, a science editor who has an uncanny ability to focus on both the little details and the big picture at once, for going over the manuscript so thoroughly. Joy Rothke kept me honest by checking all the facts. I thank Rachel Klayman for acquiring the book, and my editor, Deborah Brody, for her enthusiasm while shepherding it through.

Several magazine editors, including Lisa Davis, Karin Evans, Claire Ellis, Bruce Kelley, Mary Murray, Ilena Silverman, and especially, Peggy Northrop, contributed their ideas and red pencils to articles that eventually formed parts of this book. Leonora Wiener and Joan Walsh gave me insightful comments on the chapters they read.

Barbara Paulsen, editor of *Health* magazine, organized chapters in the air for me while we took our afternoon walks. I thank the rest of my colleagues at *Health*, including Ben Carey, Valerie Fahey, Deborah Franklin, Katherine Griffin, John Hastings, Patty Long, and Mike Mason, for sending studies my way and for helping me through scientific muddles.

Many professionals who work with people who are large or have eating disorders gave me generous amounts of their time, which deepened my understanding of the field considerably. In particular, I'd like to thank endocrinologist Wayne Callaway, health educator Pat Lyons, anthropologist Margaret Mackenzie, nutrition expert Ellyn Satter, and psychologist Susan Wooley for their wisdom and willingness to answer so many questions. Frances Berg, editor of the *Healthy Weight Journal*; John LaRosa, diet industry analyst at Marketdata Research; and Sally Smith, executive director of the National Association to Advance Fat Acceptance also provided me with a great deal of help. Others who passed along useful information to me include Ben Melnick, Ariel Sabar, Julie Wyman, Cheri Erdman, Jennifer Buechner, Marilyn Wann, and humanities professor Richard Ohmann. I also greatly appreciate the many anonymous dieters who were willing to let me interview them for sharing their often painful experiences with me.

I'm grateful to several other people for their various types of support—from good ideas to good meals—including Shelley Nathans, Vince Bielski, Cristina Taccone, Rob Waters, Katherine Weiser, Larry Bensky, Madeleine Budnick, Lauren Lazin, Lucia Ungari, Cecelia Brunazzi, Jay Rorty, and my fellow members of the Writer's Grotto. I thank my parents, Charles and Virginia Fraser, for their love and good cheer throughout (especially, my dad, a physician, for his advice on medical matters), and my sisters Cindy, Jan, and Amy, for their encouragement.

The following researchers and obesity experts generously allowed me to interview them during the course of researching this book, and I greatly appreciate their contributions:

Harvey Anderson, Ph.D.

William L. Asher, M.D.

Richard L. Atkinson, M.D.

Leann L. Birch, Ph.D.

George Blackburn, M.D., Ph.D.

Steven Blair, P.E.D.

Susan Bordo, Ph.D.

George Bray, M.D.

Kelly Brownell, Ph.D.

Denise Bruner, M.D.

Colin Campbell, Ph.D.

Karen Carrier, M.Ed.

Donna Ciliska, RN, Ph.D.

Kenneth Cooper, M.D., M.P.H.

Robert Eckel, M.D.

Paul Ernsberger, Ph.D.

April Fallon, Ph.D.

John Foreyt, Ph.D.

Rita Freedman, Ph.D.

Susan Fried, Ph.D.

David Garner, Ph.D.

G. Ken Goodrick, Ph.D.

Steven L. Gortmaker, Ph.D.

Joan Gussow, Ph.D.

Steven Heymsfield, M.D.

Jules Hirsch, M.D.

Jane Hirschmann, M.S.W.

Van Hubbard, M.D.

Marcia Hutchinson, Ed.D.

Joanne Ikeda, Ph.D.

Ron Innerfield, M.D.

Karen Johnson, M.D.

Susan L. Johnson, Ph.D.

Emily Fox Kales, Ph.D.

Allen King, M.D.

I-Min Lee, Ph.D.

Harvey Levenstein, Ph.D.

David Levitsky, Ph.D.

Hank Lukaski, Ph.D.

Andrew Lustig, Ph.D.

JoAnn Manson, M.D.

Richard Mattes, Ph.D.

Lynn McAfee

Bill McCarthy, Ph.D.

Joseph McVoy, Ph.D.

Wayne Miller, Ph.D.

Carol Munter

Thomas Murray, Ph.D.

Dean Ornish, M.D.

Patt Panzer, M.D.

F. Xavier Pi-Sunyer, M.D.

Janet Polivy, Ph.D.

Robert Pritikin

Paul Raford, M.D., M.P.H.

George Ricaurte, Ph.D.

Barbara Rolls, Ph.D.

Geneen Roth

Esther Rothblum, Ph.D.

Anthony Sclafani, Ph.D.

Lewis Seiden, Ph.D.

Harold Seim, M.D., M.P.H.

Judith Stern, Ph.D.

George Triadafilopoulos, M.D.

Varro Tyler, Ph.D.

Thomas Wadden, Ph.D.

Janet Weiss, M.D.

Walter C. Willett, M.D., Dr. P.H.

David F. Williamson, Ph.D.

Sidney Wolfe, M.D.

Richard Wurtman, M.D.

Senator Ron Wyden

Susan Yanovski, M.D.

Notes

Preface

1. "Dieting Goes 'Natural' after Fen-Phen Scare; Small Players Get Fat," by Laura Johannes and Barbara Carton, *Wall Street Journal*, September 29, 1997. Other statistics in this preface are from the *WSJ*, which did by far the best reporting on the fen-phen debacle.

Introduction: Adventures in Dietland

1. See Susan L. Johnson and Leann L. Birch, "Parents' and Children's Adiposity and Eating Style," *Pediatrics*, vol. 94 (1994), 653–61. Most kids, according to the authors, are better than adults at eating the proper amounts of food. Feed them a high-calorie snack at eleven in the morning, and most will compensate by eating less lunch. Offer them a no-calorie drink, and they'll want a full meal. The authors tested a goup of seventy-seven preschoolers and found that the kids who failed to adjust their lunchtime eating after a snack tended to be fatter. Then the researchers asked the children's parents whether they themselves dieted and, if so, whether they limited what and when their children ate. The overweight children were much more likely to have parents who controlled their kids' eating habits.

The parents' strategy to stave off a family tendency toward chubbiness backfired. "Unfortunately, when parents do things for children, the kids have a harder time figuring out how to do it themselves," says Johnson. Children may also develop a habit of rebelliously overeating when out from under their parents' watchful eyes. Johnson's advice? "Don't restrict their food," she says. "And don't worry so much."

2. See "Rating the Diets," *Consumer Reports* (June 1993), pp. 347–57. The *Consumer Reports* survey of 95,000 readers may give a more reliable picture of how many Americans lose weight on diets than medical studies. Many obesity researchers say that the widely quoted figure that nine of ten diets don't work is skewed, since the studies are done on people who enroll in medical programs, who presumably are fatter than most dieters, and have tried and failed at many other methods. Still, *Consumer Reports* found that typical dieters fared little better: "People do lose weight on these programs—but the great majority of them gain back most of that weight within two years." The survey found that do-it-yourself dieters were fairly effective at keeping off modest weight losses—10 pounds—by making their own changes in their eating and exercise habits. Overall, one-quarter of the respondents were able to keep off more than two-thirds of their weight after two years.

3. The often-quoted $34 billion figure for the diet industry comes from John LaRosa, diet industry analyst at Marketdata Research. It includes, in order of size, diet soft drinks, artificial sweeteners, fitness clubs, commercial weight-loss programs, medically supervised weight-loss programs, diet foods, meal replacements and appetite suppressants, and diet books, videos, and audio cassettes. That number, however, doesn't account for the amount we spend on weight-loss surgeries and liposuction, pharmaceutical diet drugs, the estimated $5 billion to $6 billion we spend on fraudulent diet products (according to Frances Berg, editor of *Healthy Weight Journal*), or the $1.4 billion we spend on diet books, lectures, seminars, and workshops, which is why I think the total is closer to $50 billion.

4. JoAnn E. Manson, et al., "Body Weight and Mortality Among Women," *New England Journal of Medicine*, vol. 333 (1995), 677–82.

5. See, for example, Carolyn E. Barlow, Harold W. Kohl, III, Larry W. Gibbons, and Steven N. Blair, "Physical Fitness, Mortality and Obesity," *International Journal of Obesity and Related Metabolic Disorders*, vol. 19 (1995), 541–54. In that study, lean men who didn't exercise had three times the death rate of fat men (BMI over 30) who were fit.

6. Transcript from the Endocrinologic and Metabolic Drugs Advisory Committee, Food and Drug Administration Center for Drug Evaluation and Research, Sept. 28, 1995, pp. 33–36. Another article described Manson's being paid as a consultant for the diet drug company: Seth Gitell, "Skinny on Research Doc's Connection to New Diet Pill," *New York Post*, Sept. 15, 1995.

1. The Inner Corset

1. Anthropologist Margaret Mackenzie made this observation to me.

2. See Hillel Schwartz, *Never Satisfied: A Cultural History of Diets,*

Fantasies and Fat (New York: Free Press, 1986), p. 38. Schwartz's book provided a good deal of background material for this chapter, and is an excellent resource on the history of dieting.

3. This reader, *Selections of Easy Lessons Calculated to Inculcate Morality and Piety*, belonged to my husband's great-great-great-grandfather, Henry Ezekiel Churchill.

4. Lois W. Banner, *American Beauty* (Chicago: University of Chicago Press, 1983), p. 113. Banner's meticulously researched book traces American beauty ideals, and was very helpful in preparing this chapter.

5. Clarence Day, quoted in Parker Morell, *Lillian Russell: The Era of Plush* (New York: Random House, 1940), p. 100. This book provided a good deal of background information on Lillian Russell.

6. William Bennett and Joel Gurin, *The Dieter's Dilemma* (New York: Basic Books, 1982), p. 199.

7. Grant Allen, quoted in Cynthia Eagle Russett, *Sexual Science: The Victorian Construction of Womanhood* (Cambridge: Harvard University Press, 1989), p. 43.

8. Susan Brownmiller, *Femininity* (New York: Fawcett Columbine, 1984), p. 86.

9. Russett, *Sexual Science*, p. 118.

10. Bennett and Gurin, *Dieter's Dilemma*, p. 183.

11. Joan Jacobs Brumberg, *Fasting Girls: The Emergence of Anorexia Nervosa as a Modern Disease* (Cambridge: Harvard University Press, 1988), p. 175.

12. Morell, *Lillian Russell*, p. 172.

13. Robert Howard Russell, "How Charles Dana Gibson Started," *Ladies' Home Journal* (October 1902), p. 8.

14. Ben Melnick shared his undergraduate research on the Gibson Girl with me, providing me with many helpful insights and sources.

15. Frank Presbrey, *The History and Development of Advertising* (Garden City, N.Y.: Doubleday, Doran, 1929), p. 348.

16. Quoted in Stuart Ewen, *All Consuming Images: The Politics of Style in Contemporary Culture* (New York: Basic Books, 1988), p. 179.

17. Brumberg, *Fasting Girls*, p. 239.

18. Quoted in Barry Parris, *Louise Brooks* (New York: Alfred A. Knopf, 1980), p. 130.

19. Paula Fass, *The Damned and the Beautiful: American Youth in the 1920s* (New York: Oxford University Press, 1977), p. 23.

20. Mary Ryan, *Womanhood in America* (New York: New Viewpoints, 1975), p. 69.

21. Roberta Seid, *Never Too Thin: Why Women Are at War with Their Bodies* (New York: Prentice Hall, 1989), p. 94. Seid's book contains a wealth of information on the history of dieting.

22. Ibid., p. 97.

23. Brumberg, *Fasting Girls*, p. 246.

24. Ann Hollander, *Seeing Through Clothes* (New York: Viking, 1978), p. 154.

25. Robert Sklar, *The Plastic Age* (New York: George Braziller, 1970), p. 17.

26. T. J. Jackson Lears, "From Salvation to Self-Realization: Advertising and the Therapeutic Roots of the Consumer Culture, 1880–1930," in Richard Wightman Fox and T. J. Jackson Lears, eds., *Culture of Consumption* (New York: Pantheon, 1983), pp. 1–38.

27. Stuart Ewen, *Captains of Consciousness: Advertising and the Social Roots of the Consumer Culture* (New York: McGraw-Hill, 1976), p. 160.

28. Carl Malmberg, *Diet and Die* (New York: Hillman-Curl, 1935), p. 8.

29. Brumberg, *Fasting Girls*, p. 248.

30. Bennett and Gurin, *Dieter's Dilemma*, p. 206.

31. Laurence Leamer, *The Kennedy Women* (New York: Villard, 1994), p. 150.

32. The statistics on Miss America sizes, as well as on Miss Sweden and Twiggy later in this chapter, are from April Fallon, "Sociocultural Determinants of Body Image," in Thomas F. Cash and Thomas Pruzinsky, eds., *Body Images: Development, Deviance, and Change* (New York: Guilford, 1990), p. 88.

33. Cited in Harvey Levenstein, *Paradox of Plenty* (New York: Oxford University Press, 1993), p. 136.

34. Gerald Walker, "The Great American Dieting Neurosis," *New York Times Magazine*, Aug. 23, 1959.

35. Karen S. Schneider, "Mission Impossible," *People*, June 3, 1996, p. 71.

36. Mark Nichter and Mimi Nichter, "Hype and Weight," *Medical Anthropology*, vol. 13 (1991), 249–84.

37. D. M. Garner, P. E. Garfinkel, D. Schwartz, and M. Thompson, "Cultural Expectations of Thinness in Women," *Psychological Reports*, vol. 47 (1980), 483–91.

38. Jane Fonda, *Workout Book* (New York: Simon & Schuster, 1981), p. 10.

39. Julian Guthrie, "Fast Talk," *San Francisco Examiner Magazine*, March 6, 1994.

40. Marjorie Rosen, "Oprah Overcomes," *People*, Jan. 10, 1994, pp. 43–45. See also Beth Landman, "Take It Off Like a Star," *Redbook* (September 1994), pp. 100–103.

41. Leah Garchik, Personals, *San Francisco Chronicle*, Dec. 9, 1993.

42. Steven Gortmaker, "Social and Economic Consequences of Overweight in Adolescence and Young Adulthood," *Journal of the American Medical Association*, vol. 266 (1993), 1008–12.

43. Esther D. Rothblum, "The Stigma of Women's Weight; Social and Economic Realities," *Feminism and Psychology*, vol. 2 (1992), 61–73.

44. The New England Regional Genetics Group conducted this survey.

45. See Ann M. Gustafson-Larson and Rhonda Dale Terry, "Weight-Related Behaviors and Concerns of Fourth-Grade Children," *Journal of the American Dietetic Association*, vol. 92 (1992), 818–22. Survey by Jody Brylinksy, a Western Michigan University sports psychologist, and James C. Moore, a University of South Dakota educational psychologist, quoted in *Allure* (February 1994), p. 48.

46. Brownmiller, *Femininity*, p. 26.

47. Susan Bardo, *Unbearable Weight: Feminism, Western Culture, and the Body* (Berkeley: University of California Press, 1993) is an exploration of the myths, ideologies, and pathologies of the female body; it provided helpful background reading for this book.

2. The Truth That Will Change Your Life

1. Much of the background on Graham, Fletcher, and Kellogg that follows comes from Schwartz, *Never Satisfied*. See also Bennett and Gurin, *Dieter's Dilemma*.

2. See Horace Fletcher, "What I Am Asked About 'Feltcherism,'" *Ladies' Home Journal* (October 1909), p. 20. And Donald Dale Jackson, "The Art of Wishful Shrinking Has Made a Lot of People Rich," *Scientific American* (November 1994).

3. Seid, *Never Too Thin*, provided background on Peters and on women's magazines.

4. Helen Woodward, *The Lady Persuaders* (New York: Ivan Obolensky, 1960), p. 156.

5. Lesley Blanch, "You and the New Morality," *Vogue* (April 1960).

6. Peter Wyden, *The Overweight Society* (New York: William Morrow, 1965), pp. 100–19.

7. Judy Mazel, *The Beverly Hills Diet* (New York: Macmillan, 1981), pp. xv, 14, and 55–63.

8. Orland W. Wooley and Susan Wooley, "The Beverly Hills Eating Disorder: The Mass Marketing of Anorexia Nervosa," *International Journal of Eating Disorders*, vol. 1 (1982), 57.

9. Robert C. Atkins, *Atkins' Diet Revolution* (New York: Bantam Books, 1972), p. 10; Herman Tarnower and Samm Sinclair Baker, *The Complete Scarsdale Medical Diet* (New York: Batnam, 1978), p. 151.

10. Theodore Berland, *Consumer Guide's Rating the Diets* (New York: Beekman House, 1960), provided information on the protein doctors.

11. Atkins, *Atkins' Diet Revolution*, p. 294.

12. Tarnower and Baker, *Complete Scarsdale Medical Diet*, p. 33.

13. Marian Burros, "When Diet-Book Authors Push Products with Their Programs," *New York Times*, March 20, 1996, p. C10.

14. Molly O'Neill, "Coaching the Pounds Away, Bite by Sound Bite," *New York Times*, April 26, 1995, p. B1.

15. Calvin Trillin, "U.S. Journal: Natchitoches, LA," *The New Yorker* (Jan. 12, 1981), pp. 88–91.

16. Dean Ornish, *Eat More, Weigh Less* (New York: HarperCollins, 1993), pp. 68 and 78.

3. Ten Pounds in Ten Days

1. "Dieting Goes 'Natural' after Fen-Phen Scare; Small Players Get Fat," by Laura Johannes and Barbara Carton, *The Wall Street Journal*, September 29, 1997.

2. Woods Hutchinson, M.D., "Fat and Its Follies," *Cosmopolitan* (1894), p. 395.

3. Dr. Harvey W. Wiley and Anne Lewis Pierce, "Swindled Getting Slim," *Good Housekeeping* (January 1914), p. 109.

4. Arthur J. Cramp, M.D., ed., *Nostrums and Quackery: Articles on the Nostrum Evil, Quackery and Allied Matters Affecting the Public Health: Reprinted, With or Without Modifications, from The Journal of the American Medical Association*, Vol. II (Chicago: American Medical Association Press, 1921), p. 659.

5. Paul Ernsberger and Paul Haskew, "Rethinking Obesity: An Alternative View of Its Health Implications, *Journal of Obesity and Weight Regulation*, vol. 6 (1987), 45.

6. Schwartz, *Never Satisfied*, p. 191.

7. Robert A. Kilduffe, "The Weight of the Transgressor," *Hygeia* (September 1938).

8. Theodore Berland, *Consumer Guide's Rating the Diets: Everything You Should Know About the Diets Making News* (Skokie, Ill.: Publications International, 1980), p. 223.

9. See Wyden, *The Overweight Society*, p. 184.

10. Jack Friedman, "The Cambridge Obsession," *New York*, Dec. 20, 1982.

11. Thomas Wadden, et al., "The Cambridge Diet: More Mayhem?" *Journal of the American Medical Association*, vol. 250 (1983), 2833.

12. A. N. Howard, "The Cambridge Diet: A Response to Criticism," *Journal of Obesity and Weight Regulation*, vol. 3 (1984), 65–84.

13. "Weight-Loss Doctor Under Indictment," *The Washington Post*, Nov. 15, 1988; Patricia Manson, "Diet Doctor's Insurance Scam Nets 10-Year Prison Term, Fine," *Houston Post*, July 14, 1989; "Stop Selling Weed Killer as Diet Aid, Doctor Told," *Houston Post*, March 22, 1986; "Judge Gives License Back to Doctor," *Houston Post*, June 30, 1987; "Three Lawsuits in 5 Years Result in Investigation of Texas Physicians," *Houston Post*, May 15, 1988. Texas State Board of Medical Examiners orders and complaints dated 1/26/90, 1/31/87, 5/16/86, 3/7/86, and 2/11/86. Conversation with

Texas State Board of Medical Examiners spokesperson Jeff McDonald, Jan. 17, 1995.

14. Staff memo from the Subcommittee on Regulation, Business Opportunities, and Energy, Sept. 24, 1990.

15. All testimony from "Juvenile Dieting, Unsafe Over-the-Counter Diet Products, and Recent Enforcement Efforts by the Federal Trade Commission." Hearing before the Subcommittee on Regulation, Business Opportunities, and Energy of the Committee on Small Business, House of Representatives, 101st Congress, Washington, D.C., Sept. 24, 1990 (Washington, D.C.: U.S. Government Printing Office, 1990).

16. Diana Hembree, "Over-the-Counter Diet Pills and Cerebral Hemorrhages," *Muckraker* (October 1994), pp. 10–12.

17. Rosie Mestel, "Has Chromium Lost Its Luster?" *Health* (March–April 1996), p. 56.

18. "Who Needs Chromium," *University of California, Berkeley Wellness Letter*, vol. 11 (1994), p. 4.

19. G. W. Evans, "The Effect of Chromium Picolinate on Insulin Controlled Parameters in Humans," *International Journal of Biosocial Medical Research*, vol. 11 (1989), 163–80.

20. Catherine Houck, "A 'Miracle Mineral'?" *Cosmopolitan* (May 1991).

21. "Chromium Crazy," *Longevity* (July 1994).

22. E. C. Hamilton, F. L. Greenway, and G. A. Bray, "Regional Fat Loss from the Thigh in Women Using Tropical 2% Aminophylline Cream." Presented at the North American Association for the Study of Obesity, Oct. 29, 1993.

23. Peter Jaret, "Thigh High," *Vogue* (February 1994), p. 142.

24. Paul Raeburn, "Will Lotion Reduce Fat Thighs?" Associated Press, *San Francisco Examiner*, Oct. 21, 1993.

25. Jaret, "Thigh High"; see also Janet Basu, "Dream Cream: The Thighs Have It," *Hippocrates* (January 1994), p. 17.

26. *Tufts University Diet and Nutrition Letter*, vol. 11 (1994), p. 3.

27. Judy Foreman, "Thinner Thighs? Think Again," *Boston Globe*, Feb. 7, 1994, p. 25.

28. See also William H. Dietz, "Needed for NAASO: A Code of Ethics," *Obesity Research*, vol. 2 (1994), 164.

29. Cited in Kendra Rosencrans, "Researchers Claim Key to Thinner Thighs," *Healthy Weight Journal* (May–June 1994), 53.

30. "Can You Lose Weight with Hypnosis?" *Healthy Weight Journal* (March–April 1995), 33.

31. *The Diet Business Bulletin* (Summer 1995), 16.

32. Frances M. Berg, "Herbalife—Wealthy Life," *Healthy Weight Journal* (March–April 1994).

33. Cited by Leah Garchik, Personals, *San Francisco Chronicle*, May 22, 1995, p. E8.

4. No Satisfaction

1. For the effects of smoking on weight, see, for example, Lisa M. Varner, "Smoking—Yet Another Weight Loss Strategy?" *Healthy Weight Journal* (January 1996), p. 13. Smoking does help control weight, and surveys show that 25 to 39 percent of adult female smokers smoke for that purpose. After reviewing twenty-nine studies on smoking and body weight, researchers found that smokers weighed an average of 7.57 pounds less than nonsmokers.

2. On why dieting makes people binge, see, for example, Janet Polivy and C. Peter Herman, "Dieting and Bingeing: A Causal Analysis," *American Psychologist*, vol. 40 (1985), 193–201.

3. Statistics on thinking foods are inherently good and on believing that we should eat no fat at all are taken from "Just What Is a Balanced Diet Anyway?" *Tufts University Diet and Nutrition Letter* (January 1992), p. 3.

4. Harvey Levenstein, *Paradox of Plenty: A Social History of Eating in America* (New York: Oxford University Press, 1993), p. 244.

5. Information on saccharin and Tillie Lewis comes from Madelyn Wood, "Fifty Non-Fattening Foods," *Coronet* (January 1955), pp. 88–93. The DeVoto quote is from Levenstein, *Paradox of Plenty*, p. 137.

6. Statistics from Valerie Fahey and Laura Fraser, "What Price Diet?" *Mademoiselle* (August 1995), p. 155.

7. For background on these studies, see John P. Foreyt and G. Ken Goodrick, "Potential Impact of Sugar and Fat Substitutes in American Diet," *Journal of the National Cancer Institute*, vol. 12 (1992), 99–103.

8. Warren Young, "Food That Isn't Food," *Life* magazine (June 7, 1961).

9. Marion White, *Diet Without Despair* (New York: M. S. Mill, 1943), p. 11.

10. Marian Burros, "Debate Intensifies Over Fat Substitute for Snack Foods," *New York Times*, Jan. 17, 1996, p. B6. Also interview with Barbara Rolls.

11. Barbara Rolls, et al., "Effects of Olestra, a Noncalorie Fat Substitute, on Daily Energy and Fat Intakes in Lean Men," *American Journal of Clinical Nutrition*, vol. 56 (1992), 84–92.

12. Suzanne Hamlin, "Eating in 1994: The Year Beef Came Back," *New York Times*, Dec. 28, 1994, p. B6.

13. "Just What Is a Balanced Diet Anyway?" *Tufts University Diet and Nutrition Letter* (January 1992), p. 3.

14. Philip Wylie, "Science Has Spoiled My Supper," *The Atlantic* (June 1954), pp. 45–47.

5. Were You Good This Week?

1. For studies on yo-yo dieting, see, for example, Lauren Lissner, et al., "Variability of Body Weight and Health Outcomes in the Framingham

Population," *New England Journal of Medicine*, vol. 324 (1991), 1839–44. The researchers found, in a long-term study of 5,127 people, that those whose weight fluctuated had higher rates of death from coronary heart disease. Other studies have shown that rats and wrestlers become more metabolically efficient after repeated dieting—they have a hard time losing weight each time. Recently, there's been some debate over whether weight cycling makes it hard to lose weight, but the negative psychological consequences are clear. See, for example, Kelly Brownell and Judith Rodin, "Medical, Metabolic, and Psychological Effects of Weight Cycling," *Archives of Internal Medicine*, vol. 154 (1994), 1325–30.

2. Many of the statistics on the diet industry are from *The Diet Business Bulletin*, the newsletter put out by John LaRosa of Marketdata Enterprises.

3. See "Deception and Fraud in the Diet Industry, Part I." Hearing before the Subcommittee on Regulation, Business Opportunities, and Energy of the Committee on Small Business, House of Representatives, 101st Congress, March 26, 1990.

4. "The Body of the Beholder," *Newsweek* (April 24, 1995).

5. "Long-Term Maintenance Following Attainment of Goal Weight: A Preliminary Investigation," *Addictive Behaviors*, vol. 17 (1992), 469–77.

6. Wyden, *The Overweight Society*, p. 80.

7. Quoted in Seid, *Never Too Thin*, p. 123.

8. "Fat and Unhappy," *Time* magazine (Oct. 20, 1947).

9. Seid, *Never Too Thin*, p. 125.

10. Marcia Millman, *Such a Pretty Face: Being Fat in America* (New York: W. W. Norton, 1980), p. 30.

11. Jean Nidetch, *The Story of Weight Watchers* (New York: Twenty First Corporation, 1970), p. 81.

12. Ibid., p. 138; Seid, *Never Too Thin*, p. 130.

13. Statistics from *The Diet Business Bulletin* (Summer 1995) and Weight Watchers International Inc. corporate backgrounder, 1994.

14. Kim Chernin, *The Obsession: Reflections on the Tyranny of Slenderness* (New York: Harper & Row, 1980), p. 101.

15. Barbara Brotman, "Are the Scales Tipped Unfairly?" *Chicago Tribune*, March 23, 1994.

16. Statistics from the American Cancer Society.

6. First, Do No Harm

1. John LaRosa, *Diet Industry Seminar and Mid-Year Outlook Report*, Marketdata Enterprises, Inc., June 28, 1994.

2. See, for instance, Rudolph Liebel et al., "Changes in Energy Expenditure Resulting from Altered Body Weight," *New England Journal of Medicine*, vol. 332 (1995), 621–28.

3. For a discussion of the medicalization of obesity, see Jeffery Sobal,

"The Medicalization and Demedicalization of Obesity," in Donna Maurer and Jeffery Sobal, eds., *Eating Agendas: Food, Eating, and Nutrition as Social Problems* (Hawthorne, N.Y.: Aldine De Gruyter, 1995).

4. "Increasing Prevalence of Overweight Among U.S. Adults: The National Health and Nutrition Examination Surveys, 1960 to 1991," *Journal of American Medical Association*, vol. 272 (1994), 205–207.

5. Committee to Develop Criteria for Evaluating the Outcomes of Approaches to Prevent and Treat Obesity, Food and Nutrition Board, Institute of Medicine, Paul R. Thomas, ed., *Weighing the Options: Criteria for Evaluating Weight-Management Programs* (Washington, D.C.: National Academy Press, 1995), p. 19.

6. Anne Wolf and Graham Colditz, "The Cost of Obesity: The U.S. Perspective," *PharmoEconomics*, vol. 5 (1994), 34–37. For an analysis of this study, see Frances Berg, "Obesity Costs Reach $45.8 Billion," *Healthy Weight Journal* (July–August 1995), 67–68.

7. Richard Troiano, Edward A. Frongillo, Jeffery Sobal, and David Levitsky, "The Relationship Between Body Weight and Mortality: A Quantitative Analysis of Combined Information from Existing Studies," *International Journal of Obesity*, vol. 20 (1996), 63–75.

8. Bruch, *Importance of Overweight*, p. 318.

9. Susan C. Wooley and David M. Garner, "Obesity Treatment: The High Cost of False Hope," *Journal of the American Dietetic Association* (October 1991), 1249.

10. Cheri L. Olson, Howard D. Schumaker, and Barbara P. Yawn, "Overweight Women Delay Medical Care," *Archives of Family Medicine*, vol. 3 (October 1994).

11. Bruch, *Importance of Overweight*, p. 265.

12. Jules Hirsch, "Herman Award Lecture, 1994: Establishing a Biologic Basis for Human Obesity," *American Journal of Clinical Nutrition*, vol. 60 (1994), 613–16.

13. See also Andrew Lustig, "Weight Loss Programs: Failing to Meet Ethical Standards?" *Journal of the American Dietetic Association* (October 1991), vol. 91, no. 10.

14. Diane Epstein and Kathleen Thompson, *Feeding on Dreams* (New York: Macmillan, 1994), p. 59.

15. Bennett and Gurin, *Dieter's Dilemma*, p. 217.

16. This figure comes from researcher Lars Sjostrom, of the University of Göteborg, in Sweden, quoted in Frances Berg, *The Health Risks of Weight Loss* (Hettinger, N.D.: Healthy Living Institute, 1993), p. 71.

17. "The Protein Fad," *Newsweek*, Dec. 19. 1977. See also Theodore Berland, *Rating the Diets* (New York: Beekman House, 1980), p. 190.

18. "The Liquid-Protein Controversy: Twisted Evidence?" *Newsweek* (Jan. 30, 1978).

19. Bennett and Gurin, *Dieter's Dilemma*, p. 239.

20. Polivy and Herman, *Breaking the Diet Habit*, p. 90.

21. Harold E. Sours, Victor P. Fratali, et al., "Sudden Death Associated with Very Low Calorie Weight Reduction Regimens," *American Journal of Clinical Nutrition*, vol. 34 (1981), 453–61.

22. Thomas A. Wadden, Theodore B. VanItallie, and George L. Blackburn, "Responsible and Irresponsible Use of Very-Low-Calorie Diets in the Treatment of Obesity," *Journal of the American Medical Association*, vol. 263 (1990), 83.

23. John Garrow, "The Management of Obesity: Another View," *International Journal of Obesity*, vol. 16 (1992), 559–63.

24. "Deception and Fraud in the Diet Industry: Part I." Hearing before the Subcommittee on Regulation, Business Opportunities and Energy of the Committee on Small Business, House of Representatives, 101st Congress, March 26, 1990, p. 43.

25. Schwartz, *Never Satisfied*, p. 139.

26. John LaRosa, *The Diet Business Bulletin* (Fall 1994), p. 12.

27. Michael Weintraub, et al., "Long-Term Weight Control Study," *Clinical Pharmacological Therapy*, vol. 51 (1992), 581–646. For background on dexfenfluramine, see hearing transcripts from the Endocrinologic and Metabolic Drugs Advisory Committee, Food and Drug Administration Center for Drug Evaluation and Research, Sept. 28, 1995, and Nov. 16, 1995. See also transcripts from the Joint Meeting, Drug Abuse and Endocrinologic and Metabolic Drugs Advisory Committee, Food and Drug Administration and Center for Drug Evaluation and Research, Sept. 19, 1995.

28. See, for example, George Ricaurte et al., "Dexfenfluramine and Serotonin Neurotoxicity: Further Preclinical Evidence That Clinical Caution Is Indicated," *Journal of Pharmacology and Experimental Therapeutics*, vol. 269 (1994), 792–98.

29. For more information on dexfenfluramine side effects, see "Dexfenfluramine," editorial, *The Lancet*, vol. 337 (1991), 1315–16.

30. Jules Hirsch, "Comments on 'Long-Term Weight Loss: The Effect of Pharmacologic Agents,' by D. J. Goldstein and J. H. Potvin," *American Journal of Clinical Nutrition*, vol. 60 (1994), 658–59.

31. See Sharon Marks et al., "Reduction of Visceral Adipose Tissue and Improvement of Metabolic Indices: Effect of Dexfenfluramine in NIDDM," *Obesity Research*, vol. 4 (1996), 1–7. Also Claude Bouchard, "Dexfenfluramine and Abdominal Visceral Fat," *Obesity Research*, vol. 4 (1996), 77–78.

32. See Jonathan B. Hauptman, Francis S. Jeunet, and Dieter Hartmann, "Initial Studies in Humans with the Novel Gastrointestinal Lipase Inhibitor Ro 18-0647 (Tetrahydrolipstatin)," *American Journal of Clinical Nutrition*, vol. 55 (1992), 309S–313.

33. Edward E. Mason and Cornelius Doherty, "Surgery," in *Obesity: Theory and Therapy*, 2nd ed., edited by A. J. Stunkard and T. A. Wadden (New York: Raven Press, 1993), p. 314.

34. *Weighing the Options*, p. 26.

35. John LaRosa, *The Diet Business Bulletin* (Fall 1994), p. 6.

36. Mason and Doherty, "Surgery," p. 314.

37. Edward E. Mason and Cornelius Doherty, "Complications of the Surgical Treatment of Obesity," *American Journal of Psychiatry*, vol. 144, no. 5 (June 1987), 833.

38. Berg, "Obesity Costs," pp. 74–76.

7. Thinking Disorders

1. *Crain's New York Business*, June 5, 1989, p. 28.

2. Thomas Moore, *Lifespan: Who Lives Longer and Why* (New York: Simon & Schuster, 1993), p. 148. Also press release from Sandoz Nutrition Corporation.

3. "Very Low-Calorie Diets" (National Task Force on the Prevention and Treatment of Obesity), *Journal of the American Medical Association*, vol. 270 (1993), 967–68.

4. "Methods for Voluntary Weight Loss and Control," National Institutes of Health Technology Assessment Conference Statement, April 1, 1992.

5. Molly O'Neill, "A Growing Movement Fights Diets Instead of Fat," *New York Times*, April 12, 1992, p. A1.

6. "Deception and Fraud in the Diet Industry, Part IV." Hearing before the Subcommittee on Regulation, Business Opportunities, and Energy of the Committee on Small Business, House of Representatives, 102nd Congress (Washington D.C.: U.S. Government Printing Office, 1992), p. 52.

7. "Losing Weight: What Works. What Doesn't." *Consumer Reports* (June 1993), p. 347.

8. Thomas A. Wadden, "The Treatment of Obesity: An Overview," in *Obesity: Theory and Therapy*, p. 211.

9. See Judith Rodin, *Body Traps: Breaking the Binds That Keep You from Feeling Good About Your Body* (New York: William Morrow, 1992), p. 17.

10. Kelly Brownell and Judith Rodin, "The Dieting Maelstrom: Is It Possible and Advisable to Lose Weight?" *American Psychologist*, vol. 49 (1994), 781.

11. Kelly Brownell and Judith Rodin, "Medical, Metabolic, and Psychological Effects of Weight Cycling," *Archives of Internal Medicine*, vol. 154 (1994), 1325–31.

12. David B. Allison and F. Xavier Pi-Sunyer, "Fleshing Out Obesity," *The Sciences* (May–June 1994), 38–43.

13. Karen A. Kemper, et al., "Black and White Females' Perceptions of Ideal Body Size and Social Norms," *Obesity Research*, vol. 2 (1994), 117–25.

14. National Task Force on the Prevention and Treatment of Obesity,

"Weight Cycling," *Journal of the American Medical Association*, vol. 272 (1994), 1196–1202.

15. Walter C. Willett, et al., "Weight, Weight Change, and Coronary Heart Disease in Women: Risk in the 'Normal' Weight Range," *Journal of the American Medical Association*, vol. 273 (1995), 461–65.

8. A New Paradigm

1. Ancel Keys, et al., *The Biology of Human Starvation* (Minneapolis: University of Minnesota Press, 1950).

2. Bruch, *Importance of Overweight*, pp. 12–13, 307–13.

3. Albert Stunkard and Mavis McLaren-Hume, "The Results of Treatment for Obesity: A Review of the Literature and Report of a Series," *Archives of Internal Medicine*, vol. 103 (1959), 79.

4. Polivy and Herman, *Breaking the Diet Habit*, p. 183.

5. Janet Polivy and C. Peter Herman, "Undieting: A Program to Help People Stop Dieting," *International Journal of Eating Disorders*, vol. 11 (1992), 261–68.

6. Bennett and Gurin, *Dieter's Dilemma*, p. 283.

7. Susan C. Wooley and Orland W. Wooley, "Should Obesity Be Treated At All?" in A. J. Stunkard and E. Stellar, eds., *Eating and Its Disorders* (New York: Raven, 1984), pp. 185–92.

8. Polivy and Herman, "Undieting," pp. 261–68.

9. Barlow, et al., "Physical Fitness, Mortality and Obesity," *International Journal of Obesity and Related Metabolic Disorders*, vol. 19 (1995), 541–54.

9. "Eat Your Vegetables . . ."

1. See, for example, Leann L. Birch, "Obesity and Eating Disorders: A Developmental Perspective," *Bulletin of the Psychonomic Society*, vol. 29 (1991), 265–72. Also Leann L. Birch, Susan Johnson, et al., "The Variability of Young Children's Intake, *New England Journal of Medicine*, vol. 324 (1991), 232–35.

3. Judith Rodin, "Body Mania," *Psychology Today* (January–February 1992), p. 56.

4. Kevin Thompson, "Larger Than Life," *Psychology Today* (April 1986), p. 39.

5. Sandra Birtchnell, Bridget Dolan, and J. Hubert Lacey, "Body Image Distortion in Non-Eating Disorderd Women," *International Journal of Eating Disorders*, vol. 6 (1987), 385–91.

6. Thomas F. Cash, "The Psychology of Physical Appearance: Aesthetics, Attributes, and Images," in Thomas F. Cash and Thomas Pryzinsky,

eds., *Body Images: Development, Deviance and Change* (New York: The Guilford Press, 1990), pp. 65–67.

7. Paul Rozin and April Fallon, "Body Image, Attitudes to Weight, and Misperceptions of Figure Preference of the Opposite Sex: A Comparison of Men and Women in Two Generations," *Journal of Abnormal Psychology*, vol. 97 (1988), 342–45.

Bibliography

Armstrong, David, and Elizabeth Metzger Armstrong. *The Great American Medicine Show: Hucksters, Healers, Health Evangelists and Heroes from Plymouth Rock to the Present.* New York: Prentice Hall Press, 1991.

Banner, Lois. *American Beauty.* Chicago: University of Chicago Press, 1983.

Bennett, William, and Joel Gurin. *The Dieter's Dilemma.* New York: Basic Books, 1982.

Berg, Frances M. *Health Risks of Weight Loss.* Hettinger, N. Dak.: Healthy Weight Journal, 1995.

Berland, Theodore, and the editors of *Consumer Guide. Rating the Diets: Everything You Should Know About the Diets Making the News.* New York: Beekman House, 1980.

Bordo, Susan. *Unbearable Weight: Feminism, Western Culture, and the Body.* Berkely: University of California Press, 1993.

Brown, Catrina, and Karin Jasper, eds. *Consuming Passions: Feminist Approaches to Weight Preoccupation and Eating Disorders.* Toronto: Second Story, 1993.

Brownell, Kelly D., and Christopher G. Fairburn. *Eating Disorders and Obesity: A Comprehensive Handbook.* New York: Guilford, 1995.

Brownmiller, Susan. *Femininity.* New York: Simon & Schuster, 1984.

Brumberg, Joan Jacobs. *Fasting Girls: The Emergence of Anorexia Nervosa as a Modern Disease.* Cambridge, Mass.: Harvard University Press, 1988.

Cash, Thomas F., and Thomas Pruzinsky, eds. *Body Images: Development, Deviance and Change.* New York: Guilford, 1990.

Chernin, Kim. *The Obsession: Reflections of the Tyranny of Slenderness.* New York: Harper & Row, 1981.

Chernin, Kim. *The Hungry Self: Women, Eating and Identity.* London: Virago, 1986.

Cramp, Arthur J. *Nostrums and Quackery,* Vol. II. Chicago: American Medical Association Press, 1921.

Ehrenreich, Barbara, and Deirdre English. *For Her Own Good: 150 Years of the Experts' Advice to Women.* Garden City, N.Y.: Anchor, 1978.

Epstein, Diane, and Kathleen Thompson. *Feeding on Dreams.* New York: Macmillan, 1994.

Ewen, Stuart. *All Consuming Images: The Politics of Style in Contemporary Culture.* New York: Basic Books, 1988.

Ewen, Stuart. *Captains of Consciousness: Advertising and the Social Roots of the Consumer Culture.* New York: McGraw-Hill, 1976.

Fallon, Patricia, Melanie A. Katzman, and Susan C. Wooley, eds. *Feminist Perspectives on Eating Disorders.* New York: Guilford, 1994.

Fass, Paula S. *The Damned and the Beautiful: American Youth in the 1920s.* New York: Oxford University Press, 1977.

Fisher, M. F. K. *The Art of Eating.* New York: Vintage, 1976.

Fox, Richard Wightman, and T. J. Jackson Lears, eds. *Culture of Consumption.* New York: Pantheon, 1983.

Fox, Stephen. *The Mirror Makers: A History of American Advertising and its Creators.* New York: William Morrow, 1984.

Freedman, Rita. *Bodylove.* New York: Harper & Row, 1989.

Harris, Jean. *Stranger in Two Worlds.* New York: Macmillan, 1986.

Hirschmann, Jane R., and Carol H. Munter. *Overcoming Overeating.* New York: Addison-Wesley, 1988.

Hollander, Anne. *Seeing Through Clothes.* New York: Viking, 1978.

hooks, bell. *Outlaw Culture: Resisting Representations.* New York: Routledge, 1994.

Hutchinson, Marcia Germaine. *Transforming Body Image: Learning to Love the Body You Have.* Trumansburg, N.Y.: Crossing, 1985.

Lakoff, Robin Tolmach, and Raquel L. Scherr. *Face Value: The Politics of Beauty.* Boston: Routledge & Kegan Paul, 1984.

Leamer, Laurence. *The Kennedy Women.* New York: Villard, 1994.

Levenstein, Harvey. *Paradox of Plenty: A Social History of Eating in Modern America.* New York: Oxford University Press, 1993.

Lyons, Pat, and Debby Burgard. *Great Shape: The First Exercise Guide for Large Women.* New York: Arbor House, 1988.

Malmberg, Carl. *Diet and Die.* New York: Hillman-Curl, 1935.

Millman, Marcia. *Such a Pretty Face: Being Fat in America.* New York: W.W. Norton, 1980.

Moore, Thomas J. *Lifespan: Who Lives Longer and Why.* New York: Simon & Schuster, 1993.

Morell, Parker. *Lillian Russell: The Era of Plush.* New York: Random House, 1940.

Ohmann, Richard. *Politics of Letters.* Middletown, Conn.: Wesleyan University Press, 1987.

Orbach, Susie. *Fat Is a Feminist Issue.* New York: Berkley, 1978.

Paris, Barry. *Louise Brooks.* New York: Alfred A. Knopf, 1989.

Presbrey, Frank. *The History and Development of Advertising.* Garden City, N.Y.: Doubleday, Doran, 1929.

Rodin, Judith. *Body Traps.* New York: William Morrow, 1992.

Roth, Geneen. *Breaking Free from Compulsive Eating.* New York: Bobbs-Merrill, 1984.

Russett, Cynthia Eagle. *Sexual Science: The Victorian Construction of Womanhood.* Cambridge, Mass.: Harvard University Press, 1989.

Ryan, Mary P. *Womanhood in America: Colonial Times to the Present.* New York: New Viewpoints, 1975.

Satter, Ellyn. *How to Get Your Kid to Eat . . . But Not Too Much.* Palo Alto, Calif.: Bull, 1987.

Schwartz, Hillel. *Never Satisfied: A Cultural History of Diets, Fantasies and Fat.* New York: Free Press, 1986.

Seid, Roberta. *Never Too Thin: Why Women Are at War with Their Bodies.* New York: Prentice Hall Press, 1989.

Seligman, Martin E. P. *What You Can Change and What You Can't.* New York: Alfred A. Knopf, 1994.

Sklar, Robert, ed. *The Plastic Age: 1917–1930*. New York: G. Braziller, 1970.

Sontag, Susan. *Illness as Metaphor*. New York: Farrar, Straus and Giroux, 1978.

Stacey, Michelle. *Consumed: Why Americans Love, Hate and Fear Food*. New York: Simon & Schuster, 1994.

Stunkard, Albert J., and Thomas A. Wadden, eds. *Obesity: Theory and Therapy*, 2d ed. New York: Raven, 1993.

Tyler, Varro E. *The Honest Herbal: A Sensible Guide to the Use of Herbs and Related Remedies*, 3d ed. Binghamton, N.Y.: Haworth, 1993.

Veblen, Thorstein. *The Theory of the Leisure Class*. New York: MacMillan, 1899.

Woodward, Helen. *The Lady Persuaders*. New York: Obolensky, 1960.

Woolf, Naomi. *The Beauty Myth*. New York: William Morrow, 1991.

Wyden, Peter. *The Overweight Society*. New York: William Morrow, 1965.

Index